Praise for *Tales from the Bed*

"Jenifer Estess inspired me personally, and countless others living with disease and disability, never to give up fighting for the cures that will save the lives of millions of Americans."

—CHRISTOPHER REEVE

"Jenifer Estess writes with such humor and honesty that you feel as if you know her. Her story is one that we all look at and think, What would I do in her situation? To read this story is not only to be inspired, it literally makes you see the world around you differently."

—BEN STILLER

"This wonderful book is narrative medicine at its best. Jenifer sees people as people, not as patients or as scientists. She captures the joy and love the sisters bring to one another and to biomedical science. Her story adds to a sense of excitement, teamwork, and hope that is so essential for all major advances."

—GERALD D. FISCHBACH, M.D.,
Dean of the Faculty of Medicine
and Executive Vice President for Health
and Biomedical Sciences, Columbia University

Tales from the Bed

A MEMOIR

Jenifer Estess

as told to

Valerie Estess

WASHINGTON SQUARE PRESS
New York   London   Toronto   Sydney

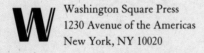

Washington Square Press
1230 Avenue of the Americas
New York, NY 10020

ISBN-10:   0-7434-7682-4
ISBN-13: 978-0-7434-7683-6 (Pbk)
ISBN-10:   0-7434-7683-2 (Pbk)

First Washington Square Press trade paperback edition November 2005

10 9 8 7 6 5 4 3 2 1

WASHINGTON SQUARE PRESS and colophon are
registered trademarks of Simon & Schuster, Inc.

Manufactured in the United States of America

For information regarding special discounts for bulk purchases,
please contact Simon & Schuster Special Sales at 1-800-456-6798
or business@simonandschuster.com.

For my sisters, our children, and my mother

Foreword

BY KATIE COURIC

I met Jenifer Estess four years ago at her apartment on West Twelfth Street in New York City. A number of our mutual acquaintances had suggested we meet. They insisted, I resisted. I had lost my husband to colon cancer just two years earlier and I was afraid I was still too fragile to befriend someone with a terminal illness. After being nudged repeatedly, I acquiesced. I headed to Jenifer's that February afternoon, and what can I say? She had me at hello. Call it kismet, call it chemistry, call it fate . . . whatever you call it, that was the first day of one of the most meaningful and powerful friendships I've ever experienced. Henry David Thoreau once wrote, "The language of friendship is not words, but meaning. It is intelligence above language." The challenge of expressing all that Jenifer meant to me is humbling and intimidating.

When I first met Jenifer, she was in a wheelchair,

ALS just beginning its insidious journey northward. We sat in the living room with Jenifer's two sisters, Valerie and Meredith, and her dear friend Julianne, and talked about this disease called ALS and their search for a cure. In a matter of minutes, I saw not a young woman with a fatal disease but a funny, vibrant, razor-sharp beauty who would quickly become my loyal friend and confidante.

How did I love her? Let me count the ways. Of course there was her amazing courage, grace, and dignity in the face of the most challenging kind of existence and most frightening kind of future. She was the personification of bravery, dealing quietly and matter-of-factly with the indignities of her disease. And she was always so present. When you were with her, you felt that you were the only two people in the world. She was sharp as a tack and had an insatiable appetite for whatever was going on in the world—whether it was a Supreme Court ruling or the latest heartthrob featured on the cover of *People* magazine. Jenifer was generous with her time and her heart. She could have crawled into her proverbial shell and shut people out, but she didn't. She remained so externally focused and completely in the moment.

She was a wonderful listener—a hip and funny Dear Abby, doling out especially good advice in matters of love. She was fiercely loyal. Pity the person who dissed a friend of Jenifer's. She wrote them off, their name never to emanate from her lips again, except in a hilariously catty remark. Most of all, Jenifer was about love. That was her greatest gift. She enveloped you in love and made you feel so special that you sometimes forgot how special she was.

But if loving others was her greatest gift, her sense of humor had to share top billing on her already remarkable résumé. Jenifer took the elephant in the room and turned it into a circus act. Her remarkable and, yes, deadpan humor (she would have had a field day with my choice of words) got so many of us through a very unfunny situation. I wish I had written down all the "Jeniferisms" I heard over the last four years. "Hi Jenifer, how are you?" "Great, except for this ALS stuff." "Jenifer can I call you right back?" "Sure, but can you give me a few hours? I'm going to run a marathon."

She even proposed a sitcom featuring her beloved nurse Lorna, complete with a theme song sung to the tune of *Three's Company*: "Lorna, please move my leg . . . can you give me a drink?" Jenifer dealt with an outrageous situation by being outrageous herself. And when she could no longer go to the party, the party came to her—up until the end, sitting on her bed, surrounded by legions of friends and the nieces and nephews she adored, Jenifer remained the high priestess of love, laughter, and light.

ALS robbed Jenifer of so much. But through it all,

she continued to appreciate the beauty of life even when her ability to live it was so cruelly curtailed. ALS couldn't take away her brilliance, and the one muscle it could not destroy was her heart.

Jenifer cannot be described without mentioning her two sisters, Valerie and Meredith. They so reminded me of the powerful and motivating combination of fear, desperation, and love. I, too, was motivated by those same things when my husband was diagnosed with colon cancer. But while I could cling to a sliver of hope as Jay went through chemotherapy and radiation, there were no such options for Jenifer—no treatment and certainly no cure. Yet, somehow, from this terrible abyss of hopelessness, sprung a thing of beauty: the love, loyalty, and power of this sisterhood.

They say good things come in threes. Pythagoras, the Greek philosopher of the sixth century, called three the perfect number. Man is threefold: body, soul, and spirit. The world consists of earth, sea, and air. And in Greek mythology there are three fates, three furies, and three graces. These three sisters should be added to that list. I will always think of them as a perfect triangle, providing each other with strong, steady, unconditional support. Take one away, and all that is left is a plain, straight line. Jenifer was taken away, but she'll forever be the apex of that triangle, the pinnacle of courage and grace to which we can all aspire.

Jenifer and her sisters had a favorite expression.

Whenever anything seemed unattainable, like being asked out by a ridiculously handsome guy, they'd say with an air of bemused resignation, "Hopes!" But Jenifer's life raised ours, and thanks to the Estess sisters, finding a cure for ALS is no longer unattainable.

My friend Jenifer Estess made everything seem possible. While it now may not be possible to call her, to see her, to laugh with her, it is still possible to love her. I do and always will.

Tales from the Bed

Chapter One

MARCH 17, 1997, was a very windy day in New York City. Walking up Amsterdam Avenue to the gym that morning, I wanted to turn around and go home. The old me would have. My apartment was dark and inviting, my bed was warm, and the gym would be there tomorrow. But then I thought of the Muffin Shop, which was opening in an hour. If I worked out for an hour, I could stop by on the way home for a muffin and coffee to go. One of the great pleasures for me was sitting at my new kitchen table with my muffin and coffee, planning the day. I had a big day ahead of me, so I kept going.

I'd been listening to Annie Lennox a lot on my Walkman. She was instrumental in some of the recent changes for the better I'd made in my life. Annie didn't sing—she spoke to me. "Please get your butt on the treadmill, Jenifer," she said. I always loved that English accent. *Right-ee-o, Annie.*

After six months, I had worked up to thirty minutes of running at 5.0 on the treadmill. Then I'd stretch and do a hundred, make that seventy sit-ups on the mat. I looked around the gym for my friend Billy Baldwin, who did sit-ups with me, but he wasn't there. The sit-ups were harder that morning, which was strange because I had a pretty strong stomach. I had to stop a few times. A handsome trainer walking by asked if I was okay. I said that I certainly thought so. He winked at me and kept going. *Sixty-seven . . . sixty-eight . . . Talk to me, Annie.* I dripped sweat. Hard-core athletes dripped sweat like this. I thought I was getting into some kind of shape. My sister Valerie would be proud.

Back at home I sat at my new table, feeling its smooth, sturdy contours. It had been a major purchase for me, the perfect Williams-Sonoma starter for a woman on the verge. I had my whole table in front of me, my blueberry muffin in hand, and a boy in my eyes. I hadn't met the boy yet. That would be happening tonight at Raoul's, a popular restaurant in Soho. My friends Martha and Merrill were going to spy on my date and me from another table. If it felt right, I'd give Martha the high sign, and the four of us would go dancing from there. Dating was something I didn't do much of in my twenties. I think people were a little worried about me. I kept saying I wasn't ready, I wasn't ready.

Then, when I realized I'd never be ready, I told my friends to fix me up, and suddenly there was an all-points bulletin out for an eligible guy for me. On some level, I still thought that blind dates were for losers, but I was learning to keep my eye on the prize. What I wanted most was to love someone and to have children. Maybe tonight was a step in that direction. It probably wasn't going to be *West Side Story,* but maybe it would be. *Could be . . .*

I sipped my coffee, forever my drink of choice. It was all about this kind of loving self-discipline: one muffin at a time, not two, eaten like a human being sitting at my gorgeous new table, not out of the bag on the run. Most of my friends were married and having babies or inviting me to showers or lamenting not getting married. I was starting to bask in self-reliance—I was working hard, step-by-step, to make my dream life a reality. My design for living was simple: I drew on the lessons of my girlhood. I was taking good care of my body. I was making a safe, comfortable home for myself. I was on a roll work-wise. The ideas came fast and furious: *Maybe for my next birthday I'd register at Bloomingdale's. Why should I have to wait for a fiancé to get a couch?*

"Oofah," I said, pushing back from the breakfast table. I was really late for work. I suddenly remembered the loofah brush and lavender soaps I'd picked up from Crabtree & Evelyn for my date. They were still in a shopping bag on the floor in my closet. When I bent down to get it, I got stuck in a crouch. As I got to my feet, and it took a minute, my burgundy silk shirt hanging from above fell into the Crabtree bag. Surely that was a sign. I'd do the burgundy silk shirt tonight, with my black jeans, and the brown suede jacket . . . or my black Donna Karan coat. The coat was dressier, a three-quarter length, and gorgeous. *Keep him guessing with the combination of dressy on the outside and totally casual-comfortable underneath.*

Running for the shower, I waved to my new Fiestaware plates stacked on the kitchen counter. I hadn't cooked a meal in years, but I would cook soon. I'd start with something simple—a pasta, maybe? Then came my really weird shower experience. As I unwrapped my loofah and my bathroom filled with steam, I imagined my date—rumored to be very handsome—watching me walk oh so elegantly through the steam toward the shower. Like those showgirls through dry ice in Las Vegas. But that wasn't even the weird part. Suddenly I felt oh . . . so . . . bogged down, as if I were wearing a wet wool blanket. I went into slow-motion showering, loo . . . fah . . . ing, and drying off. The towel was heavy, too, a second wet wool blanket. Was there such a thing as working out too much?

I blow-dried my hair in a hurry, never a problem. My hair was my calling card—thick chocolate chunks of

4

excellence, very Marlo Thomas in *That Girl*. My hair had gotten me through a lot in life. When I was posing for my head shot in second grade, I brushed my hair carefully around my slightly chubby face. I knew instinctively how to use my hair to create illusions of lankiness and great beauty. For as long as I could remember, I led with my hair.

As I ran down Columbus Avenue to catch a cab, I had my own *That Girl* moment. I saw my whole life coming toward me: I saw him and them, a husband and children, as true possibilities. I saw my sisters Valerie and Meredith walking in stride with great purpose. There I was between them, walking confidently. I looked pretty good. *Diamonds, daisies, Broadway*—wow. The wind really kicked up. It was so strong it pushed me backward. I sweated and slowed down on the sidewalk just as I had in the shower. I tried to fight the wind. I tried accelerating on the human highway of tourists walking to the St. Patrick's Day Parade, but there was nothing in my tank. I was alone in a sea of Kelly green. I wanted to tell everyone it was a great day for the Irish—and me, too—but they just kept passing me. I wanted them to know I was going to Raoul's that night. I wanted to tell them that I was lucky, and that I had my whole life ahead of me. Did I mention the wind? It was really blowing. It had a personality now—it wanted me dead.

I felt instant relief at the office with my feet up on the desk. My office was absolutely gorgeous, a dramatic departure from the alternative spaces I'd worked in as an off-Broadway theater producer. It was twenty marble-appointed floors up in a luxury midtown high-rise with great air-conditioning and a view of Central Park—salary *so* not commensurate. The job itself was a little disappointing. I was doing public relations, which I didn't care for, but in the end my office was the perfect front. Behind closed doors, twenty floors above Central Park, Valerie, Meredith, and I were planning a creative coup. Since high school, my sisters and I had had the idea of starting our own movie studio, and I was finally putting that plan into action. After years of hard work, Valerie, Meredith, and I were finally pursuing our best laid plans of childhood. It had taken us a while, but I felt sure that our hard work was about to pay off.

Meredith walked into my office for one of our top-secret working lunches just as my boss, smiling and totally unsuspecting, was walking out. My boss was a nice enough person. I knew one day she'd forgive me for the empire I was about to create. From across the desk, I watched Meredith lean in to her lunch, a tuna sandwich from Mangia, one of the best places in the city for tuna.

This was the moment I'd lived for, relaxing with my little sister over perfect tuna before an afternoon's worth of hard work. I reached for my sandwich feeling proud not only of Meredith but of my evolving perspective on food. I ate when I was hungry, that was all. I kicked my legs back up on the desk and started writing a few overdue checks.

"I see your legs," Meredith said.

"Who doesn't?" I said.

"No, seriously," she said, and she was right. The twitches in my legs that Valerie, Meredith, and I had seen occasionally over the last few months were going wild. My thigh muscles moved like snakes under my black slacks. They undulated and piled up on one another. I agreed it was bizarre. Meredith put down her sandwich. She saw twitches in my arms, too.

"I don't like it," she said. It was scary when Meredith weighed in. My little sister always meant what she said.

"Maybe I should see a doctor," I said.

"Like now," Meredith said, but I wanted to work. After lunch Meredith and I talked about a movie treatment that Valerie had written. I still felt the twitches in my legs, but I didn't want to look down at them. I wanted to look anywhere else. I wanted to look at my Fiesta plates and start the day over. *Don't look down.* I wanted to look out of my window at the thousand Kelly green dots of people marching, gliding, walking, running, pushing, strolling, kissing through Central Park. *Keep working.* I wanted to look at Meredith like this forever, an amazing woman in the prime of her life. Just like me.

Look down. My heart talks, I listen. The muscles of my legs and arms were rolling like the sea. As usual, my heart knew what my head would learn. Against the backdrop of my picture window, against the eagle's view of New York, my city, the impossible truth was announced: Something was seriously wrong with me.

The doctors invited me to a square dance. My first partner was my internist. I called him Undershorts. Undershorts was so tiny he could have fit under my exam gown. When I pulled up my gown to show him my twitches, he blushed and looked away. Then he climbed up onto a ladder and examined my ears, eyes, and throat. Undershorts didn't find anything wrong, so he swung me out to my second partner, Dr. Hainline, a sports neurologist at the Hospital for Joint Diseases. I bowed to my partner.

"Benign fasciculations," pronounced a busy Dr. Hainline, whose dance card was full. He said *fasciculations* was the clinical term for the muscle twitches I'd been experiencing. Apparently, my fasciculations had resulted from an unremarkable misfiring of nerve cells. I was fine. Good to go. That deserved a do-si-do.

That next week, I had trouble walking up the stairs

when I was with my friend Nicole at the theater. "You didn't say anything about stairs," said Dr. Hainline, during my second visit to his office, and he danced to the left. "I'm going to run one test," he said, "but I know it'll come out negative." Negative was positive, I remembered from my days watching *Medical Center*.

What's a square dance without a good psychiatrist? After I booked my appointment for the test, I placed an emergency call to my shrink, Karen. She reminded me of Sally Field. I loved Karen, I really did. She had been one of my clear-thinking, commonsense beacons in the last couple of years, mentoring me item by item down the having-it-all checklist: weight loss (check), dating (check), landing a better-paying job (half-a-check). The Zoloft didn't hurt, either.

When I rolled up my sleeve to show her my arm muscles moving, Karen fidgeted, she crossed and uncrossed her legs—she was all over the dance floor. My commonsense beacon was having a neurotic break with reality. Our repartee, which had always been verbal and jokey, filled up with more pauses than a Pinter play.

"Karen," I said.

"Jenifer," she said.

I placed my palms on the Abercrombie & Fitch jeans that she had helped me fit into. Karen was a medical doctor. I wondered, *Didn't she want to mosey on over and examine me?*

"The twitching is getting really bad," I said.

"The twitching . . . ," she said.

"You remember . . . the twitching." Was this an echo chamber? "The neurologist thinks it's all in my head," I said.

"Do *you* think it's all in your head?" Karen asked. That was all I could stand. I swung my partner and let go, quite frankly. For all I know, Karen's still reeling down Central Park West.

On March 26, I went for my EMG, the one test that Dr. Hainline had said would show nothing. The EMG measures how well your nerves talk to your muscles. I wasn't sure what that had to do with me. The EMG room was small and filthy, with a big computer. My mother sat next to me in a folding chair. Valerie was next to me on the exam table, as a tall woman taped cold foil discs all over my body, turned to the computer keyboard, and tap-tap-tapped with her back to us for about ten minutes. The tall woman rose, wished me luck, and left the room. Then a very pregnant radiologist came in. She had a thick Russian accent. My ancestors were Russian, or at least I thought they were.

"Weren't our ancestors Russian?" I asked my mother, swinging my legs off the side of the table.

"Who knows? Who cares?" she said. My mother wasn't exactly the family historian. Our family didn't really have a historian.

The pregnant radiologist asked me to lie down for the second part of the test. She stuck long, sharp needles into different muscles in my arms, legs, and torso. It hurt a little. Each time she stuck me, the computer recorded data. After about fifty sticks, she rose. "Please wait," she said, pausing at the doorway and exiting stage right. People came and went so quickly here.

Minutes passed. Fifteen minutes. Valerie was losing her temper. She looked down the hall and saw a huddle of white coats. The huddle broke and a third doctor came in. With a Russian accent so thick you could cut it with a scythe—radiology must have been all the rage in Moscow—he introduced himself as the director of the department. He asked me if I had taken any prescription drugs lately. There was the Zoloft and an occasional Advil. He asked me if I used cocaine. I was always too scared to try it. The doctor scratched his five-o'clock shadow. He inserted two last needles, one into my neck and one into my tongue. That hurt a lot. I saw my mother grab Valerie's arm. The doctor wrote on a clipboard for a long time. Then he wheeled around in his chair to face us.

"Well, there *is* something," he said. It was the moment of truth in a made-for-TV movie. I went numb. As for the earth, it shifted 180 degrees. "I'd say it's fifty-fifty."

"*What's* fifty-fifty?" I asked.

The director shrugged and sent us downstairs to Dr. Hainline, who had prescribed the EMG, the one test that was going to come back negative. We sat for hours waiting for Hainline. For kicks, nothing beats a neurologist's waiting room, especially after a preliminary diagnosis of *fifty-fifty*. A middle-aged couple, the man's head wrapped in yellowed gauze, held each other and wept. A limping child hurtled scarily toward a pile of toys. A woman with an evangelist's stare looked only at the ceiling. A receptionist finally appeared.

"I must say I'm surprised by the results of your EMG," Dr. Hainline said. He buried his head in my manila file. "You seem to have some kind of motor neuron disease."

"What the hell is a motor neuron disease?" Valerie asked.

When I heard *motor,* I immediately thought of going somewhere, of getting up and running out, and never stopping. I thought of movement. The phrase itself—*motor neuron disease*—didn't conjure up anything specific. But I knew it was bad. Instinct ordered me to leave my body and supervise from above. My spirit hovered over the scene, trying to make sense of a new phrase—and what I sensed was going to be a whole new life.

"Will I be able to walk?" I asked.

"We'll keep an eye on that," he said. Dr. Hainline spoke in tongues, ancient doctors' tongues.

"Is it a virus?" Valerie asked.

"No one knows for sure," he said.

"Will I be able to play tennis?" I asked.

"I've been at it for thirty years and I still can't play," he said, laughing and blushing. I pictured Valerie smashing a ball down Dr. Hainline's throat, but she and I pressed on responsibly with our twenty questions. So far, motor neuron disease hadn't qualified as animal, vegetable, or mineral. We looked for answers, even grains of answers.

"Will this situation clear up? Does it come and go?" Valerie asked.

"Need a more definitive diagnosis first," said the doctor.

"I've been working out a lot lately, maybe too much," I offered.

"Agreed!" declared my mother, jumping in bravely. "If I may . . . Dr. Hainline . . . what my daughter does to her body at that gym is dangerous, with the weights and the running and the going and the coming. It's too much for any one human—too much."

"Hmmm," said Hainline, closing my file, blushing crimson.

"Can you give us anything to hang our hats on?" Valerie asked.

"I can give you a wonderful referral," said Dr. Hainline, heading for the door. "Up at Columbia," Hainline said. "He's a giant in the field." I pictured the

Jolly Green Giant on a box of frozen baby peas. I ate a lot of those peas when I was a girl. I liked the butter sauce.

I had a motor neuron disease and a giant at Columbia University was going to tell me what that meant. Maybe he could take it away. I felt my arms and legs disappearing right then and there. *I must have a fast-moving case,* I thought. Dr. Hainline's receptionist handed me a card with the giant's phone number on it, and my mother, Valerie, and I left the hospital.

It was a black-and-blue night in New York. I was changed from before. I was a different woman hailing a taxi. My mother dropped us off at Valerie's house in Greenwich Village. Valerie, Scott, and their baby boy, Willis, lived in an ancient brownstone on Jones Street, a quiet street. Their house was my haven. After work, I loved hopping in a cab and going down to see them. Willis was my little blond duck. The house always smelled so good, like Valerie's chicken or her pasta cooking. There was always a place set for me. That night I wanted to stay and never leave.

We didn't do much crying or talking that night. Everyone just got busy. Scott set up my foldout cot in the living room. Valerie asked what we thought of spaghetti and a salad. Willis ran around in his diaper. Once, when he was eight months old, Willis and I pressed our foreheads together and laughed like no one had ever heard. We knew how to reach each other. That night, after

Valerie and Scott had gone downstairs to bed, Willis and I started our sleepover. We were the night birds of the family. I opened a box of animal crackers, and we sat on the cot changing channels and laughing at everyone until midnight. We settled on a Hercules serial dubbed in Spanish, and Willis fell asleep in my arms. As I held him, I watched Hercules picking people up, throwing them down, and carrying them to safety. Maybe Spanish Hercules would save me. But in all likelihood, that job was going to be mine.

In April, after that horrible March madness, I finally had my appointment with the giant in the field, Dr. Lewis P. Rowland, the director of the Neurological Institute of New York at Columbia University. Dr. Rowland was a happier version of my grandfather George, a kind, handsome, incredibly successful Chevrolet dealer from the Bronx, who never smiled. Dr. Rowland was old-school all the way, right down to the threadbare Oriental in his book-lined office and his wardrobe of bow ties. In fact, Dr. Rowland had been around long enough to have actually attended the Old School.

On the day of my appointment, I asked Meredith and Valerie to "answer phones at my office," code for moving our fledgling movie studio to the next planning stages. When they found it impossible to concentrate, my sisters went to St. Patrick's Cathedral and prayed. I'd asked my mother and oldest sister, Alison, to take me to Dr. Rowland's office at the Neurological Institute. The institute was a huge brick fortress that looked like a prison. I got the feeling that you checked in to a place like the institute, but you didn't check out.

"What brings you here, Miss Estess?" asked Dr. Rowland as I approached his mahogany desk the size of a ship. Maybe I left my legs in the cab. I couldn't feel them.

"I have a motor neuron disease," I said. I was Dorothy facing the Wizard.

"You don't have motor neuron disease," Dr. Rowland boomed, my file from Dr. Hainline sitting closed on his desk. Dr. Rowland's friends called him Bud.

"Oh my God, I don't?" I said.

"No, no. You don't have motor neuron disease," he said again.

Oh, Bud. I swooned. The other doctors were such amateurs. Just like that, Dr. Rowland commuted my sentence. They didn't call this guy the giant for nothing. My mother wept for joy. Alison ran out to call Valerie and Meredith. I was going to be okay. That meant I'd live to dance at my mother's weddings.

Then Dr. Rowland opened my file from Dr. Hainline, for the first time, I guess. As he reviewed the file, his face screwed up into a ghastly seriousness.

16

Bud, you've changed. "Step out, please," he said to my mother, ushering her out of the office in a hurry. So much for peas in butter sauce; color drained out of the world.

"I'm sorry, Miss Estess. You'll forgive me," he said gravely as he and I sat alone. "I hadn't seen the results of your EMG or your spinal tap," Dr. Rowland said. "I saw you . . . and I spoke out of turn. I've not done that before. Of course, I'll want to run my own tests."

Dr. Rowland gave me a neurological exam right there in his office. He followed my eyes with a flash-light. He hit my knees with a giant rubber hammer. He dragged a foot-long Q-Tip across the soles of my feet. For diagnosing motor neuron disease, the giant in the field used clown props.

"May I ask you to sit on the floor, Miss Estess, and then stand up?" *Tumbling?* All these weird tests, these Rube Goldberg variations, seemed so unscientific. But I was determined to win Bud over. If this was the extra-credit test, I felt sure I could ace it, charm him, and change his mind back again to *you don't have motor neuron disease.* After all, I could be very persua-sive. I ran my fingers through my hair and settled onto Bud's Oriental like a lotus flower. I was great. I was graceful. I made good eye contact. Then I tried to stand up. I gave it my all—I used my arms and legs, and the stomach muscles I'd worked on at the gym— but I couldn't get off the floor. Dr. Rowland extended

17

his hand, helped me up to a chair, and kneeled before me.

"You probably have ALS, Jenifer," he said, resting his hand on my knee. "Let's take a walk." Dr. Rowland and I walked arm in arm down an endless beige hallway. He told me that ALS was amyotrophic lateral sclerosis, a neuromuscular disease that destroys cells in the brain and spine called motor neurons. Without motor neurons, the brain can't tell the muscles what to do. Without directions from the brain, muscles can't function. Without muscles, a person can't walk, speak, swallow, breathe. . . . It was all getting a little confusing.

"Will I be able to have children?" I asked.

"You can have them," he said. "I just don't know if you'll be able to keep up with them." I started crying.

"We will have no tears," Bud said. He put his arm around me. I think Dr. Rowland assumed that because I'd walked into his office that afternoon young, confident, and self-possessed, I was also healthy. Poor Bud.

The only thing I remember after the beige hallway was collapsing into Valerie's arms. She held me like a mother while I made sounds I didn't recognize. They were animal sounds, sounds from nature, unplanned sounds. *This is what a dying woman sounds like.* Then Meredith moved in close and we three huddled as one. Silently, Valerie, Meredith, and I renewed a sacred girlhood pact: *Nothing, no one will stop us.* Over the next months, I would come to reject conventional wisdom, the books and TV shows advising me to let go as I died. For my sisters and me, dying, as living, wasn't about letting go. Holding on to each other was what we knew. Holding on like this and reaching.

Dr. Rowland admitted to making a terrible mistake that day, one that I forgave. But as I soon learned, ALS was much less forgiving. The Yankee baseball legend Lou Gehrig died from it, and so did every single one of the hundreds of thousands of other people who got it. No one survived. There was no medicine for ALS, and nothing Dr. Rowland could give me would slow it down or stop it. I was thirty-five years old. My cells were dying. I was dying. Dr. Rowland didn't say that exactly—he gave that job to his nurse and a bunch of pamphlets.

But for some weird reason, Dr. Rowland kept hanging around me after that first day. As I fought for my life, he taught me to buck up and be strong. He listened to me. He had my back. From that day on, Bud Rowland became the father I never had. I'm still trying to make him proud.

Chapter Two

MY REAL FATHER'S NAME was Gene, ironic given that a gene on chromosome 21 is responsible for one form of ALS. I didn't have that form of ALS per se, but scientists believe that I and others with so-called sporadic ALS are genetically predisposed to it. In other words, my DNA, or the genetic blueprint I was born with, made me a prime candidate for the disease.

I don't remember much about my father, but in his case a little goes a long way. Gene Estess grew up the favorite child of Adolph and Lillian Estess, a Jewish couple who lived in a pretty house on the banks of the Mississippi River, in Rock Island, Illinois, deep in Mark Twain country. My father was a shapely man, not like a farmer or a machinist, the kind of guys you saw around Rock Island. He was large and curvaceous. I thought he was handsome in his own special way. "Your father is *great*-looking," my mother always said, loud enough for him to hear. I took her word for it. My mother was a major tastemaker of her time.

My father wore a toupee. There's no question he would have looked better bald, but he opted instead for the three inches of cheesecloth. My father's toupee was a real presence in our house. It was a regular member of the family, with its jet-black hair, double-stick adhesive strips, and its own personal Styrofoam stand in the shape of a human head. Eventually my father's toupee came to symbolize much more to our family—cover-ups. Gene Estess was the Richard Nixon of fathers. I loved him; I looked up to him; I was onto him. My sister Valerie said I always knew things first. I suspected from a very early age that my father was an unfaithful person.

One of my father's outstanding features was his sense of entitlement. Lore has it that as a sophomore visiting home from college, Gene marched into the Star Restaurant, a Rock Island burger joint, and demanded an immediate change in the menu. He wanted a beef tenderloin sandwich added to it. Sliced beef tenderloin had become my father's favorite sandwich back East at the University of Pennsylvania, and he expected Rock Island to get with the program. My grandpa Adolph made a call to the owner of the Star and it was done. A beef tenderloin sandwich became the first menu addition in the history of the place.

Thanks to my dad, you could now order a hamburger, a cheeseburger, or a beef tenderloin sandwich there. My father was a big man with big appetites. He expected them filled.

In 1957, at the age of twenty, Gene had an appetite for my mother, Marilyn. He fell in love with her at a college mixer. I knew he fell in love because I found his old letters to her in my grandma's attic. Those letters don't lie. My mother said my father was "sick drunk" the night they met. From there, her account of their courtship gets murky.

"Was it love at first sight, Mommy?" I asked over coffee.

"How should I know? He was passed out and vomiting," she said. My mother and I talked over coffee a lot. I was her Rock Island confidante. As she drank black coffee and painted complicated word pictures, I looked at her and listened, captivated, as if I were watching a movie. My mother, who was a master at using her imagination to transport herself to better places, told me many secrets over coffee. She told me that our family was special. We were spectacular, she confided, and gifted. "You'll see," she said. "You'll see." I learned the power of the imagination from my mother. From our time together, I learned to love listening. I found I was good at it. I was good at listening, probing, and advising.

"But, Mommy," I persisted, "you had so many

boyfriends. There was that football player from Stamford—"

"*Stanford,*" she said, dragging deeply on her Salem cigarette.

"And that nice boy from Dartmouth," I said.

"Your father was the right person at the right time," she said, exhaling.

My parents got engaged two months after they met, then married lavishly at The Plaza hotel in New York. I thought they made a handsome couple. In fact, I still measure the elegance of a wedding by my parents' black-and-white photo album, a fairy-tale scrapbook that I memorized as a girl.

My mother was without a doubt the most beautiful woman in Rock Island, the Bronx (where she was born), and maybe the world. I'm talking drop-dead gorgeous. She was Faye Dunaway before there was a Faye Dunaway. I idolized her face and perfect figure, her clothes, and her sense of style, all of which she trucked out to Rock Island dutifully, right after the wedding. It's safe to say that my mother's many gifts, her deep intelligence and artist's eye, were lost on greater Rock Island. She roamed the cornfields dressed in Pucci, size 0. I felt protective of her. Some days, when I sensed that my mother was in danger and needed my protection, I would make myself sick and stay home from nursery school. I sensed danger as a girl. I had a built-in radar for it.

No house in Rock Island ended up being quite right for my parents, so they built their own Camelot, on a hill. My mother put everything she had into designing our new house, the oddest, most modern structure Rock Island had ever seen. I was proud when the local newspaper came over to interview my mother about her "architectural influences." That was my mother—she could have written her own ticket as an architect, a clothing designer, an artist, a lawyer, anything. I think she really wanted to be an actress.

My mother taught me that there are no small parts, only small actors. She had one line in her senior play at Skidmore College. Her job was to stand on a wooden log and say: "He went thataway." On opening night, as my mother delivered the line, her log began to roll stage right. He went thataway, all right, and so did my mother. She rolled right off the stage. It brought the house down. That was the power of one line, she said, delivered with *umph* to the back of the house. My mother seemed like a happier person when she talked about theater.

With all that talent and nowhere to put it, my mother ended up doing what she claimed every other woman of her generation did at the time—she got pregnant. The first in her family to graduate from college, my mother received her diploma from Skidmore while carrying her first baby, my sister Alison, in a sling. Then in the next six years, at Moline Hospital near Rock Island, she had the rest of us: Valerie, Jenifer, Meredith, and Noah—four girls and a boy. Sometimes I think my mother endured the girls just so she could have a son.

"Don't be ridiculous," she always said. "There's nothing like a girl."

Noah was born sick with a serious form of epilepsy that kept him and my mother in a Chicago hospital for the first year of his life. Doctors couldn't figure out how to control my brother's grand mal seizures, which were happening at the crazy rate of several per hour. I went to Chicago once to see him. I wandered off to where I shouldn't have been and saw my brother's swaddled silhouette through the darkened window of a room filled with sick babies. He bent in half like a billfold, opening and closing, over and over, uncontrollably. What the hell was happening, and why weren't the doctors doing anything to help my brother? It doesn't take a brain surgeon to connect the dots. My family had its neurological issues: Noah's epilepsy, which would take him years to get under control; my grandfather George's debilitating depression; assorted migraine and anxiety disorders; my ALS. Brain-wise, rather than drawing from a gene pool, my family drew from a gene cesspool.

Once my mother had five children, she had to figure out what to do with us. We definitely looked good. She sent for outfits from New York by the exclusive children's designer Florence Eisman and dressed us up. I loved my white gloves and my pretty patent-leather purse to match. Noah wore knickers, scalloped collars, and saddle shoes, just like John-John Kennedy. He was cute like John. Lending new meaning to the phrase *all dressed up and nowhere to go,* my sisters, brother, and I milled about Rock Island, visiting local wildlife amusements like Fedge-a-very Park, where a bored family of goats stood in a pen while we ruined our dresses with ketchup and ice cream. One of my favorite Polaroids is of my mother looking devastatingly gorgeous at Fedge-a-very Park, despite the five of us hanging on her like monkeys.

We children spent most of our time in Rock Island with our babysitter, Kaka. Her name was Kathleen, but baby Alison couldn't say that. *Ka . . . Ka,* Alison said. And it stuck. My Kaka smelled really good, like apples and honey. She used to make brownies—if anyone sold them now she'd be very wealthy, but the recipe is lost. The brownies would come out of the oven, and as Kaka stood there with a spatula in her hand, my sisters and I would eat them hot, right out of the pan.

My parents traveled to New York a lot in those years. At least they told us they were going to New York. I had a feeling they were really just dropping us off at Kaka's house and going back home for a rest. Sometimes my sisters and I lived at Kaka's little salt-box for weeks at a time. Kaka had long, long hair the color of hay that she wore up in a perfect bun. Her skin was soft and felt like peach fuzz when she held me to her. Late at night, after she tucked Meredith and me into our beds, I'd sneak into the hall outside her bathroom and watch her put her teeth in a glass. I could never tell how old she was. Kaka was one of the last surviving pioneers, strong as an ox—and so resourceful. From the grapes in her backyard she made jelly. From the flour in her kitchen she made golden crust for pies. From the yarn in her wicker basket, she knitted fisherman sweaters for my dollies.

"I feel exhausted just watching you," my mother said to Kaka, during a rare appearance in Kaka's kitchen. At night, my sisters and I watched TV with Kaka and her husband, Ed, a retired Navy man and machinist for International Harvester. I think they considered us their children. Ed sat with Valerie in his remote control recliner. Kaka rocked in her chair, sewing and knitting. I was on the floor, my head on my hands, as close as I could get to the huge black-and-white set. I loved television deeply. As an emotional, slightly chubby girl of five, I flung myself into the dramas of the small screen. I watched them all, *Ed Sullivan, The Wonderful World of Disney,* anything Hayley Mills. Once when Ed hooted at a barmaid on *Bonanza* who had just had her heart broken by a cowboy, I told him, "You leave me alone—and you leave that lady alone, too," and I stomped out of the room. Kaka always got a kick out of that line. She quoted it until her death. Ed just laughed at me. But he'd see soon enough. They'd all see. I was secretly grooming myself to be *someone,* a personality, a star—and big, big, big. The fact that I could eat a box of Twinkies at one sitting didn't exactly hurt my chances.

When I was six and my mother told me that we were leaving Rock Island to live in New York, I told her I supported that. "I love you, Mommy," I said, and I went right to my room to pack. She told me that through family connections, she'd helped land my father a job as an account executive with Gray Advertising. My mother felt that my father could grow in advertising. The seven of us would live temporarily with her parents, my grandma and grandpa Rosenberg, in their spacious new house in Harrison, an affluent suburb north of Manhattan. Once in Harrison, we'd find a special house of our own, she promised me, a bigger, better Camelot.

"Will I have my own room?" I asked.

"And then some," my mother said. "And then some."

I was going to miss Kaka and the simple pleasures—the smell of the vinyl seats of her creaky old Corvair on a hot day, her singing "Peace in the Valley" to me as we fished together for catfish in the Mississippi, and the brownies. I was too young for nostalgia, though, and ready for adventure, so I put my dolls and their sweaters in a suitcase and said good-bye. We packed the station wagon, plugged our portable TV into the lighter socket, and drove away. After I toasted my future with one last frosty mug at the A&W Drive-In, as night fell, my family merged with the open road. One by one, my sisters and brother fell asleep. I sat in the way-backseat, glued to the TV. It was sending me private black-and-white messages, comforting messages, exciting ones. The broken horizontal lines, the muted audio, the grainy faces of the world's biggest stars—it was all a secret code telling me I was about to enter a new world. As my father drove, the messages came through the television, through the night, through Illinois, Ohio, Pennsylvania, and New Jersey. And they were all good.

Chapter Three

"GO DEEP." Valerie gripped the football in her left hand as Meredith and I ran out across the huge front lawn of our new house, Trilarch, named by its previous owners for the clutch of three unremarkable larch trees that welcomed visitors to the three-acre property. Trilarch was a lavish expanse for Harrison, New York, and it was all ours, sort of.

"This one's for . . . Jenifer." Valerie called my number and threw long to within inches of my chubby, outstretched fingers. Desperate to make contact with the ball, I went horizontal and hit the ground hard. The pass was incomplete. I cried into my hair and the dirt. People made fun of my crying. They compared me to the famous actress Sarah Bernhardt, except, they said, I was more like Sarah *Heartburn*.

"Uh-oh, here comes Coach," Meredith said.

Meredith had nothing to worry about. She had already caught three bombs, the long throws that Valerie used to test our running and catching skills.

"What seems to be the problem?" Valerie asked, standing over me on the ground. My sister Valerie was one scary eleven-year-old. She looked like a tree with her stringy brown hair for branches and a pretty scowl. Valerie told me to stop crying, but that wasn't happening. I'd been very honest with her: I didn't like football or baseball or any of the other sports she made us play. I liked ice-skating. At least there were outfits and a snack bar, and my legs looked great in those nude opaque tights—

"Get up and do it again," said Valerie. Life with Valerie was well defined. She was the Coach. Meredith and I were her players. We did as she said.

"What about Meredith?" I asked.

"Did Meredith catch a bomb?" Valerie was up in my face.

"Yes," I said.

"Did *you* catch a bomb?" she asked.

"No, Coach, I didn't catch a bomb," I said, hanging my head.

"Don't hang your head," she barked. "Ever." I looked to the sky. My tears fell on the ground.

"Do you want to achieve your personal best on the field, or do you want to cry in your room?"

"Is that a rhetorical question?" I asked.

Valerie wasn't amused. She took Meredith's and my education very seriously. After school and before dinner, Valerie made our every minute count. After supervising our sports, she marched us over to our playhouse in the backyard. Our playhouse was nicer than some people's real houses. It was an FAO Schwarz exclusive—a sturdy cabin with a white picket fence and its own lookout tower, where I watched for enemies. Valerie would change the personality of the playhouse periodically to suit her interests. The first year, our playhouse was the Monkees Fan Club of Harrison. Valerie appointed herself president and plastered pictures from *Tiger Beat* of Micky Dolenz, her favorite Monkee, all over the walls. My job, as I saw it, was to love the Monkees' lead singer, Davy Jones, with my whole heart forever. My job, as Valerie saw it, was to keep the clubhouse clean at all times. Meredith and I were expected to wait on Valerie's friends when they came over for Monkees meetings. We served the older girls snacks that we ran over from our real house.

The second year, Valerie turned our playhouse into the Science Lab. She made Meredith and me watch while she dissected grasshoppers and butterflies with a scalpel. "Don't you find this fascinating?" she asked, slicing into the pale white stomach of a frog.

"I do," said Meredith. Yeah, sure she did.

"I gotta be honest, Valerie. This just isn't me," I said.

"We appreciate your honesty," said Valerie, pulling back the frog's belly to reveal a gut filled with surprisingly vivid reds and blues. "But the world isn't about you, Jenifer."

Valerie educated Meredith and me across disciplines. She taught us science, sports, the latest music. She taught us survival techniques on the nature trail, an overgrown part of our property. I'd be lying if I said that I loved the daily lessons. But basic training wasn't meant to be fun or easy. Basic training was something you hated being in the throes of and appreciated later on. I paid my dues on the field every day. I tried my best, listening and learning until dinner was over. Then it was my turn. When Valerie finally retired to her room for homework, I closed the door to my own room and warmed up to Frank Sinatra. I loved Frank. If my father and I shared anything, it was our deep admiration for Sinatra. I felt cool liking the same singer as my father.

Nighttime was my time. In the privacy of my bedroom I worked on improvised monologues in my vanity mirror. I transformed myself into Cher and Barbra Streisand. I listened to my parents' Judy Garland records until my close-and-play gave out. Okay, maybe I was a gay man trapped in the body of a nine-year-old girl, but who cared? I was too busy performing, working, getting out the kinks—life in the spotlight of the moon was my destiny. And there was no way I was going to face my destiny without Meredith, my little football star. That was the picking order—Valerie picked mostly on me, I picked on Meredith.

"And five, six, seven, eight . . . ," I said, tapping out time. Whenever I wanted, I dragged Meredith through the halls of Trilarch by her beautiful black hair and locked her in my room. I hadn't raised a fool—Meredith knew she'd have to dance her way out.

"Relax the feet," I said from my vanity table, as Meredith attempted a stiff soft-shoe that fell way short. I told her I'd be over to demonstrate the proper technique the moment my nails dried. My new nails were real beauties—pink, frosted, and fake—a new arrival at Polk's, Harrison's superior five-and-dime store. Jumping beans, sewing kits, the largest conceivable selection of fake nails and eyelashes—these were Polk's specialties, and I was a preferred customer. The smell of the greasepaint was one thing—the glue fumes from my new Sally Hansens were a pure shot of energy. I jumped up from my vanity, ready for work.

"All right, let's go right into the big number," I said, swinging Meredith around by the hair. Meredith hated the big number. It was my equivalent of the bomb. "It's for your own good," I assured her.

"I really don't see how it's for my own good, Jenifer," said Meredith, in a rare insubordinate outburst.

"Ahhh . . . time will tell," I said, fanning an invisible crystal ball with my elegant fingers. Whereas Valerie was more definitive with her threats—*Do it or I'll punch your lights out*—I went for witchy and ominous. Sufficiently convinced that I could predict her future and alter it mysteriously, Meredith sailed into the blocking for "You Are Woman, I Am Man," the romantic turning point in *Funny Girl*. In my book, *Funny Girl* beat the Bible for wisdom and life lessons. I'd been to Sunday school. I'd played a hamantasch in the Purim parade, and although I genuinely admired them, I never really connected on a gut level to Ruth and Esther. Was there a Rachel? As far as I was concerned, Barbra Streisand's performance in *Funny Girl* contained every life lesson a girl needed to know. I considered it my God-appointed duty to pass on this wisdom to the Younger.

"Do I have to wear the mustache?" Meredith asked. Meredith played Nick Arnstein, Streisand's movie husband, a greasy cheat.

"You disappoint me, Nicky," I said, tapping my nails against the door frame. Meredith fetched the Nick Arnstein mustache from my vanity and sighed as I lowered the needle of my close-and-play onto the movie soundtrack. We did the whole number without stopping, mouthing the lyrics in a precise karaoke duet, kiss included. It went off without a hitch. When we were done, I released Nicky from my clutches, and

Meredith flew as fast as she could down the hall. "We're all alone in the end," I called after her. For me, it was back to the vanity, my drawing board, where I rehearsed improvised lovers' confessions until bedtime.

As my sisters and I grew into early adolescence, my parents struggled to keep up appearances. They couldn't afford our English Tudor–style mansion in the first place—not its acres, its man-made ponds and nature trails, or its elevator. My parents had borrowed money from their parents for the down payment on Trilarch, then never stopped going to that bank. This put pressure on my mother, who was so overdrawn on her fantasy of us as the Jewish Kennedys—perfect house, powerful husband, and charmed children—she didn't have a penny left for reality shopping. And the reality was my father seemed to change jobs a lot. The guy may have had a decent toupee on his shoulders, but to me he didn't seem to know much about work. Entitlement had been the ethic of his upbringing. On some level I think my parents believed that my father was the anointed—that success would fall around him like a glitter storm if only he wore the right seersucker suit from Paul Stuart or if they shipped their children out to the most prestigious overnight summer camps in Maine.

My mother was the one who should have been wearing seersucker, but she continued to put it on my father. My mother was the one who should have run a stock options firm on Wall Street, but that was my father's expertise, she insisted, over coffee in the kitchen after school.

"I thought Daddy worked in advertising?" I said once.

"He's much too talented for advertising," she replied. "Dollars and cents are his expertise."

As far as I could tell, my father's only expertise was marshmallow fudge. Sometimes late at night, I found my father in the kitchen boiling Marshmallow Fluff together with Hershey bars. Then he'd pour it all in a pan and watch it harden.

"Want some fudge, little girl?" he'd ask, standing in his bathrobe.

"No, thank you, Daddy," I'd say, making off with a Twinkie or two.

Putting my father first—living for him—had left my mother with a deep need to talk. I was her go-to girl. After school, I tried teaching her the new math: *Take one hundred percent of a mother's greatness and project it onto the father—that leaves how much for Mother?*

"Why don't you go to law school, Mommy?" I asked, echoing a dream I knew she had for herself.

"It's too late for me," she said.

"Are you happy being married to Daddy?" I said, sipping coffee, swallowing grounds.

"It's better than a poke in the eye with a sharp

stick," she said. *Wuthering Heights* my parents' marriage wasn't, I'd realized. I knew my father's type, but I loved him anyway.

It all came down to pot holders in September. A few weeks after I started eighth grade, my parents, sisters, brother, and I began campaigning in earnest for my father's election to the Harrison School Board of Education. Saturday mornings we stood like the First Family in front of Vaccaro's grocery store, dressed in our navy blue turtlenecks and gray slacks, handing out pot holders stamped with VOTE FOR GENE to shoppers. The pot holders had been my father's idea—an ingenious political device, he thought.

"Every time someone reaches for a pot or a pan, they'll think of me," he explained during our ride to the shopping center. It was the kind of subliminal advertising a candidate couldn't buy, he said.

"Hello, Mrs. Kelly," I said, extending a pot holder to Mrs. Kelly and her son, my friend Timmy, who came out of Vaccaro's pushing two huge carts full of groceries.

"Well, hello, Jenifer. What have we here?" asked Mrs. Kelly.

"A pot holder," I said.

"My, my, isn't that something? Look, Tim, a pot holder."

"Oh, yeah, just what I always wanted," he said, rolling his eyes. I loved Timmy Kelly. He was the most popular boy in my grade. His mom was my friend, too. When I went to Timmy's house to play, I usually ended up in the kitchen, where Mrs. Kelly asked me to call her Shannon and we talked about marriage over coffee.

"And who are you going to vote for next week, Mrs. Kelly?" I asked her.

"Well, now, Jenifer, I haven't quite made up my mind," she said. "I sure do wish you were running for the board of education." Now, that was strange. Shannon Kelly and I were pretty close. Why was she so reluctant to show support for my father? I was about to ask her when my radar picked up a strange frequency. I turned my attention to a small, deserted area, a tiny patio set back from the main entrance to Vaccaro's. My father was there, locked in an intense, whispered conversation with a woman I'd seen before. The mole on the woman's face looked very familiar. It was the kind of mole you couldn't buy at Polk's. *Right,* I thought, she was that reporter for *The Harrison Independent,* our local newspaper weekly. *Hmmm . . .* and my father had gone to the *Independent* offices the three previous Sundays to answer her questions about his political platform. He'd been there all day. I wondered, could her questions and his answers have possibly filled up three long Sunday afternoons when, with all due respect, I could have summed up my father's political platform in a haiku?

I think I was born with supersonic vision, kind of like those submarine radars. I couldn't help seeing beyond the parameters of normal. *Deet-deet-deet. Deet-deet-deet.* That autumn morning in front of Vaccaro's, one whole horrible panorama came into focus. I saw my mother smiling in a Chanel suit like Jackie, putting voters at ease. I saw my sisters, Alison, Valerie, and Meredith, and my brother, Noah, handing out pot holders for a man they believed in. I wondered if my father was having an affair with that lady. Valerie always told me that I saw things first, knew them first, and did them first. She wondered if I knew how lucky I was to possess such gifts. I wondered if Valerie knew that all I ever wanted was to catch a bomb.

Over the next months, Valerie's obsession with Honda minibikes reached a crescendo. After school, privileged neighborhood kids would ride their minibikes and go-carts around Trilarch in a wild, unsupervised motocross. Although I was deathly scared of Valerie's minibike, which was basically a motorcycle for children, I promised her that I would test-drive our neighbors' less intimidating go-cart. It was a shot heard round the world when on my first run I crashed the go-cart head-on into a tree, transforming Trilarch into Bilarch in an instant. Meredith was first on the scene.

"Are you okay?" she asked.

I stared straight ahead for minutes, they told me, silent and unblinking. They say I sat motionless under my white mushroom motorcycle helmet until twilight came, long after our friends had gone home. There was the undeniable impact of girl meeting tree. But the sight of a more serious accident up ahead threw me into shock. *You know things first.* I knew that my father was going to leave my mother. I didn't know what my mother was going to do about that. Neither did my grandmother Rosenberg.

The familiar whiff of L'Air du Temps mixed with peppermint Chiclets told me that Grandma Rosenberg was in the house early one Sunday morning. I followed my nose down our grand front staircase to the third step from the bottom, where I settled in for some serious eavesdropping. My grandma and my parents were hunkered down in the library, a wood-paneled room right off the entryway, where we watched TV. By the time I had adjusted my supersonic hearing—*come in, please*—they were deep in conversation. The cadence of my grandma's voice was different from usual—a clue. She was being very forceful. My mother was crying. That was always tricky—my mother had different cries for different occasions. This was her most heartbreaking, the Desdemona, clue number two.

"I need time, Eleanor," my father said. "I need my

own space. Not permanently—just for now." His voice was tinny and weird. He was definitely lying to my grandmother, clue number three.

"That's crap, mister. You can't fool me," Grandma bit back. "There's only one thing that takes a man away from his family—"

"Gene is thinking of leaving, Ma. He wanted you to know first," my mother's voice wavered and cracked. Then I lost transmission. *Come in, please. Come in.* Nothing. But I had a lot of material to work with. There was the scene on the patio behind Vaccaro's . . . and now three more clues. I did as I felt I must. I made the call: It was Gene Estess in the library with a candlestick, in a reporter girlfriend, perhaps? I ran like Paul Revere up the stairs and through my sisters' rooms. "Divorce . . . divorce . . . divorce!" I yelled. I ran through Alison's room looking for Valerie.

"Maybe you could knock first," Alison said. Our oldest sister was easily annoyed by my histrionics and mad that I'd recently broken her prized Chinese wind chimes. A daughter of the counterculture, Alison spent the vast majority of her time kissing, and more, with boys; sketching in her Hippie Notebook, 1975; and filling out forms for her early admission to Brandeis University, the Angela Davis school. Alison always had one foot out the door.

"What's up?" asked Valerie, meeting me outside her room. Joni Mitchell played on her stereo.

"Divorce," I said, trying to catch my breath. "Daddy's leaving."

"Really?" Meredith met us there.

"I heard it. I knew it. I heard it. I knew it—" I was hyperventilating. It was my first anxiety attack since I was eight, when I thought my father was fooling around with the babysitter. I had made myself throw up that day so I could stay home from school to be near my mother.

"Get ahold of yourself," said Valerie.

"That's what you get for eavesdropping, Jenifer," said Alison, who had joined us in the hall. She was crying.

"Get in the car and wait for me," Valerie said. "Everyone, now." Alison complied, Valerie grabbed Noah, and the five of us piled into our gray Chevy Vega. Valerie ordered Alison to drive, Alison put the pedal to the metal, and we escaped from Trilarch. We had an emergency picnic. Alison made the requested pit stops according to our every desire along the way: tuna on a bed from Milk Maid, turkey on a roll with Russian and coleslaw from Butler Brothers, hot dogs from Walter's. We parked across the street from Walter's in Larchmont and headed with our food up a hill to the grassy knoll where we made family history. No one had seen the bullet hit, but we children had been blown away by the news of our parents' divorce. I loved my parents being together. It was hard to imagine my world any other way.

As Alison practiced transcendental meditation on her private patch of grass—"I have to get home for a five o'clock date," she reminded us—our baby brother, Noah, wandered off to gather rocks. That left the three of us together on the hill. As the sky darkened, Valerie, Meredith, and I made an eternal pact there. We swore that nothing would ever break us apart. No divorce or hurricane, no national emergency or act of God. No one would break our will or our bond.

"We'll march our band out, we'll beat our drum," said Valerie. It gave me chills hearing Valerie quote from *Funny Girl*.

"And if we're fanned out?" I asked.

"You get up to the plate and try again," Valerie said. "Or I bat for you, or you bat for Meredith, or Meredith bats for me. Whoever can step up, steps up."

The old hierarchy that had Valerie beating on me and me beating on Meredith had suddenly outlived its usefulness. On the grassy knoll, it occurred to us that if we were to survive, let alone succeed, we'd need to become one another's hearts and minds, mentors—not tormentors—mutually and unconditionally. Each of us would have the other two checking in at all times, making sure, protecting, and inspiring. This dinghy wasn't going down.

"We have to go out into the world and prove we're still a family," said Meredith.

"That is correct," said Valerie, beaming.

Valerie retired her coach's whistle that day and, at age fifteen, set about the more complicated job of raising Meredith and me. After my father moved out and my mother lay down for a long rest, after Alison drove north to Brandeis University and Noah turned into a Ping-Pong ball ending up far away in my father's court, Valerie took over our care and feeding. She drove Meredith and me to school and out for dinner. She gave us money from her waitressing jobs and helped us with our homework. She did my homework when I played her right.

When my father packed up his Styrofoam toupee stand, I knew he was leaving for good. He left us without any way back to him. He grew a beard, bought a pea green Cadillac, and drove into his next life. It was like he was in the witness protection program. I was crushed when he left. He was the only man I'd known. My mother depended on him, and I loved her so much. My mother took the divorce the hardest. She spent most of her time the next year wearing Lollipop underwear and smoking in bed. She took a lot of Valium. Still, I was struck by her uncommon beauty. No one, not even Diane Keaton in *Annie Hall,* looked that good in an undershirt.

I tried coaxing her out of her room for meals, but she was seriously depressed. My mother's Kennedy dreams had exploded in her face. Her Camelot had collapsed like a house of jokers. Her magnificent clothes hung in her closet like corpses, constant reminders of her failure as a wife. She didn't deserve that rap, not for a second. The turn of events had been unfair. The burden he left her, the children he left her, the house on the brink of foreclosure—all of it was unfair and unjust. But there wasn't a court in the land that ruled on this sort of thing. Unfairness was a fact of life. Still, I wished my mother would put on some lipstick.

"Jenifer, please bring me my medicine and a glass of water," she said as I sat on the edge of her bed.

"There's pizza."

"All I want is to pull the covers over my head," she said, sliding into her ocean of a bed. She was unavailable for further comment for about two years.

By that time, my sisters and I were deep into high school. Valerie was president of the senior class. My sisters and I had taken after-school jobs at the local meat market and my favorite, Clover Donuts, a coffee shop. You should have seen me flipping those donuts, boy. I was pretty good at eating them, too. If food was a comfort to my family before the divorce, it became a savior now. My sisters and I didn't do drugs—we did the twenty-four-hour Pathmark in Yonkers, where we set land-speed records for consumption of Entenmann's chocolate chip crumb loaf at four o'clock in the morning.

By the age of fifteen, I was making decent pocket money at three Clover Donuts locations in White Plains, managing the counter and the grill. Just as Valerie had taught us, the work and resulting paycheck made me feel really accomplished. I probably could have lived without the two-a-day Bavarian cremes—where was the "a" in *creme* anyway, Valerie wanted to know. Learning to make good coffee, keeping a clean store, developing friendships with the truly handsome cops who were Clover regulars—all of this felt satisfying. I had taken my personal best from my room to the road, only now I was being paid for it. I was a working girl now, a Clover Girl. While Cover Girl was my first choice by far—no question I had the skin for it—I was grateful for my gig.

Meredith didn't last long at the meat market. The guy who owned it was kind of a maniac. Scrub as she did, Meredith couldn't quite clean the slicing machine to his liking. She quit after two weeks. Meredith was growing up to be so beautiful—she had that Linda Carter–TV miniseries look about her that I respected so much. Valerie and I were the waitresses, the heavy lifters of the family. Meredith became our princess.

The princess and I became best friends. We ruled the breezeway, the hallway in our high school that separated the women from the girls. I taught Meredith hair. She taught me Frye boots, huge hoop earrings, and Levi's corduroys. Meredith became my absolute last word on The Look. Her fashion instincts may have even surpassed my mother's. The up-and-coming designer Calvin Klein was Meredith's idol. She followed Calvin like I followed Frank Sinatra. A great day for me was taking Meredith to Bloomingdale's and buying her a little—very little—something Calvin with my Clover money. Meredith and I had all the same friends. The front door of Trilarch, which had been closed to all but the occasional delivery from Harrison Chemists, was flung open for a never-ending party with our mutual friends, who quickly became family. Trilarch became *the* party house, as supervised by Valerie. She or I would often arrive home from work to find the action in full swing.

High school was the best time of my life. You'd think that one of my parent's taking a powder and the other one's swallowing it in pill form would've been a setback. It did take a piece of my heart. Life with Father and Mother had been exciting. There was Angela Lansbury in *Mame,* car trips to Washington, D.C., and Boston, Bette Midler at the Palace, dinner at La Caravelle when we were the only kids in the restaurant. But when the bill came due, no one was there to pay it. Now that I was working, I wanted to make a lot of money so I could share it with my sisters. I decided I was going to buy us all a huge house in Malibu one day for our husbands, our children, and friends passing through. My boyfriend Michael told me that his uncle Harold had bought himself quite a house on the beach in Malibu.

"One day we're gonna live in Malibu, my treat," I announced to Valerie and Meredith one night, as Valerie sat at the kitchen table writing my latest English report, "The Forest as a Symbol in Shakespeare's Comedies." (She came up with the idea for the paper, too.) *I saw things first*: I was probably going to act in plays, I thought, make some movies—maybe one day my sisters and I could start our own movie studio.

As my basic training came to an end, I felt a new energy. My childhood and early education had left me with a well-earned excitement for the future. The lessons I'd learned about love, work, and what it meant to be a family gave me direction. They were lessons in granite, true lessons. I'd always had big, big dreams— now I had the means for achieving them.

"So, what do you think, Valerie—a house on the beach—?"

"I'm working here, do you mind?" she said.

"Do you think I'll get us a place in Malibu?" I asked.

"I know I'm counting on it," said Meredith. She was waiting for Valerie to write her a note explaining to the homeroom teacher why Meredith had missed the previous two full days of school. Valerie had written many notes excusing Meredith and me from school. They were all lies, of course. But Valerie was really mad about this one. Without asking Valerie, Meredith had taken the family car and spent two days camping in the forests of northern Westchester with Peter Hulbert, a gorgeous West Point cadet who would capture our little sister's imagination forever.

"I bet I know what happened in *that* forest," I said. Meredith laughed. Valerie didn't laugh.

"You want a house on the beach?" Valerie said, rising from the kitchen table and coming toward me. She was so mad. "You want to live your own life and call your own shots? Do you want to make a difference in this world?" She was up in our faces.

"Yes, Valerie," Meredith and I said in unison, mockingly. We were teenagers now. We were going our separate ways, together.

"Then go deeper," she said. Valerie stormed out of the kitchen, ran up the stairs, and slammed her door closed.

Chapter Four

YOU HAVE TO LOVE what you have in the time that you have. Okay, so it wasn't Malibu, but the Westhampton Beach rental my mother treated my sisters and me to that summer in 1997, two months after my diagnosis, wasn't chopped liver, either. It was a pretty house with a swimming pool and a short drive to the beach—and I loved it. In my heart I knew that Westhampton was the last time we would be free as a family. It was the last summer I'd pass as another lucky thirty-five-year-old loving the Hamptons.

The hammer of my ALS diagnosis had fallen in April, but I still wasn't showing overt signs of physical loss. To look at me you couldn't tell anything was wrong. Walking had become a little harder, but I still ran errands on Main Street. Getting up from low patio chairs around the pool was hard, but I still got right up from every other kind of chair. I began noticing subtle physical changes when I was alone. ALS was a real creep that way. It waited until I was alone so it could whisper in my ear. It whispered to me when I was shaving my legs.

The downstairs bathroom at Westhampton was one I would have designed for my dream house. It had a big glass-enclosed shower and marble tiles. I couldn't wait to steam things up in there. I shampooed and sang. I shaved my left leg. It was tan and elegant and so smooth. Truth be told, the muscle atrophy caused by ALS had my legs looking so very slim. Boy, did I ever love my left leg, all of a sudden. When it came time for me to swing my right leg up onto the marble shelf, I couldn't—quite—do it. I tried kicking it up again, but no go. Okay, so . . . I wouldn't shave my right leg. European women didn't shave either leg and everyone still loved them. This was where having a degenerative disease got a little tricky. ALS would take away something relatively small—shaving my right leg—knowing that I would immediately rationalize the loss. Nature designed human beings to rationalize loss. We are programmed to make comforting excuses for ourselves when painful things happen. Without rationalization, we'd all go off the deep end.

I rationalized my experience in the shower. Although I couldn't shave my right leg, I figured I still looked healthier than ever. My hair, my tan . . . I didn't *look* sick. People said I'd never looked better. I probably had a slow-moving form of ALS. There was such a thing, I'd been told. Even if there wasn't, I knew that if anyone could set a new precedent for the disease, I could. The brochures from Dr. Rowland's nurse didn't begin to describe the woman in *my* mirror. They had photographs of people tilted back in wheelchairs with tubes and machines coming out of them. They had oatmeal recipes for patients who couldn't swallow solid food, and line illustrations of clawed hands. The printed materials were so "complete dependence." They didn't describe me for a second, and they looked like they were printed in 1950. After a glorious summer in the sun, my sisters and I would find other brochures, consider new medical perspectives, and gather second and third opinions.

In the meantime, I was loving every moment. *No one, nothing, will break us.* I swam with the kids in the pool all summer. I held them in the water. I ate Meredith's guacamole, the best on earth, and I put on lipstick. I drank hot coffee by the pool in the morning and danced with the kids at night. I didn't have children of my own, but my sisters gave me theirs. The children and I were so in love with each other. The guys, Jake and Willis, were a midget Butch Cassidy and the Sundance Kid, with Jake, Meredith's oldest, the sultry five-year-old leader, and Willis, the sunshine. There was a girl on the scene now, Jane, who would be Meredith's middle child. Jane was two. I watched Jane play on a brilliant orange beach towel. Her eyes were the color of purple Tootsie Pops, just like her mother's. The colors that summer: Jane's eyes, the red of tomatoes, the blue sky and the pool, the greens and chocolate browns of lettuces that had just been pulled from the ground. Colors stood out as never before. This was what I stood to lose, the amazing colors of life.

My friends were all over the Hamptons that summer. Martha, Geoffrey, and Merrill came by for a visit in their red rented convertible, top down. Martha brought the world's freshest salmon to cook that night. The guys wanted iced coffees. Jane watched Martha prepare foil packets of salmon and summer vegetables while Geoff, Merrill, and I drove into town. I wanted to pick up something for the kids. I loved getting them a little something from town.

"Are you crazy, Jenifer?" said Meredith, when she'd see the daily shopping bags from town filled with candy and toys for them.

"It's just a little something," I'd say. "Relax."

Driving with Geoff and Merrill on a sunny, breezy afternoon in Westhampton made me feel powerful, as if a miracle could happen at any minute. My guys looked buff in the front seat, with their tank tops and their tans. I was the babe in the back. My dark hair blew proud like a flag in the breeze. We had our sunglasses on. Someone should have taken a picture.

It was funny. I was definitely different from my friends—I was building an individual life for myself. I was creating my own way. But being with Martha, Geoff, and Merrill reminded me how much I loved being part of the crowd. Pursuing individuality was important. It was crucial to my happiness. But I felt proud blending in, too. I loved being a part of things, playing in all the reindeer games. I loved participating. As Geoff and Merrill hopped out of the car for coffee, I struggled to get out of the backseat. My legs were like posts. A wave of exhaustion washed over me. I thought that I was going to faint, so I waved the guys on and stayed in the car. I saw the candy store and the toy store a few feet away from me. They were so close yet so far away. I wanted to hop out of the car and shop, but I couldn't.

"Come on, Jen," said Geoff. He felt scared to see me still sitting there when he came back to the car with his coffee.

"I feel a little weird," I said.

"Walking might be good for you," he said, offering me his arms. I didn't think so. I had started wearing plastic braces for walking. They were supposed to prevent my feet from dragging on the ground. The braces didn't work very well. All they seemed to do was make my calves sweat profusely. I felt the plastic rubbing against them in the heat.

"Tomorrow's another day," said Martha, rationalizing my trip to town over salmon and chardonnay. I loved my friends. They loved me so much. I worried about tomorrow. I went shopping with Valerie and Meredith at our favorite fruit and vegetable stand. The uneven ground presented new obstacles to my walking and balancing. But Martha had been right. Tomorrow was another day. I was able to get out of our car. I relied on my inner Valerie, Jenifer, and Meredith to get me through. *Steady,* I thought, approaching the stand decked out in luscious fruits. *Just get to the avocados. Walk over to the avocados slowly and pick one up. Good girl. Excellent.* I brought my bag of avocados over to Meredith, who had chosen sensational peaches and nectarines. Valerie paid. The whole thing went off without a hitch. We bought. I blended in. As far as the world was concerned, I was just another woman shopping for her family. I loved that.

For two straight months, Scott manned the barbecue. It was hard for me to picture him anywhere except hovering over sea bass or thick steaks grilling. He cooked every single thing perfectly to order. There were fights that summer, and wine, and a lot of laughing. We watched fireworks from the patio as the Fourth of July came and went. Jake swam in the deep end for the first time. One night, after Meredith had run from the dinner table nauseated, she announced that she was pregnant. Then in August the waves started coming regularly. The weird wave of exhaustion that I'd experienced in town that afternoon with my friends came back. The waves drove me to my bed, where they broke and washed over me. My bed was no longer a place for sleeping or watching TV or making love. It was my hiding place.

Rationalizing became all the rage that summer. Everyone was doing it. Valerie and Meredith were determined to spin gold from Dr. Rowland's diagnosis. They were sure I had a remarkably slow-moving case, and they heartily endorsed the program of physical therapy that had been prescribed by the same nurse who'd given me the brochures. Physical therapy didn't make much sense to me. The nerve cells in my spine and brain were dying. My muscles were drying up. I didn't need to work out. I needed medicine, fast.

"Georgia says you're the strongest ALS patient she's ever seen," said Meredith as I lay on my bed, completing a series of leg lifts prescribed by a jaunty physical therapist who was well-meaning but knew nothing of ALS. I had always wanted to have a daughter and name her Georgia. Instead, I got a physical therapist named Georgia. My muscles shook and fasciculated as I lifted the light weights strapped to my ankles. The kids watched, fascinated.

"Go, Jen Jen," Jake cheered. I dripped sweat.

"This is totally stupid," I said, lifting my ton of bricks. "You can't get better from what I have." I couldn't blame my sisters for believing that a course of exercise might buy me a little time. No evidence to the contrary existed. But I was starting to feel frustrated. The general perception out there, especially among people who love you, is that if you try very hard, you can make yourself better. But there are things in life and death that are beyond our control. The power of positive thinking extends only so far. Walking on burning coals, for example—I could see where that was totally doable, at least during the first year of ALS. Overcoming a fatal, totally untreatable illness through exercise and eating right seemed like a bit of a stretch.

"Peter says you've never looked healthier or more beautiful. You *know* he doesn't lie," said Meredith. My little sister and her West Point cadet had married. Meredith and Peter were our family's version of Elizabeth Taylor and Richard Burton, our resident jungle cats. They fought and made up like nobody's business. Peter was air for Meredith to breathe. I've felt that way about a couple of guys in my life, but Meredith was married to it, body and soul. Peter was my brother. We had known each other for a long time.

"Let's go to the beach, Jenny," he said one afternoon as I held my iced tea glass poolside. I had navigated much of civilized Westhampton successfully, but I was scared of the beach, mostly because of the sand. And the bathing suits. "Nonsense, Jenny. Let's go see the sunset."

I leaned on Peter as we walked from the parking lot to the edge of the beach. "Look at the sun," Peter said, turning his face to catch the last few rays. We settled onto the sand.

"You realize it's gonna take a miracle to get through this," I said.

"What would life be without miracles, Jenny?" Peter said, and the sun was gone. I couldn't get up. Peter lifted me partway, then I pitched forward onto my knees. Sky, sand, and water merged, then separated into distinct bands of color. I knelt before the totem of colors and prayed for a miracle. It was getting cold.

"Let's go home, Jenny," said Peter. He picked me up and carried me in his arms to firm ground. We had to get home for dinner. Meredith was making sea bass. Scott was grilling.

Princess Diana died that summer. I remember watching television late one night when the news broke. I was the first one in the house to hear about the tragedy, and I was Paul Revere again, waking people up, telling them about a woman who was my age, whom my sisters and I had admired, who had died in a terrible car accident. I loved Diana's face. I felt a strange twinge of relief at the news of her death. The tragedy comforted me, in the same way my friend John Kennedy's death did later on, and not in a misery-loves-company kind of way. I felt that if Diana and John were brave enough to go to the other side, I was, too. I gained strength thinking about them. If I was going to be blending in with a new crowd one day, I could do worse than those two. I imagined what it would be like meeting them on the other side.

The summer was over in a second. The last night, from my bedroom just off the patio, I could hear my family all around me. Jake and Willis were laughing. My sisters and their husbands talked logistics for the trip home. Although I longed to be a part of the conversation, I was drawn to rest. For the first time, I felt a distance between my family and me. The disease was whispering to me again. The next morning, I put on my lug-soled Gucci loafers, the only footwear I felt safe wearing, and walked down the front steps for the drive home to Manhattan. I went down with a bang. It was a bad fall. Meredith came running and screaming.

"Oh my God, you tripped on the avocado," she said.

"What?" I said, dazed and totally confused.

"You tripped . . . the avocado," she said, indicating a dried-up avocado peel in a gutter on the other side of the driveway.

"You don't trip on an avocado, you slip, and I didn't slip, I fell because I can't walk," I said.

None of us was ready for the fall. When my family dropped me off at my apartment after the summer, I could have been any other single woman coming home from her Hamptons share. As I stepped out of Meredith and Peter's car, I noticed the colors change: Summer red turned into sidewalk gray; sky blue turned into taxi yellow, and Tootsie-Pop purple, the color of Jane's eyes, became the drab fluorescent white of my vestibule. This was the light that would guide me from the car and my family's unforgettable summer into the autumn. Valerie and Meredith stayed in the car as I walked into my building. We were starting to realize that there were journeys I'd have to take alone. I pulled myself up by the banister, step-by-step, to my apartment. I didn't look back. *No hurricane, no act of God will break us.* I was already focused on the job ahead. In my heart I knew that in order to fight ALS, I'd have to come up with a force at least as strong. That force was my love with my sisters, my best thing.

"I still think we can get out of this," Meredith had said as I'd struggled through Georgia's grueling physical therapy regimen that summer. And that became my sisters' and my mantra: *I still think we can get out of this.* As my body changed, my sisters and I would say it over and over. But the truth was that even if my sisters and I didn't get out of ALS, we'd get out of it. Does that make any sense? It made sense to me my first night back on Seventy-first Street, as I walked carefully to my bed and lay there in the dark fantasizing and fasciculating for hours. This was what I wanted to say to my sisters and what I hoped they would always remember: Even if I died soon, our love would roam the earth like a kind, three-headed monster. I wanted to tell them that we would prevail, as family, as one, eternally. It may sound queer, but I knew I was born to love. Love had gotten me through my first summer of ALS, and I was betting my heart it would take me further. All I had to do was go deeper.

Chapter Five

I WAS NEVER that great a student, academically speaking. When September rolled around, my best thing was buying new notebooks with my sisters at Big Top and sticking Wacky Packages on them. I remember being very hardworking the first days of third grade. I arranged my pencils and sharpener in a new carrying case and carefully laid out my next day's outfits on top of my bureau. I listened hard in class and wrote down everything my teachers said. I was adamant about completing my homework with precision and neatness.

"Wanna play Barbies?" asked Meredith, a mere second-grader. She stood at my door with our black patent-leather Barbie carrying cases and her mop of black hair.

"Sorry, Pigpen, I have more important things to do," I said, closing the door in her face.

My passion for academics generally lasted about two weeks. I think I started each grade *pretending* to go to school, like I was starring in a movie *about* school. Then, when reality set in, and I recognized that third grade—a.k.a. pure drudgery—was my fate, I totally tuned out.

"So where's my Barbie case?" I asked Meredith, who had been staring blankly at the TV for two weeks, and we ran upstairs for an afternoon of international fashion. I'd like to see my social studies notebook from third grade now, with its first two pages of meticulous notes and the rest totally blank.

By the age of thirty-five, I had accepted that drudgery was a part of every life. But staying in the game and taking notes—no matter what—definitely had its payoffs. I wasn't crazy about my current job in public relations, but it was helping me pave my way to my next project—the production company I was starting with Valerie and Meredith. Autumn had become a time of year to reassess my goals. The cool snap in the air was a starting gun: Make the meeting; buy the shoes; call him. But when the starting gun went off that September after my diagnosis, I couldn't get out of a taxi by myself anymore. I couldn't run out for a client meeting or a tuna sandwich. I couldn't run. Elevator rides to my twentieth-floor office had become surreal. Half of me went up while the other half stayed in the lobby. The leg braces I'd started wearing at the end of the summer remained more of a nuisance than a help. I started calling in sick a lot. Then I quit my job. My best friend, Simon Halls, came from Los Angeles to console me the day I told my boss I was gravely ill and I'd be packing my office to leave immediately.

"You're out of there, Kitty," said Simon, raising a glass of champagne over roasted chicken and mashed potatoes, our favorite, at Cafe Luxembourg. Simon called me "Kitty." He'd borrowed the nickname from Peter and Meredith, who had started calling each other "Kitty" when they fell in love in high school. Simon and I might as well have been married—our chemistry was that complex. I'd met Simon when he lived in New York. He'd hired me for my first job after Naked Angels, an off-Broadway theater company I'd helped run. Before Simon, I had worked for next to no money. Simon introduced me to the notion that I could make a career *and* money for myself in entertainment. He'd encouraged me to take the public relations job I'd just quit.

"It wasn't the perfect job, Kitty, but it was a total step up," he said. As Simon spoke, I took in his chocolate brown eyes and boyish hair. Even when he was rumpled, Simon was elegant. "An elegant human being," my mother had dubbed him. I found him intoxicating at times. Simon was the champagne of men, and he was brutally honest with me. We hadn't seen each other since my diagnosis. I was afraid that he was going to notice a big change in my walking and say so.

"Look at you, Kitty. You're doing so well," Simon said as we made our way back to my apartment, arm in arm, after dinner. He pulled me close to him.

"I can't walk, Kitty," I said. I called Simon "Kitty," too.

"What do you call *this,* Kitty?" he said.

"Walking," I said, "v-e-r-y slowly."

"Slow is good, Kitty," he said, laughing. "Silly Kitty."

Simon and the night air smelled so good. After he dropped me off, I collapsed on my couch. But the night was young. Buoyed by champagne and Simon's encouraging words, I decided to run a few neurological tests of my own. I'd been playing games with myself most nights to see how fast my ALS was moving. I stood on my tiptoes reaching toward the high cabinet over my refrigerator. I touched it. I filled a coffee mug with water and carried it back and forth across my living room floor without spilling it. I sat down at my table and got up and sat down and got up. If a chair wasn't too low to the ground—my dining room chair wasn't—I was still okay getting to my feet. Maybe I had what Dr. Rowland said we were hoping for, a quirky case. I prayed nightly for the quirkiest, slowest-moving ALS case in history. Unfortunately, I failed the tweezers test. For the first time, I couldn't grip them. *Good-bye, tweezers.* ALS forced me to say good-bye to at least one thing every week. This week it was my job and tweezers.

The next morning I headed out with my new cane to deposit my last paycheck. Canes work fashion-wise, if you're Simon Halls or Fred Astaire. With its shiny black metal shaft and rubber-tipped bottom, mine had an undeniably orthopedic look about it, but if I wanted to avoid a repeat of the phantom avocado incident in Westhampton, I had to use it. Navigating my neighborhood had become quite an adventure. I suddenly had trouble opening the front door to the Muffin Shop, where I'd developed a satisfying flirtation not only with the muffins but with a guy named Phil from my block. That morning, Phil's rosy face screwed up with concern as I struggled with the door. He didn't know what to make of the cane.

"Hey, Jenny, how ya doin'?" Phil asked, making room for me at his table. I will never forget the warmth of the Muffin Shop, the mixture of steam from the coffee and hot muffins that always pulled me in from the cold. The Muffin Shop was our kind of sauna, Phil and me.

"Flu's got me," I said. "Some kind of weird flu." I grabbed my bag to go and headed for the exit. "Bank time," I said.

"You gonna rob one?"

"You and me, Phil," I said.

"Take care, Jenny," said Phil, winking. I never saw him again.

Something bad was happening. My inalienable rights to life, liberty, and the pursuit of errands in my own neighborhood were being violated by ALS. I crossed Columbus Avenue to the dry cleaners, where I picked up my favorite black suit, a sleek, stunning creature. I was so happy to see it. Gripping my cane and bag in my right hand, I slung it over my left shoulder. "All right, let's do it," I ordered my body, which ignored me. Like me at a school dance, my body seemed unable to initiate anything. I stood motionless on the sidewalk for minutes, not knowing how to make the first move toward Citibank, my last stop before going home. *Put one foot in front of the other.* By the time I got to the bank entrance, my Guccis felt like cement blocks. Because the muscles around my feet had weakened, I was having trouble lifting them for my next steps. It took me a good hour to snake my way through the bank line, but the teller finally handed me my pink deposit slip. It was like getting a medal at the Olympics.

Since when do muffins weigh a hundred pounds? As I turned onto my block, my dry cleaning weighed down on me. I hoisted the hanger into the crook of my neck as I fought on, but I wasn't going to make it after all. My street was deserted and Phil was nowhere in sight, so I unburdened myself. As I continued unsteadily toward my apartment, I let go of my muffin bag, I let go of my suit in its plastic wrap, I let go of my deposit slip. Piece by piece, my morning fell to the sidewalk like leaves. By the time I got inside, it was dark all around. I fell on my bed. New York was my city. My sisters and I worked there. My friends and I had closed it down a few times. New York was where I had made some big mistakes and where I was making my mark as a producer, a mover, a shaker, and as a woman who was ready to move with her family to a quiet apartment overlooking the most incredible city in the world. I dialed Valerie.

"I can't live alone anymore," I said. "My city . . ."

"That's okay," Valerie said. "Everything's going to be okay." We stayed on the phone a long time, just listening.

Valerie and I packed the things I'd be needing into boxes, and I moved back to Harrison, the town of my youth. I had always fantasized about returning to Harrison one day. It was a high school reunion fantasy with my fellow graduates collectively gasping as I whisked into the hotel ballroom at the top of my game. I'd be more beautiful than they had remembered, and verging on fame. Between bites of bad beef Stroganoff, I'd entertain them with photos of my children and stories from the set of my latest production, a comedy about sisters. Then I'd whisk out, more beautiful to my classmates than when I had whisked in.

My actual return to Harrison wasn't as auspicious by half. Meredith, Peter, Jake, and Jane lived in Harrison in a modern ranch-style home. It seemed so perfect that Meredith and Peter had moved back to Harrison when they married. It was the place where they had first laid eyes on each other. Meredith and Peter had returned to Harrison to build something of their own. And now I was moving in. My biggest fear was burdening Meredith and her family and basically ruining their lives. ALS was a family disease. It wanted to cut everyone down. But you don't cut Meredith down so easily.

Meredith was my little sister, but in many ways she grew up being the toughest of us. Unlike Valerie and me, Meredith didn't talk up, down, and around a subject. Valerie and I had the gift of gab—Meredith had the gift of go. She landed the plane. Plus Meredith was just plain great to look at. No one knew how she did it—maybe she shopped when everyone was sleeping—but Meredith always managed to walk in with that one great new shirt or those pants or boots that made you notice. There she was in the driveway to meet me the day I moved in. She looked like the Statue of Liberty, with her upright, broad-shouldered frame and eyes that could cut diamonds. From the car I could smell dinner cooking.

I would hit my emotional bottom during my stay at Meredith's house, probably because it was the safest place on earth for me to do it. If Martha Stewart ever does a roundup of the most fashionable rooms for facing down one's mortality, she'll want to feature my room in Meredith and Peter Hulbert's house in Harrison. The Hulberts converted their storage room into a private bedroom and bathroom with pretty pastel soaps just for me. Meredith put in carpeting and a firm new bed, and dressed it in Ralph Lauren and puffy pillows. She had made sure that if I was going to be spending more time in bed, mine was fit for a queen.

My sisters and I had always taken care of one another, but I was about to rely on Meredith big-time. I felt inhibited being so needy. As the older sister, I felt much more comfortable taking care of her, giving her advice when she and Peter fought, and devising business strategies together. Now I was going to be waited on by my younger sister, who had two young kids with another on the way. My body started tanking as soon as I got there. It was as if it had been waiting for me to get to a safer place before it fell apart. Meredith cooked healthful meals for me. She cleaned my room every ten minutes, she held my arm as we walked up and down her street together, and she kept me in fresh flowers.

"I feel like I'm living in a hotel," I said to her. She

provided me with every conceivable comfort and convenience around the clock.

"Some hotel," she said, rolling her eyes. Meredith worked hard at being a wife and mother, and she had the kids to show for it. Jake and Jane were fine children, just great human beings. They would be my saviors over the next ten months. The way they looked and smelled and walked and talked—they satisfied my senses. They made me feel alive with love. I worked to stay strong so that I could make them proud.

"Jane, get off the bed!" Meredith screamed, running in with a knife from the kitchen. She'd been chopping vegetables for a stir-fry.

"No, Mer, I love it," I said. The kids were my air. They were like puppies jumping on my bed and nuzzling me. I held them and they held me back.

"Stay here forever, Jen Jen," said Jake.

"Stay here forever, Den Den," said Jane. When Scott, Valerie, and Willis came up to Harrison, I'd have the three kids in my room. Jake, Willis, Jane, and I would go shopping on the computer. I bought them toys. I bought them a lot of toys. Those afternoons were educational, too. I taught the children how to order anything they wanted online using my credit card.

"Are you crazy, Jenifer?" asked Valerie, surveying the latest shipment of cartons from Toys "R" Us.

"It's just a little something," I said.

"Do you think there are worms when you die?" I asked as Meredith and I sat cross-legged on my bed eating turkey sandwiches with Russian dressing for lunch one day. "Like, do you think they crawl into your eye sockets?"

"I try not to think about worms," she said, rising from the bed with that look in her eyes. "Gotta go."

At roughly the same time that I started becoming obsessed with worms and skeletons, Meredith developed wicked morning sickness. She could be seized at any moment by a volcanic nausea. We'd be deep into a conversation when Meredith, suddenly overcome, would bolt.

"See ya," I said. I felt guilty: I was sick because something was dying inside me. Meredith felt guilty: She was sick because life was growing inside her. Oy, the guilt of the sisters . . .

Despite my efforts at staying positive, my days took on a troubling shapelessness. Before I got sick, it was the momentum of my routine—working out, eating healthfully, working my butt off, and dating—that propelled me forward and gave my life meaning. Without that structure, I slid into depression. I sat on my bed, looking out the window at a big tree in Meredith's backyard. The tree had lost its leaves. Its brittle branches moved in the wind. At night the tree turned into a swaying skeleton inching toward me, arms outstretched. Thoughts of death wrapped them-selves in my Ralph Lauren sheets. My pillow became a tombstone. I would fall asleep to the sound of me dis-appearing, all except the bones. Worms crawled through my eye sockets—

"Jen Jen," said Jake. When I woke up, Jake was sit-ting on my bed in his red devil costume for Halloween. If this was the devil, I suddenly wasn't scared of dying.

"I love your costume, sweet baby," I said. He smiled. Jake was the oldest of my nieces and nephews. If Simon and I had ever had a son, he would have looked like Jake.

"Are you coming trick-or-treating tonight?" he asked.

"Maybe," I said.

"Please . . ." I was tempted by the devil, but we decided I'd be better off staying in and handing out candy to visitors. Speaking of Halloween thrills and chills, my walking had gotten so bad that I'd started using an aluminum walker to get around. I had never seen a young person using one of those things. I stared at my walker parked in the corner of my room. The cold afternoon sun reflected off its aluminum sides. It was the scariest Halloween I could remember.

"Bubble gum," said Jane, waddling in. "Bubble gum."

"You want bubble gum?" I asked.

"Bubble gum," said Jane.

"Where's Mommy?"

"Bubble gum kitchen bubble gum kitchen bubble gum kitchen—"

"I get it, honey. I'll get it." Meredith had run out to the store for candy for me and the trick-or-treaters, and my baby girl wanted her gum. Balancing with my walker, and with Jane and a curious Jake in tow, I ventured out to the kitchen. The sound of that walker was really something: click-click-click, click-click-click. It was an old metal horse—a three-legged thing—probably headed for the glue factory. I made it to the kitchen counter, where I released the walker and grabbed marble. Suddenly I was Clint Eastwood hanging on to one ledge while trying to get to the next building. From there I reached up to a cabinet holding Jane's shocking pink gum dispenser and some glasses. One wrong move from me and those glasses were coming down.

"What is this stuff?" I said, handing the gum to Jane.

"Bubble gum!" said Jane, triumphant. I felt triumphant, too. Giving the children what they wanted meant everything to me.

"Say thank you," said Jake.

"Thank you, Den Den," Jane said, unraveling yard after yard of strawberry gum. We three spent the rest of the morning chewing bubble gum on my bed.

Whenever I was alone—when Peter wasn't bringing me coffee and a muffin from town, or Meredith and I weren't talking about Valerie, or Valerie and I weren't talking about Meredith, or the kids weren't playing football on my bed—the creeping thoughts returned. I thought a lot about never having children. I thought about never running my own company. The notion of *never,* which I had often fought against, made its way into my mind. The waves of exhaustion from the summer had returned and were more frequent now. I hibernated. I started sleeping later into the mornings. The sounds of the Hulberts would awake me momentarily: Peter's polished shoes against the kitchen floor before work, the garage door going up, Jake and Meredith fighting about his backpack, Andrea, the nanny, getting Jane down the front steps—clunk, clunk—in her stroller for nursery school. The sounds of my family heading out into the world were like an extra blanket that sent me back and deeper into sleep.

My friends tried to break the door down. They had been so easygoing in Westhampton only a few months before. But now they seemed impatient. I listened to their pet theories of why I had gotten sick in the first place and what I needed to do to make myself well again. My friends became guerrillas on a mission. They came up to Harrison from the city in shifts and tried to scare me into action.

"Life is a river, Kitty," my friend Merrill said, illustrating in the air. He called me "Kitty," too. "Picture this big rock in the middle of the river. The rock changes the course of the river. *You* are that rock, Kitty. *You* change the course of your illness."

"I think you've been watching too much public television, Kitty." I called Merrill "Kitty," too. He was starting to sound like that guy with the beard on Channel 13 who talked about the miracles of broccoli. Merrill and I had produced many a play together in our heyday at Naked Angels. We'd made names for ourselves turning young plays into hot, sold-out happenings. He and I had willed the masses to our theater on Seventeenth Street. As far as Merrill was concerned, we were going to will away my ALS. Other friends tried coaxing me out to dinners and parties in the city. They felt my returning to New York was the best medicine, but I couldn't bear going back. New York was the crime scene now, the place where my dreams had been shot down.

Everyone who came to visit me in Harrison brought me a book either about broccoli and being, rivers and rocks, or death and dying. One book was about stages of dying—Chapter One: Anger; Chapter Two: Denial; Chapter Three: Acceptance—as if there was a particular, predictable order to the whole process. There wasn't a word in that book about worms, nothing about the inability to reach out and hold a guy or never seeing your nephew graduate from high school. When people came to my bed with books, I asked them to please place them on the stacks on my floor. I had collected about a hundred books in short stacks. They made a great doorstop.

I started reading the obituaries instead, scouring them for mentions of other young people. Everyone in the death section was older than me: A physicist died from heart failure at ninety-three; a shipping magnate lost his battle with cancer at eighty-seven; a woman who had discovered a hidden meaning in birdsongs stroked out at seventy-six. One day I read about a young woman who had died in her early thirties from a rare form of lymphoma. She was quoted as saying that being sick was like drifting farther and farther away on a raft. She said she felt that she lived in another country. Her I could relate to.

Valerie wanted to make me better in one fell swoop. When she wasn't in Harrison helping Meredith, or psyching me up for the medicine we were somehow going to find, she was on her computer, on the Internet, learning about the latest in ALS research.

"The problem here is that the experts know nothing," she said, after she had spent three days straight visiting useless neuroscience websites. She stayed in the game, though. She kept taking notes and researching the research. Then she discovered her one fell swoop. His name was Jeffrey Rothstein, and he was an accomplished ALS researcher and clinician at Johns Hopkins University in Baltimore. Valerie had made an appointment for us to see Dr. Rothstein.

"This guy's the maverick," Valerie said. I'd already seen the giant in the field. I had nothing to lose in meeting the maverick. Valerie rationalized that there was no definitive, beyond-a-reasonable-doubt diagnosis for ALS. Maybe Rothstein's second opinion would differ from Dr. Rowland's first one. Plus, Rothstein had medicine—apparently, plenty of it—cooking in his lab. Something called *growth factors* that Valerie felt might help me.

My sisters and mother and I went to Johns Hopkins on the Amtrak. While Meredith and I ate pretzels from the bar car, Valerie laid out our dream scenario: Rothstein would examine me and tell me I didn't have ALS, or, worst case, he'd tell me I had ALS and that he was going to give me something to slow it down or stop it. Then we'd celebrate in the restaurant of the luxurious Harbor Court Hotel, where Valerie had made reservations.

"My treat," said Valerie.

"My treat," said my mother. "And pass me a pretzel." The hotel part worked out. We got a lot of great room service at the Harbor Court before my appointment at Hopkins the next morning.

In bed that night, I felt hopeful. I was a very hope-ful person. I thought about high school, when my friend Timmy and I had gotten a really good laugh from that word: *hope*. It was one of those words that was so corny to say out loud: "I *hope* you're coming to my house after school, Tim." So Timmy and I made up a little play on it. When we didn't think there was a hope in hell of something happening, we'd say *hopes* or *many hopes*. If Timmy asked me if I was going to pass the geometry Regents, I'd say, "Hopes." If I asked Timmy if he was ever going to marry Nancy (my best friend who was in love with him), he'd say, "Hopes." Then my sisters started doing it. The cult of hopes fol-lowed me into adulthood:

Me: You remind me of Cary Grant, Kitty. Simon: Hopes.

Simon: You're so much prettier than Catherine Zeta-Jones, Kitty. Me: Many hopes.

I was all sarcasm when it came to hopes, but in my heart I was high on a hill, hoping that Dr. Rothstein would set me free.

"I like what he's wearing," Meredith said, as Rothstein whizzed past us in the waiting room at Hopkins. Dr. Rothstein was my age and well put together, but there was something about him that gave me a queasy feeling the instant I met him. Where Dr. Rowland had been gentlemanly, Dr. Rothstein seemed aggressive, like he couldn't wait to share the hard, cold truth with me. My whole family jammed into the tiny exam room, waiting for Jeff Rothstein to commute my sentence. He rolled over facts and figures of ALS like a lawn mower, using the paper on my exam table to illustrate the deadly pathways of the disease. His exam was different from Dr. Rowland's but just as bizarre. Dr. Rothstein used circus equipment, too—pulleys.

"No question you have ALS," said Rothstein as I closed my gown around me. He confirmed Dr. Rowland's diagnosis immediately. He was unequivocal. "Your motor neurons are dying," he said, "and they'll never be replaced."

"I don't understand," I said. "We can replace damaged hearts and kidneys. Why not motor neurons?"

"Cell transplants? That's science fiction." He smashed our questions like bugs.

"But you're developing therapies to block glutamate, right?" asked Valerie, who was starting to use words and terms that none of us had heard before. "You and your colleagues are doing important work with growth factors."

"Oh, that's all early stages," he said. Dr. Rothstein said that a cure for ALS was twenty years down the road. "People come in with questions," he said. "Unfortunately, we just don't have answers." We were stunned. I asked my family to leave the room. I had to know the effects ALS was going to have on my love life.

"Emotionally, the love might deepen," he said. "Physically, everything will change."

"What should I do?"

"Travel maybe. I had one patient who went to Paris. Some people max out their credit cards." No matter what the future held, Dr. Rothstein and I would always have Paris.

"I want you to go on with your lives," I said to my family back at our messy suite in the Harbor Court Hotel. It was way dark outside and way past checkout time. "Nothing will be the same now, but you must promise me you'll go on with your lives. If you don't live now, I'll feel worse. Everything will be worse." There wasn't much to say. The only sound was tears falling on the carpet. It had been raining in Baltimore, a cold, driving rain, from the moment we'd gotten off the Amtrak from New York the day before. I would always remember Baltimore in the rain and the sight of my sisters' defeated faces after we got our second opinion. It was a long train trip home. My sisters and I got drunk on M&M's.

I was back at Meredith's hibernating again when a tornado blew in from the East. It settled over the house and stayed for a while. It was rare winds—something

I'd call a tornado of the absurd. My sisters and I got caught up in it but good. After our visit with Dr. Rothstein, with no Western solutions or any true medicine in sight, Valerie, Meredith, and I got caught up in healing options from the East. Two afternoons a week, we three devoutly Western girls drove to Long Island for my meetings with Caran (emphasis on the second syllable, naturally), a self-described psychic minister. Seriously, the woman had business cards. Caran had a healing hut, which was really just a warped toolshed behind her clapboard house. Walking to the healing hut, I could see my minister's family's underwear drying on the line.

"I hate talking about money," Caran said when she met me.

"Yeah, it's a drag," I said, leaning on my walker.

"But if you want me to rearrange your cells, it's gonna cost you," she said. Basically, Caran was a masseuse. She wasn't a bad person. The woman had kids to support.

"It's something to do," I admitted as Valerie, Meredith, and I flew down the Long Island Expressway for my twice-weekly Caran treatments. Meredith said she noticed that I might be getting a little stronger from my sessions with Caran. Valerie agreed.

"At seventy-five bucks a pop, you'd like to think so," I said.

———

"Hey, Caran, ya gotta lose the stoop," I said after a couple months of seeing her. I couldn't get up the cement stoop to the healing hut anymore, even with my walker.

"Stand in your legs," said Caran. "You can do it."

"I'm gonna fall on this stoop, Caran. I'm gonna fall on my ass." When we first met, Caran promised she would cure me. She sure changed her tune as I got worse.

"Only *time* will tell if you'll heal," said Caran.

"I thought *you* were gonna heal me."

"Time is wiser than I," she said. "And speaking of time, Jenifer, when might you honor your outstanding balance for November?"

Tornado-force winds knocked us back and forth. Meredith blew into my room with an open jar of truly foul-smelling paste. There had to be a dead moose in that jar.

"Are you trying to kill me?" I said as she waved it under my nose.

"Give it a chance," she said. The paste was called Amrit Kalash. It was an ancient blend of herbs from India that balanced the body and the mind. Forget what it did to your digestion.

"Get out of here with that crap," I said. Meredith

cracked up. She'd been mixing it into my daily smoothies for weeks.

There was a homemade battery advertised on the Internet for stimulating my muscles. We bought that. There was the purported medicinal power of burning sage. We burned bundles. Valerie came home with bags of vitamins. I took them. One woman, who had apparently saved serious heart patients with a laying on of hands, laid her hands on me. She looked like a lemur. She jumped around on all fours on a couch. She scared me. My sisters and I were desperate. We drove everywhere, sent away for everything, anything that would make me better. We were dizzy and desperate. We were broke. There was snake oil and swamis and healers galore, and everyone took MasterCard.

I needed a Diet Coke. As I walked to the kitchen on my walker, I fell backward and cracked my skull against the hardwood floor. Meredith ran in and cradled my head in her hands. "You're fine," she said. "I promise you." She lifted me into my room and onto my bed. I'm surprised she didn't give birth right there.

"I think I gotta get a wheelchair, Merry," I said, my head spinning from a slight concussion.

I called Dr. Rowland's nurse, the one who had given me the brochures. I tried relating to her woman-to-woman. She wasn't part of the tornado. She was more the Wicked Witch flying through it.

"Maybe I'm not using the right shoes," I said when

we met in her office. "Maybe there's something with a negative heel—something in an Earth Shoe—that would be safer." The nurse was eating a tuna sandwich with her mouth open. *Good-bye, tuna.*

"I'm gonna say the dirty word, Miss Estess," she said. "*Wheelchair* . . . I don't want you ending up in the emergency room with broken bones." She seemed about as genuine in her concern as Nurse Ratched. "If you want Medicaid to pay for a chair, ya gotta order now," she said. She fanned out more brochures for me on her desk. They featured huge gleaming wheelchairs with knobs and trays and scaffolding. She recommended a custom-made chair, one that could accommodate the progressive weakness, eventual paralysis, and a respirator.

"But I don't need that now," I said.

"You will," she said. "You will."

"I want to die," I said, riding shotgun as Meredith drove home.

"Not yet," Valerie said from the backseat.

"I'm ruining your lives. I'm infecting . . . everything," I said. "It's in my body . . . everywhere. I want to stop while I can still remember what everything looked like. I want to remember colors the way they were."

"So remember colors the way they were," said Meredith.

"What if I can't?"

"You wanna die?" Meredith asked.

"Yes," I said, and the tears came. "Please."

"You wanna die," Meredith said, confirming.

"I wanna die. I wanna die."

"Let's do it," said Meredith, slamming the gas pedal to the floor. We went from twenty to eighty, fast.

"What's your fucking problem?" asked Valerie from the backseat.

"Jenifer wants to die, we'll die," said Meredith, hitting ninety. When I said Meredith had the gift of go, I wasn't kidding. The world flew by.

"Oh my God!" Valerie screamed.

"Maybe I don't want to die," I said, but it was too late. Meredith swerved and we skidded sideways across the Major Deegan Expressway. We came to rest safely at the far edge of the right shoulder. It was quiet for a long time.

"We're fine," Valerie said.

"Are we?" said Meredith.

"Good. I'm good," I said.

"Good," said Meredith.

Valerie, Meredith, and I drove back to Harrison. We inhaled burnt rubber the whole way. It had burning sage beat by a mile. There wasn't much left for us to say. My sisters and I had almost violated our life's pact of eternal oneness on the Major Deegan, but we didn't, so there was no use talking about it.

After dinner Meredith turned off my light and I fell into a dream of the Century, the grand railroad train that once traveled back and forth from Chicago to New York. I loved that train. We had ridden it when we lived in Rock Island and my mother wanted to go home to New York to see her parents. Once, my mother took the five of us children into the dining car for breakfast. It was a very proper dining room with starched, pressed linens and fine silverware on the table, and the smell of freshly brewed coffee in the air.

My mother noticed the talent impresario Ted Mack at a table near us. He was reading his newspaper, minding his own business, but not for long. On the count of three, my mother made us stand and sing for Mr. Mack—"Take Me Out to the Ball Game"—as loud as we could. Ted Mack was very polite. He waited until we had finished singing, nodded his thanks, and left the dining car. He probably wanted to run. My dream that night took place on the Century, but it had a different ending. In my dream, when Ted Mack stood up at the end of our song, he didn't leave. He clapped for us. He stood and clapped a long time for a kid group that he honestly believed was going places.

"I'll see you very soon, Jenifer," he said, writing down his phone number for my mother.

"On the big show?" I asked.

"On the big show," he said.

I hit bottom that winter at Meredith's, but I was still

dreaming of a better life. My sisters and I had survived the tornado of the absurd, but we remained hungry for answers. It occurred to us that we had been looking for answers everywhere *outside*. In our sadness and desperation, we had forgotten our own true strength. Then we stopped looking outside and turned our attentions in.

Chapter Six

I DIDN'T KNOW if I would ever have a baby, but I was sure starting to feel like one. Valerie and Meredith spent more and more time caring for me in Harrison. I couldn't stand up by myself for any length of time. They had to help me shower. Scott came up with his tools and an armload of lumber one weekend and built me a cedar bench for the shower so that I could be more independent. Meredith and Valerie grabbed me under each arm and helped me from my walker up over the lip of the shower stall toward the bench.

"God, I love the smell of wet cedar," Valerie said, trying to divert everyone's attention away from the fact that she and Meredith were dragging their totally naked sister to a bench in a shower.

"Is there any way you guys could close your eyes and do this?" I asked them.

"I think we've seen naked people before, Jenifer," said Meredith.

"Not each other," I said.

"Speak for yourself. I'm a total nudist," said Valerie, the liar. It felt okay when the water came, but I just couldn't—bathe—with my sisters there. They tried to respect my privacy: Meredith stood outside the shower staring straight ahead like a butler holding a bottle of shampoo, while Valerie washed me with a soapy washcloth, pretending not to.

"Do you smell the cedar?" Valerie asked.

"I smell the cedar," I said.

"It's enough with the cedar," said the butler, rolling her eyes.

I really hated asking my sisters for certain hygiene-related help. They had their own children to take care of. I had heard that you could call Medicaid for assistance with these things, so I did, and Memory came. Memory was my first home health aide. She didn't know anything about ALS.

"You have a car accident, honey?" she asked, coming toward the bed.

"You're the nurse?" I said, peering at her from over the edge of my comforter.

"That's me, Memory," she said, smiling. Memory was right up there with the giant and the maverick in her grasp of ALS. At least she had a pleasant smile. Memory had pretty gold rims around her front teeth.

"Your sister says you want to take a shower," she said.

"Yes, but I have ALS."

"I have a car accident one time."

"Yeah, well, I didn't, okay?" I said.

"Still you want a shower, honey," said Memory. "Trust Memory."

It was a relief when Memory took over, although it was totally humiliating being dressed and showered by a complete stranger. In my view, a woman should only ever have to utter the words "Can you get this button?" to a romantic prospect. The last time I'd said it was to Jeff Sherin, the best kisser on this green earth, bar none, whom I'd wanted to give me a hand—in a hurry—with my Anne Klein evening dress. But I had to hand it to Memory. She made a concerted effort to know me and my needs. She turned death-defying acts of grooming into predictable routine.

"Upsy, little daisy, and away we go," she'd say, standing next to my bed with my walker and our handy new travel pack of toiletries. Memory and I had gotten showering down to a science.

In bed at night, I started thinking less about skeletons and more about what Dr. Rothstein had said. He had told me my motor neurons were dying and they'd never be replaced. He'd said there was no medicine and to max out my credit cards. How did doctors get away with it? Doctors were supposed to make you well. I started taking the whole thing personally—and politically. I felt that my country had let me and millions of sick people down. If you had ALS, Alzheimer's, or Parkinson's, you weren't a citizen of the United States. You were strictly Third World. Why wasn't America declaring war on disease? It seemed to me we could be more efficient and aggressive in fighting brain disease, and not just by throwing money at it. Where was the game plan? Maybe a little violence would do the trick.

Violence was an option, I guessed, but for me it was just a Band-Aid. When Valerie was applying to college, it had dawned on her that waitressing wasn't going to cover her tuition. Our father had left us with nothing emotionally—the financial reality had never occurred to us. Valerie was right. We had no savings. We were forced to move out of Trilarch. Alison had already taken out gargantuan bank loans for her sophomore year at Brandeis, and my mother had just entered the workforce. She was selling advertising space for the local yellow pages. Alison, Valerie . . . how would any of us get through college?

"We'll find the money," I had promised Valerie as she paced the kitchen of our new house on Fenimore Drive one Sunday.

"Bastard," she said, opening the refrigerator and

emptying its contents on the counter: cartons of eggs and a couple cans of Tab. "Help me with this."

"What are you doing?" asked Meredith as we gathered the eggs and Tab.

"Let's go," said Valerie. Before we knew it, Meredith and I were in the backseat of the Vega, speeding on Route 287 toward my father's new house in Armonk. My father was living there with his new wife, the reporter, and her children. Valerie pulled up to the curb near their house and cut the engine.

"When I say go, start throwing and don't stop," Valerie said. Valerie hadn't taught me the art of bombs for nothing. Meredith and I loaded up on eggs. My adrenaline pumped. *And five, six, seven, eight—*

"Go." We tore out of the car and up the driveway. Valerie launched the first eggs rapid-fire, hitting my father's new car.

Meredith flung eggs at the house. "Big, fat idiot!" she shouted.

I threw the bombs of my life, hitting my father's front door with one egg, two eggs, three bull's-eyes in a row. "Big fat idiot!" I shouted.

"Let's get the hell out of here!" screamed Valerie. We ran to the car, fell in, and tore away, hooting like marines all the way home.

"I've gotten a disturbing call from the Harrison police," said my mother, later that morning, as we sat debriefing in the kitchen. "Your father's wife has registered a complaint—something about eggs, desecration, and daughters."

"That bitch ain't seen nothin' yet," Valerie said, swilling a can of Tab.

"I believe you'd get farther faster, Valerie, if you refrained from speaking like a truck driver," my mother said. And she left the room. My sisters and I cried laughing.

But after the Tab ran dry, I felt dissatisfied. Egg throwing wasn't my way, ultimately. Neither was violence. Messing up my father's new house with eggs had been thrilling in the moment. But if I could grow up loving, working my hardest from morning until night, and protecting my family—all the things my father hadn't done—well, that would be my statement. I never saw my father again. I grew to accept that his leaving was good for everyone. It made me a much more responsible person. I felt proud taking responsibility for my own actions. Pride, I realized, was the ultimate revenge.

I felt very responsible and mature—very nonviolent—picking out my first wheelchair. Did I want to throw eggs at every neurologist from here to Tibet? Yes, but that wasn't going to get me anywhere. If I wanted to get anywhere, I was going to need some wheels. Dr. Rowland's nurse referred me to

Homecare Solutions, a store in White Plains. It was a Wal-Mart for the elderly, disabled, and dying. The salesman took Valerie, Meredith, and me on a tour of the wheelchair showroom. It was a nightmare version of my grandpa Rosenberg's University Chevrolet showroom in the Bronx, where my sisters and I had hopped in and out of '68 Novas and Corvettes just off the assembly line. We would fake-drive to exotic locations.

"Where may I drop you, madam?" Valerie, my chauffeur, would ask.

"Hollywood Boulevard, please," I would say, sliding into the backseat of a brand-new, gray-blue Monte Carlo. "I'm late."

"Right away, madam," Valerie would say, and we'd drive in place until lunch, when my grandfather would take us for grilled cheese sandwiches and egg creams at our favorite soda fountain off University Avenue.

It's a seller's market when you're dying. Our salesman was nice enough, but those chairs were gonna run us. The sheer scope of wheelchairs for sale was staggering, with one uglier and more expensive than the next.

"This is the Breezy," said the salesman, stepping back from one of his bestselling manual models. "Have a seat," he said, holding the chair for me. Sitting in a wheelchair for the first time was terrifying. There was a point-of-no-return permanence about it.

"So?" asked Meredith. I was in a state of shock.

"Do you like it?" asked Valerie. "Or, I should say, do you hate it less than you hate the other ones?"

"I think I'm a dead duck," I said.

"Maybe she wants more independence," suggested the salesman, hopping on an electric cart and riding it toward me. "Try the Jazzy." He looked like an idiot. There was no way I was going out in that thing.

"If you wanna spend a little more, there's always the Celebrity," he said. The Celebrity was displayed rotating on an Astroturf pedestal, basking in its own private spotlight. I had always dreamed of celebrity, but the possibility of experiencing it in wheelchair form made me want to run out of the store. It was bad enough being in a wheelchair. Why did they have to give them these names?

"Who comes up with these names?" I asked the salesman.

"It ain't Elizabeth Browning," said Valerie, folding up my new Breezy and putting it into Meredith's car.

I was heading toward a new acceptance. I was ready to use my walker, my wheelchair, whatever it took, to get me where I wanted to go. I wanted to go to new places. I was ready to work.

"What stinks?" asked Jake, coming home from kindergarten one day.

"Memory's fish," said Meredith, who had given over the kitchen to Memory during weekdays. The smell of Memory's daily fish fries was enough to knock you over. It made us long for a whiff of wet cedar. Who knew you could cook with that much oil at that high a heat and not burn down the house?

"Mommy, I think I'm a vegetarian," declared Jake right then and there. Thanks in large part to Memory, which they say works in strange ways, Jake became our family's healthiest eater—fruits, vegetables, and grains, all the way.

"You want fish, Jenifer?" Memory asked over the sound of boiling oil.

"No, really, you eat it." I said, pumping my wheels toward the dining room. My Breezy and I joined Meredith, Valerie, and my friend Julianne Hoffenberg around the dining room table. It was a week before Thanksgiving and they were talking menu. Meredith had invited Julianne and Geoffrey to join us for Thanksgiving dinner.

"What should I bring, Mer?" asked Julianne, who had worked beside me at Naked Angels. I called her "Jules."

"Yourself," said Meredith, engrossed in her shopping list.

"Well, I'm gonna bring *something,*" Jules said.

"Bring me some medicine, why don't you," I said.

"Okay," said Jules. I had been somewhat of a mentor to Julianne. She had become a dear friend. She always aimed to please. "Seriously—what if *we* find the medicine?"

"Great," I said. Willis had told me that he and his friends had dug for medicine for me in the sandbox at Washington Square Park. Maybe Julianne wanted to dig in the park with Willis. They'd probably find medicine faster than Dr. Rothstein.

"Jules has a point," Valerie said.

"She does," said Meredith. "I mean, we couldn't do much worse than anyone else."

"There's enough brain power out there—enough raw intelligence. But no one's working *together,*" said Valerie.

"Or working efficiently," said Meredith.

"Maybe we could make them work together—" said Valerie.

"And meet deadlines," Meredith continued. "I mean, what happens to us when *we* don't meet deadlines?"

"Fired," I said.

"Fired," said Jules.

"They fire your ass," Meredith said.

"These doctors need to collaborate like we did at Naked Angels, don't you think, Jen?" said Jules.

"I'm thinking," I said. "I'm thinking." It was a big Andy Hardy moment. Gathered around the pre-Thanksgiving table, it occurred to us that we kids could do better. We could bring our business skills to bear on science, which seemed so all over the place. Effective management skills were effective management skills. We possessed those skills in spades. Heck, I'd produced plays before—why not a cure for ALS?

"Let's put on a show," I said. "Seriously, you guys, we could raise money—and use it to leverage these doctors to work harder," I said.

"This is what we do—we lock the smartest scientists in a room, and put a gun to their heads until they come up with a plan of action, kind of like the Manhattan Project," said Valerie. I didn't know what that was. "They invented the atom bomb fast. There's precedent here. We created the atom bomb. Why not medicine for ALS? We could call it . . . the A.L.S. Project."

"That sucks," said Meredith.

"How about Project A.L.S.?" suggested Jules.

"Project A.L.S. . . . Project A.L.S. . . . Hmmm, I like that," I said.

We all did. We got to work. I went back to my room to call friends in the business that might be willing to help. We decided to inaugurate Project A.L.S. with a star-studded fund-raiser in New York. We had two aims: educate people and raise the first bribe money for our Manhattan Project researchers.

I called Ben Stiller. He and I had worked together at Naked Angels, but our association went further back. His sister, Amy, and I had been friends as girls. I'd attended Anne Meara and Jerry Stiller's legendary New Year's parties since my teens. Amy, our friend Vicki, Ben, and I had made our own kind of music at those parties. We were like the junior brat pack within the senior one.

"I'm there, Jen," said Ben. "Name the time and place." Ben agreed to host our first event. Project A.L.S. was in business.

Our first office was my room in Meredith's house, where Jules, Meredith, and I worked the phones. We made lists and files. We took risks asking corporations to sponsor the event and celebrities to participate in it. Jules was brilliant at production. She called her old vendors and got commitments of goods and services at a discount. Meredith said our goal should be putting on a great show for no money and walking away with plenty of it. She crunched numbers while I called Kristen Johnston, another colleague of mine, an Emmy Award–winning actress from *3rd Rock from the Sun,* who agreed to join Ben as our cohost. Forget Valerie. She turned into that girl from *Poltergeist.* She went into the light of her computer and didn't come out. She continued researching the research relentlessly and set up first appointments with scientists at Harvard, Columbia, and Johns Hopkins.

"I don't know why you girls are starting something new," said Dr. Rowland as Valerie, Meredith, and I sat in his office. "There are too many organizations as it is."

"Don't worry, Bud, I won't embarrass you," I said. It was going to be hard convincing Bud or anyone else that Project A.L.S. was going to make major changes. ALS research had been chugging along for two hundred years, and no one else had found anything. Project A.L.S. decided to worry about the critics later. We had too much work to do. The first order of business was asking Bud Rowland to act as our research advisor. He accepted.

A harsh winter gave way to glorious spring. Acceptance of my own mortality had led to the birth of Project A.L.S. and an opportunity for me to work hard again. Meredith's house overflowed with activity. Valerie and Julianne worked the phones. My friends Geoff and Michael ran up Krispy Kremes from the city. I never saw Meredith without a calculator. Her baby was due in two weeks.

"Jenny, the First Lady of the city of New York wants to meet you," said Sue, a dear friend who had jumped in right away to help. Sue was close with Donna Hanover, then the wife of New York mayor Rudolph Giuliani. I knew of Donna as an actress, a journalist, and an activist. She was intrigued by Sue's description of Project A.L.S. Donna and I hit it off right away. She offered to give Project A.L.S. a press conference at Gracie Mansion before our event, and she invited me to speak at it. I asked Donna if I could sit next to my friend, colleague, and former sit-ups partner, the elegant Billy Baldwin, on the dais. I knew from experience that the press was more likely to show up when and where famous actors did. My sweet Billy. If the Estess sisters and the Baldwin brothers ever did a remake of *Seven Brides for Seven Brothers,* I know which brother I'd pick.

Meredith couldn't come to the press conference. She would be giving birth that day. Her doctor wanted to induce labor and had no other availability. I missed Meredith the morning of the press conference in more ways than one. I was afraid that without her, I wouldn't look my best. It was my big return to New York. With all due respect, Memory didn't quite cut it in the fashion- and beauty-advice department. I was going to be seeing my friends for the first time in my wheelchair. I wanted to look pretty and as confident as possible. My mother put on my lipstick. That was an adventure. Memory laid out a couple of horrific outfits at first, but we eventually settled on a decent pair of slacks and my burgundy blouse. I could still blow-dry my hair, but I had to use two hands.

"I have to use two hands now," I said.

"So did Chrissie Evert," my mother said. "And look how far she went." I really missed Meredith.

The first person I saw when I rolled into Gracie Mansion was my friend Martha. I took her in. She took me in. We both started crying. "You look so beautiful," she said and hugged me for a long time. My fear of being seen by the people I'd hidden away from in Harrison disappeared. I talked to a lot of people. Then it was time to start. My mother sat at the back of the room. Valerie watched from the side of the dais. Billy wheeled me to my place next to him. He kissed me.

"You look great, Jen," he said. I spoke into the microphone. As I described that first twitch in my leg that Meredith had noticed, I saw the reporters in the audience look down at their legs. When I talked about making ALS a topic of national concern, I saw them write in their notebooks. My speech was effective. Of course—Valerie had written it. After the press conference, Billy wheeled me to a terrace off the south side of Gracie Mansion. The sun was on us, brilliant and warm. I looked downtown toward NYU Medical Center, where Meredith and James, who had just been born healthy at nine pounds, were resting comfortably. No drugs for Meredith. She had pushed a few times and that was it. "Done," as my most efficient sister is fond of saying.

I was done with the better part of the scariest year of my life. Project A.L.S. had developed almost instant momentum. My sisters, friends, and I had worked our butts off. I was working harder than ever in my life. Our inaugural benefit at the old dance hall Roseland, in New York's theater district, was a great success. It raised hundreds of thousands of dollars for research. Valerie, Meredith, and Jules were in the car the next day, delivering research grants to scientists whom Valerie had found.

The night at Roseland was spectacular. Nancy Jarecki, who was the first person to join the Project A.L.S. board of directors, and her husband, Andrew, greeted me at the entry ramp. I was so nervous to go in there in my wheelchair. I was scared that people I hadn't seen would view me as a marked woman whose days were numbered. But Meredith and I got me looking quite good. The Jareckis coached me up the ramp and inside. Everyone was so happy to see me and so gracious, my nerves went away. The food was good. The wine was good. The messages from the stage were direct and moving. People gave me checks for Project A.L.S. It was my wedding, basically. As a producer, I had always prided myself on creating entertainment that had emotional impact. Otherwise, why bother? I think that Project A.L.S. achieved that its first time out. The eight hundred people in attendance that night became a family that would grow— and work together—to change the course of a river.

———

It was time for me to leave Meredith's house. Watching baby James on my bed, I was sure of it. I looked at James's round face and his smiling eyes. He was a tiny swaddled Buddha.

"What would your best day look like, James?" I asked him. "Your very best day . . ." He looked past me to the tree outside my window. The haunted tree from last winter was now covered with buds and new leaves. It was bursting with life.

"Is that what you want, James?" I said. James just stared at the tree, vibrating. "Well, we'll just have to work for it. You and me," I said, touching his cheek with my hand, which felt weaker than I wished.

The Hulberts were in the driveway to see me off: Meredith with her arms around Jake and Jane, baby James sleeping in his stroller, Peter crying, and Memory. As Valerie and I loaded into the car, I was sad and excited to be returning to New York City, this time to a wheelchair-accessible building near Valerie's house in Greenwich Village. I smelled summer in the air. It was my favorite season. In a few weeks an acquaintance of mine named Reed would be coming to New York from Los Angeles, where he lived and worked as an actor. I don't know why, but I'd picked up the phone early on to tell Reed that I had ALS. I didn't know Reed that well. He was handsome. He had made me feel safe the times we'd been together in health. So I called him.

Reed had already visited me once at Meredith's

house. I don't know how to describe it: There was something about the way he put his hands around my waist that I loved. There was undeniable energy between our bodies. It was weird being on a walker and being attracted to a guy at the same time, but at the end of the day, anatomy was anatomy. Reed and I had the anatomy thing going.

My life, in its unconventional way, was falling into place. I had a new job, Project A.L.S., a new apartment in a doorman building in Greenwich Village, and a cute guy coming into town to see me for the summer. As I waved good-bye to the Statue of Liberty, and to all she'd taken in, I looked forward to my New York homecoming.

Chapter Seven

MY NEW APARTMENT in New York was on West Twelfth Street in an elevator building. I was an uptown girl by nature, but I felt safer being downtown, only a few blocks away from Valerie. If there was an emergency, she could get to me in minutes. I was right across the street from St. Vincent's Hospital. Everyone said how great that was, though there wasn't much St. Vincent's could do for me. Ambulance sirens screamed day and night: *Dying people stuck in traffic.* That took some getting used to.

I found that with every move, I had less to unpack. Jeans and sweaters, winter coats, anything made out of wool or leather or layers, was too much for my body to bear. Gravity was pulling me down, so I shed my clothing. I brought only a couple of boxes with me from Meredith's to Twelfth Street, lightweight sweatpants and T-shirts mostly, and photographs in frames.

I bought a new electric queen bed that, as advertised on TV, made sitting up and lying down easier. Through the Visiting Nurse Service, Medicaid sent over my new home health aide, Lorna Cofield, a quiet, caring woman my age who worked weekdays. Twelfth Street had wide doorways for my wheelchair and a roll-in shower. For a few hours each day it got good sun.

With the success of the first Project A.L.S. benefit behind me, as scientists dug deeper in the sandbox to find medicine, I got sunnier. My friends insisted on taking me out in my wheelchair for walks in the scenic West Village. One time Geoffrey took his eye off the road—someone caught his eye on Perry Street—and he ran me right into a tree. Geoff, Jules, Bradley, Jace—they all played down the perils of going out for an ice cream cone. No one wanted to admit that taking me out in the wheelchair was a life-or-death proposition. Our gang didn't know from wheelchairs. We knew from the Keystone Kops. That's who we were, pushing me over cobblestones and hauling me up the warped curbs of Greenwich Village.

I started staying inside, where I was still able to use my walker for short trips to the bathroom, living room, and kitchen. The more I stayed in, the more my mind wandered to Reed, who was due in town from L.A. any day. Why was I so excited to see Reed? He and I had met years earlier in the theater program at New

York University, and again at Naked Angels. He was one of those guys who camped out occasionally on the periphery of my vision. He wasn't a focus. I always assumed that Reed wouldn't like me *that way*. So I never bothered liking him *that way*. I never invested in Reed. But we definitely hit it off as friends. When Reed and I were out in a group at dinner, we would always manage to find each other around the table. When he stayed with me at my Seventy-first Street apartment a few times on his way through New York, we did some serious laughing. Reed and I actually made love one night in Nantucket. We snuck into a hotel room during the Nantucket Film Festival, which I had helped to produce. It was a great time, but in the morning he wore sunglasses to breakfast. It was like *Invasion of the Body Snatchers*. He pretended not to know me. From then on, Reed always made a point of telling me about this or that girlfriend. It was never simply Natalie or Caitlin. It was always "my girlfriend Natalie" this, or "this girl I've been seeing, Caitlin" that.

I didn't know if Reed was coming to New York that summer just to see me, but I decided not to question it. He was planning to stay at his friends Billy and Maura's town house on Charles Street. I figured if I saw him once in a while that would be great; if not, great. Mostly I was excited to see the guy because I sensed he knew how to protect me physically. He had strong hands and perfectly chiseled . . . everything.

Reed knew the human body, all right. When he wasn't acting, Reed was running or swimming. He was like a large dog. Give him a yard and a ball and he was happy. Reed's body was a textbook illustration of health and vitality. Mine was another story, although I still thought I looked pretty decent.

"Seriously, how do I look?" I asked Meredith and Valerie, who were hanging out on the floor in my new room one day.

"Better than you have in a year," said Meredith.

"What if Reed hates the wheelchair?" I asked.

"Screw him," said Meredith.

"He can kiss my ass," said Valerie. My sisters and I were beyond protective of one another in love matters. If two sensed that the other was about to have her heart broken, they closed around her like the Mob. *You come near my sister, I'll kill you.* It was a bit over the top. Valerie and Meredith never thought I had the best taste in men. They accused me of going for the cheesecake. Granted, I was attracted to cheesecake in many forms. When it came to romance, I definitely had my own style. I started with dessert. I wanted a husband and children like my sisters, but my pursuit of the dream wasn't as linear as theirs. Starting from childhood, I had made my way in love as in so many other things, without the benefit of a road map.

———

I was married once for a brief time to Robert Redford. We wed in an ultraprivate ceremony in my bedroom with the door closed. I was thirteen and he was an eight-by-ten glossy taped to the wall over my bed. As I touched his golden hair, I vowed to have and to hold—

"Through sickness and in health," he said. We were already finishing each other's sentences. I had met Robert Redford at the Rye Ridge Cinema, where I saw *The Way We Were* seventeen times during an extended run. My mother, who was just divorced from my father, was glad to drop me off for afternoons alone at the movies.

"Don't worry about me, Mommy," I called after her. She was already halfway to the light. They all knew me at Rye Ridge.

"The regular, Jenifer?" asked the smiling woman in a paper hat.

"Plus a Junior Mints today, Josie, please," I said.

"So, how is . . . he?" she asked, topping off my popcorn with an extra shot of butter.

"I tell you, Josie, the man is a lifesaver," I said, walking toward my love in the dark. Who is as gorgeous as Robert Redford playing Hubbell Gardner in *The Way We Were*? Nobody. The man knew his way around a carrot stick. His crunching wasn't annoying like other people's. His smile, his hair, his fisherman's sweater—

"It seems like all you care about is what a guy looks like," said Valerie.

"Is that so bad?" I asked.

"If he's a horrible person it is."

"Hubbell isn't horrible. He's beautiful."

"He's a character in a movie," Valerie said. People were always so quick to judge. That's why Hubbell and I cut off from the world. I was fascinated by Hubbell's relationship in the movie with Barbra Streisand. This time, Barbra played Katie Morosky, an outspoken Jewish girl who wanted Hubbell more than life. Katie bent over backward cooking Hubbell the perfect steaks, ironing the kinks out of her hair, getting him a writing job. She made all the first moves. But Hubbell never loved Katie *that way.* He thought she pushed too hard, the ultimate turnoff for a guy like him. Life according to Hubbell wasn't about pushing. Pushing was messy and desperate. *Wait a second* . . . I pushed a lot. I was a big pusher from way back. Wasn't that the way to get things done? *Hmmm,* I thought, *does a girl push or should she be craftier?* What was that phrase . . . *feminine wiles?* Instead of calling Hubbell, maybe she waits for him to call her once in a while. Dial the phone or sit by it? It was a disturbing dilemma for a girl.

"Another Junior Mints, please." I was back at the concessions stand.

"Is there trouble in paradise?" asked Josie. She was getting on my nerves.

"We're fine, thank you," I said curtly. In the end, of course, I'd married too young. I realized I needed seasoning, other experiences. Robert Redford stared straight ahead unblinkingly when I told him I thought we should see other people. I don't know if he believed me, but I swore to return someday, if only to run my fingers through his hair one last time.

After the breakup, I had a hard time getting started with boys. My best friend, Nancy, was so frustrated with me that she started pimping me out at parties. She made me sit next to her in the circle for Spin the Bottle. I wanted to run out of the room. I kept thinking that when the bottle came to me, the guy would say, "Ewww, I'm not kissing her." Those boys weren't even kissing anyway. They were banging their heads against the girls' heads. A few boys had their mouths open. I couldn't figure out where they were going with that. The girls didn't seem to be enjoying themselves at all. My ex had spoiled me. I decided to hold out. I was looking for a certain skill level, a certain carrot crunching.

"You need to be kissed," said Nancy, who was obsessed with getting me my seven minutes in heaven. Nancy loved Timmy Kelly, the David Cassidy of our grade. He was adorable and funny and a good athlete. Nancy told me to shadow her. She said if I did exactly as she did in her cunning pursuit of Timmy, I'd land myself a whopper, too. My life changed abruptly when

Timmy took me aside and told me that he was in love with me. It was a real eye-opener. The most popular boy in the school loved me. I loved Timmy, too, but not *that way*. Maybe my loyalty to Nancy prevented it, but there was no way I was getting involved with Tim. But just knowing he loved me made all the difference during a confused time. I fit in suddenly, and without all the muss and fuss of adolescent groping. Timmy landed on his feet, too. He and Nancy got together for about seven minutes. Everyone was happy.

"There's a new guy in tenth grade," said Valerie one day as we sat in the cafeteria cutting class. I was more interested in my Linden's butter crunch cookies than just about anything. I knew what to expect from those cookies.

"Listen to me," said Valerie. "He's a man in a boy's body." And in he walked, on cue. Michael Dwyer, a tanned boy in clogs wearing overalls without a shirt. He was a teddy bear with muscles, a great head of curly brown hair, and granny glasses. My heart stopped. I had to figure out the best way to meet Michael Dwyer. I made Valerie drive by his house at night.

"This is so idiotic," said Valerie, turning into Michael's narrow winding driveway. As we reached the house, a floodlight flashed on.

"Oh my God, he sees us!" I screamed, and Valerie slammed into reverse. This went on for about a week.

"And the point of this exercise would be?" asked Valerie, who would've rather been watching the Knicks game.

"I don't know. I don't know what to do," I whimpered.

Valerie did. "Why don't you go up to him and start talking." After all the hemming and hawing, it made sense. Talking—it was a rational strategy somewhere between tackling and teasing, somewhere between Streisand's Katie Morosky and a Harrison High School cheerleader. It worked. My first real kiss was with Michael Dwyer, when I was fourteen and sitting cross-legged on the front stoop of my house. He leaned down and took my face in his hands. *Soft,* I remember thinking. Then he put his lips on mine. *Warm,* I remember thinking. The guy had tremendous potential—carrot-crunching quotient, off the charts. As we kissed I felt the cold of the cement through my jeans. *Right,* I remember thinking.

Maybe on some level I knew I'd die young and that if I was going to have a long-term relationship I'd better get down to it. Michael and I fell in love and were together for five years. As products of broken homes, we slid through the regulatory cracks. No curfews or drug testing for us. Michael and I were free to love each other like mad. It was poetry. Picture a slightly less attractive Romeo and Juliet.

Michael's mother lived in a rambling old house in

Katonah, a pretty suburb north of Harrison, where he and I stayed for long, snowy weekends in the winter. The Katonah house became ours. Michael and I grocery shopped and argued politics. We wore sweaters together. We socialized as a couple, were known as a couple, and lived in my mind as a couple. Thanks to advice from my sister Alison, who at seventeen became the youngest student in the history of Brandeis University to serve as president of the Student Sexuality Information Service, I approached sex responsibly. I came of age with my diaphragm in my purse.

"You were born older," Valerie said. I felt that Michael was born older. We were a woman and a man living the best years of our lives together a little ahead of schedule. When Michael and I decided to make it official, his father took a sudden, passionate interest in me. Michael's father liked me, but he felt that Michael was too young for marriage. I guess he had sway. The day after a rip-roaring fight, I saw Michael's yellow Beetle convertible parked in my neighbor's driveway. My neighbor was younger than I was. She had a boring face and legs for days. I went crazy on Michael. He went away.

For most of my early twenties I was like an Italian widow. I swore off men for mourning over Michael. He had been my life. Now he was gone. There were others in time: Eddie, Tico, Phil. Each hinted to me of love the way it ought to be. But no one was meant for me, not in the way Michael had been in his prime. Meredith and Peter were meant for each other. That's what I wanted, and I was going to wait for it. Jeff came close. Jeff Sherin, a stranger in a tuxedo, walked into my crowd's annual New Year's Eve party, and the whole room fell in love with him. I was the only one who got to go home with him. I was free in my Anne Klein dress and my Donna Karan tights. I was free out of my dress and tights. Nights with Jeff were some of the best, but when the sun rose on us I never felt relaxed with him. Jeff wanted me to join him in his parents' hot tub. I wasn't the jump-in-the-Jacuzzi type. I wanted us to take our time over coffee and current events. Besides, I wanted to lose a few pounds before I got into anyone's tub.

"When will I see you again?" I couldn't resist asking Jeff.

"When you see me again," he said, which meant minutes, months, I never knew. Then Jeff disappeared completely. A friend told me he'd married and divorced a Singapore model. Jeff and I saw each other a few times in the years after that. He was a wolf, I realized, one of those men who kisses and talks to you and makes love to you so expertly and gently and generously that you think he's in love with you. I still had vague notions of taming the wolf and of our ending up together down the line. Then Jeff died. His young heart gave out on a snowy mountain. I cried hysterically when I heard. I wanted to be with him. A month later, I was diagnosed with ALS. My friend Kathie said that my diagnosis was Jeff summoning me to him.

"I like this bed, Jen," said Reed, lying next to me on my new shift-o-matic, sending us up and down with the clicker. He had stopped at my new apartment straight from the airport.

"Thank God," I said, and Reed laughed hysterically. Reed and I had a verbal chemistry. He provided the setup, something benign and flat as a wheat field like "I like this bed." And I came back with sarcasm, the murder weapon. I could slay Reed with the slightest intonation. Reed and I were very Nick and Nora, platonic, of course.

Reed arrived at my bedside in June looking perfectly tanned and coiffed. (I think that Freud would have been proud of me. Every single guy I ever pretended to date, dated, or thought of dating had amazing hair, which probably meant that I wasn't trying to marry my father.) Reed wore his army fatigue shorts just so. His T-shirt fit him perfectly, and his sandals revealed flawless, tanned toes.

"The guy's a doll," Valerie said. There was something Ken-dollish about Reed, but for my sisters, I think that his perfect looks were an easy target. Outwardly, they were defensive of me, but in their heart of hearts they were praying for Reed and me to fall in love and get married, and for Reed's love to be the medicine that would make me better. As far as I was concerned, Reed presented a safe way out of the house. He certainly looked safe—and dangerous.

"Lorna!" I shouted.

"Coming," said Lorna, who helped me dress, prepare meals, and turn in bed when I couldn't, which was more often now. Lorna was my lady-in-waiting.

"What do you think of this lip gloss?" I asked.

"It's nice," said Lorna. To Lorna everything was nice, good, or fine. When my sisters asked Lorna how I was doing, it was always, "She's real good."

"What do you think of Reed?" I asked.

"He's good, real nice," said Lorna.

Lorna got a big dose of Reed and me that summer. Reed was either on his way out for a shower back at Billy and Maura's—he was very Lady Macbeth with the washing—or on his way in with a take-out dinner and movies for us to watch. Reed came and went with the wind. That summer, I was along for the ride. Reed was a Zen master with the wheelchair and my body. He knew how to nudge the chair, lift it, carry it. I never felt bumps. We never derailed. With Reed at my back, it was all smooth sailing. He made me forget I was sick.

Our first night out he pushed me along Seventh Avenue. Women stared at me. What was someone their age and outwardly healthy-looking doing in a wheelchair? And was it contagious?

"Such a beautiful night—my husband and I couldn't resist," I said to one. "We just had a baby boy. Give her a cigar, honey."

"I'm all out," said Reed.

"Then let's haul out," I said, and we took off.

"Congratulations!" the woman called after us.

Reed and I pushed westward to the edge of the Hudson River. The black water lapped up against Manhattan. Our hair blew in the breeze.

"When will I see you again?" I asked.

"Tomorrow," Reed said. We saw each other day and night for two months. Reed and I tread where few New Yorkers had dared—the edges of sidewalks, the steepest subway stairs—all with me in the wheelchair. An actor who was also a terrific photographer, Reed was determined that we see the city through a convex lens, starting with Fellini. He pulled out his perfectly folded movie listing with Fellini's *Nights of Cabiria* at eight o'clock neatly circled. I hoped he was in the mood to push the wheelchair for about six hours, because it was playing way uptown at Lincoln Center Plaza.

"We're taking the bus, Jenny," he said. I didn't do mass transit when I was healthy. It seemed crazy to start now. "Do it for me," Reed said. The idea of doing it for him suddenly appealed to me. The guy had sky blue eyes. I took a deep breath and prepared to board my first Sixth Avenue local. The bus driver opened his doors, took one look at me in the chair, and closed the doors, but not before Reed forced them open again. He got right up into the driver's face. Within minutes I was strapped into my appointed cranny on the bus with Reed next to me. I think that we both felt triumphant. We got to the movie theater early. Reed got me onto a stone bench in the courtyard of Lincoln Plaza. To look at us then, we were a normal man and woman—stunning, I might add—just waiting to see a movie. Later, in our theater seats, Reed fed me Cadbury cookies. His crunching was positively Redfordesque. People walked past us in the aisles. I smiled at them; they smiled at us. I felt so proud. Thanks to Reed's persistence, I was back in the land of the living.

At the end of the night, Reed transferred me from my wheelchair to my bed. It was our first time. The transfer with Reed was unlike any physical experience I'd had. My friends, Lorna, my sisters, no one knew how to get me out of the chair without a major planning discussion first. Reed knew instinctively. As he held me tight around my waist and pulled me up and toward him, I felt beautiful. He looked pretty good, too. We were heart-to-heart, as close as two people could be in a thrilling, wordless dance over to the bed. From that night on I didn't want to let go of Reed. I was deep into my Summer of Love, my last chance to have love with a man. My heart rushed to get everything in.

"Lorna."

"Coming," said Lorna, balancing my wicker basket full of cosmetics with my morning coffee. Lorna and I had gotten used to getting ready for Reed. We'd already changed outfits five times that day. Meredith had bought me some new shirts, and Lorna and I were plowing through a bag of them. The drawstring pants worked, finally, with a scoop neck, light blue tee. It was a look—not my first choice—but one I was determined to perfect for Reed and me. Meredith also threw in some Annick Goutal, a fragrance that drove me wild. Lorna doused me. I looked pretty damned good, if I do say so, in the scoop neck and my new lipstick from Chanel, a gossamer shade. I couldn't wait to see Reed.

"I like me a man, Lorna," I said.

"That feeling is a fine feeling," she said. "It's a real good feeling." I kicked into high gear. I called my old friends in the beauty business. They generously made house calls—hair color and cut, manicure and pedicure. My friend Martha gave me dangling earrings. I was back. Reed arrived smelling like soap. We were ready to go.

"I'll pray for you," said Lorna, a deeply religious woman.

"That may not be necessary," I said, feeling especially confident, as Reed rolled me out the front door. We went downtown to the World Trade Center, where small outdoor concerts during the weekdays were a well-kept secret. A few Wall Streeters lingered during their lunch as the music started. It was jazz. I got the beat, baby, instantly. So did Reed. He lifted me onto his lap in the chair, and he wheeled us back and forth to the music. I leaned back into him and wrapped my arms around his neck. The sun was warm on my face. People stared at us dancing in the wheelchair. I think they saw my love.

Women worry about a pimple. Women worry about ten extra pounds, or whether they're smart enough or pretty enough to be loved. I used to have the same worries. They kept me very busy. Then I got ALS. Leave it to me. It took a deathly disease for me to realize that if I wanted to love someone I could, with no restrictions, no matter how I looked or who I was. Love was my right as a woman, my responsibility, my manifest destiny! Love was my best thing. I was a Love Girl. I wanted to love Reed with everything I had in the time that I had. It didn't matter if he felt the same way. My love was my love. I was ready to pursue it.

My heart may have been ready for love, but my body wasn't. Each first experience with Reed was clouded by a ghostly awareness that it was my last—my last dinner with him in a restaurant, my last time swimming with him in the pool on East Houston Street, my last dance. I felt a Donna Summer song coming on: "It's my last chance for romance tonight." For the first time in my adult life I was ready for a thousand sunsets, but I had time for only one. It happened on the roof of Billy and Maura's brownstone. Somehow Reed had gotten me in the wheelchair to the top of the steep narrow stairway. When he got us to the roof, Reed paced like a proud father, his T-shirt drenched in sweet-smelling sweat. Getting me around New York had become Reed's extreme sport. We drank Absolut and cranberry juice as the sun went down.

"Do you see the Empire State Building, Jenny?" he asked, taking pictures. It was kind of hard to miss. I took it all in, especially the subtler Village skyline. To the east I thought I saw Valerie's house. I pictured Valerie and Scott and Willis safe inside. I loved them so much. Up the river to the north I saw Meredith and the Hulbert house, which had been a harbor to me during my most difficult days. I looked to the river. How many more times would I see it? I was getting quite a buzz on from the cocktails. I needed that kind of help saying good-bye to the skyline. *Good-bye, New York.*

"Watch the sun and the water," said Reed. It was the end of another New York day. The huge burning sun, hot and tired from work, was about to cool off in the Hudson, or so we thought. Right before the sun fell into the water, it disappeared behind New Jersey. That was surprising.

"I love you, Reed," I said.

"I love you, Jenny."

The summer was already ending. Reed's duffel was halfway packed. He asked my advice about flights back to Los Angeles.

"It's July," I said. He already had one foot out the door. Valerie put a couples' dinner together. Meredith and Peter, Scott and Valerie, and Reed and I met at Bar Pitti, for wine and pasta and sautéed spinach. From there, Reed and I were going to the theater. We all sat in the middle of the restaurant, three sisters in love. How Reed got me to the heart of that crowded restaurant I don't remember. How he got me to the theater at the height of the theater rush I'll never know. Or down into the subway, or surfing an escalator at the Loews Cineplex, or into the basement of the Village Vanguard. I can close my eyes and see Reed on Rollerblades pushing Willis and me fast, faster, mind-blowingly fast down to the ends of the city. The man knew my body. He knew how to be with me at a time when no one else did. Reed knew my needs and he anticipated every one of them.

The Summer of Love was *my* love story. My feelings drove the narrative. But let's face it, I wanted Reed to return my love in every way, shape, and form. I wanted us to get married and for him to see me through to the end. Maybe I pushed too hard, for Reed showed not the slightest hint of changing his plans. He would return to Los Angeles as scheduled on Labor Day weekend. On one of our last nights together we sprawled out on my bed watching *The Silence of the Lambs*. Reed had his back to me. It was a scary movie. I longed for him to hold me, not in a treacherous stairwell or on top of the Empire State Building, but in the way a man holds a woman when they're watching a scary movie. I wanted to reach out for Reed. But I couldn't reach him—I literally couldn't reach out with my arms to hold him. That was even scarier.

The day Reed left was my last day of walking on earth. It was a Sunday. He was on my bed watching a preseason football game. I was contemplating getting to the bathroom using my walker. The scene was a fast-forward glimpse of what Reed and I would be as an elderly couple.

"I don't think I can walk anymore," I said.

"Don't be ridiculous," Reed said. He was eating a sandwich and talking to the quarterback. "Just use the walker."

I didn't want to disappoint him. I wanted to keep walking. I wanted to walk to Los Angeles. I pulled myself up in bed. I knew I was going down before I took my first step, my last ever. "Reed . . ." I crashed to the floor. Reed was at my side. He held me.

"I'm sorry, Jenny," he said. "I'm so sorry." What was he sorry for? I had done things with Reed that summer that I never would have done as a healthy person.

Reed and I transferred one last time. Lorna and I had dressed my bed in satin sheets and a cashmere blanket for the occasion. I sat next to my bed in the wheelchair. Reed faced me. For us, the transfer had become an art form. My friend Martha said she learned everything she needed to know about love between a man and woman from watching Reed and me transfer that summer. Reed put his arms around me and lifted me to him. I smelled his soapy smell. I cried hot tears into his neck. For those weeks Reed and I had been as close as two people could be. As I held my face against his, I wanted to kiss him. *My last kiss.* I could have, but I wasn't quite ready to say good-bye to kissing, or to Reed. That one I'd save for later. We held each other for a long time, rocking. Then he put me down onto the bed. He sat looking at me, then staring off. Hubbell, my Hubbell. I had sworn to return to him, if only to run my fingers through his hair one last time. I ran my fingers through Reed's hair. He was crying. He picked up his duffel, promised to call, and left for the airport.

About a week later, photos arrived in the mail. Reed had captured the essence of the summer with his camera. There were beautiful pictures of New York, of my family and me. In my favorite, I am sitting on the grass with the World Trade Center behind me. I am smiling and looking healthy, looking at Reed.

Chapter Eight

IT WOULD HAVE BEEN NICE if Reed had gotten down on his knees at the end of the Summer of Love and asked me to marry him, but he didn't. He *so* didn't. When he sashayed out of my room for the airport, my heart shattered. I started dreaming about him. I didn't want to dream about Reed. I wanted to throw fruit at his head. But every time I closed my eyes, I saw us racing down Seventh Avenue or eating cookies with Fellini. I spent the first few weeks after he left crying into my pillow and talking my sisters' ears off about Reed, Reed, my Reed.

"This is so sick," said Meredith as I talked compulsively about Reed in his shorts and sandals. "I hate those sandals," she said.

"Awww, don't be mean to my baby with his little shoes," I said. I was out of control. In my heart I knew that no one would touch me again the way Reed had.

What does a woman do when a man breaks her heart? One plots revenge. Another vows never to make the same mistake again. I ate candy. Late one night, after a nightmare starring Reed in truly unattractive sunglasses, I called on my bedside stash of Rolos, the genius chocolate and caramel candy that gave me solace. But reaching for midnight snacks wasn't so easy for me anymore. I was horizontal. My outstretched fingers were inches from the Rolos and victory. I channeled Reed for one final push. *Oh, Reed.* It didn't work out—as I lunged for the Rolos, I fell out of bed. I fell and I couldn't get up. I had two options: stay on the floor until morning when Lorna arrived, or somehow get to the phone and call for help. *Stupid Rolos... Hey, wait a minute,* I thought. *Rolos. Roll ... over. Roll over.* With everything I had, I rolled once, twice, toward the phone, which was up on my nightstand next to the candy. I pulled the cord as hard as I could, the phone came crashing down to the floor, and I dialed for help. Within minutes, Valerie and my friend Michael were picking me up and dusting me off.

"Such ingenuity, Jen," said Michael, who is the hardest-working actor I know.

Ingenuity was part of it. I had good ideas. But my true salvation after that heartbreaking summer with Reed was my other great love in life, work. Reaching, rolling, falling, fighting, holding on, speaking out—hard work had been my salvation as a girl and it was my only hope now. I had said it in health, and I was saying it again, louder: Love and work are the most important things in life. Without love and work, a woman is a shambles. She's a Rolos-eating mess.

Just as I had known that Reed was my last chance at romance, I believed that Project A.L.S. was my last stop on the work train. I was using everything I had to make Project A.L.S. unique and compelling. I turned away from Reed and focused like a laser on the work. My self-doubt and the occasional fears of failure that had plagued my earlier efforts in the working world were gone. Fueled by the lessons of my past and facing what was very possibly my last chance to work, I became my most efficient self. Along with my sisters and friends, Project A.L.S. and I began a methodical, thrilling, epic chase for robbers who were stealing lives. I couldn't run after the robbers anymore. But I knew that with ingenuity and hard work, I might catch them.

My sisters and I were already building Project A.L.S. from shitdust—you'll excuse the French—into a young, respected force against disease. That's because we were taking on the problem of ALS for the first time as a team, as a family. Scientists thought that our "family approach" was novel—or new. I didn't think it was new. I thought it was as old as the hills. It was absolutely essential that scientists and doctors and corporate leaders and government officials work together to make sick people better. I also believed that if we continued executing our plan, Project A.L.S. could become to disease research what MGM had been to the movie musical. We could become the best at what we did.

I had always wanted to be the best at something. When I was seven, I could do the Hula Hoop better than anyone in my family. Even my mother was impressed. Since then, I had made an effort to try to do my best at every job. It wasn't always easy. I got fired a couple of times. But at the end of the day, I could always say I had worked—that I had put in a good, honest day of work. I could always say I'd earned my night's sleep.

As my body weakened, though, I wondered if I was going to have enough energy left to push Project A.L.S. over the top. The company was off to a great start, but we needed to grow. In order to grow right, we needed to impose a structure on ourselves. I thought for a long time about whether I could say yes when Valerie, Meredith, and Jules offered me the job of Project A.L.S. CEO. It took me about two seconds. I finally had my own company. Project A.L.S. was in the business of finding medicine for an incurable disease, or, as our closest advisors might have said, accomplishing the impossible. I believed that my sisters and I were as qualified as anyone to make that happen.

———

My best work had always come from passion and love. As a senior at Harrison High School, I was already building a respectable résumé. After two years at Clover Donuts, I was promoted to head grill girl. I flipped donuts *and* burgers. I had a steady boyfriend. That definitely qualified as work. On the home front, my mother got her first paying job. After she moved us into a smaller house in Harrison, she started selling gigantic ones. Of course, my mother thrived as a real estate broker. Better than anyone, she understood a family's dream of living in a modern-day castle. My mother's dream had come true for about five minutes with Trilarch. She was helping her clients hold on to their dreams for a little longer. I felt proud that my mother was finally doing what she'd spent her best years motivating my father to do.

At a certain point, my working in the food business was like an alcoholic tending bar. Most of what I earned at Clover or Butler Brothers delicatessen was canceled out by my tendency to eat the profits. Help was on the way. My humanities teacher, Mr. Toppo, approached me one day after class to say he thought I should audition for the Declamation Contest, an annual event at Harrison High School that featured students acting out monologues. The contest was sponsored by the local outpost of the American Legion and was judged by a panel of Legionnaires, teachers, and independent experts in diction and public speaking. I auditioned for the Declamation Contest and was selected as one of the final six contestants.

I fell in love with acting the moment I tried it. I also fell in love with Mr. Toppo. I was seventeen at the time—he was about 110. This was to become a pattern—my falling head over heels for any man I worked with intimately, regardless of his age, availability, or sexual orientation. Mr. Toppo and I worked for weeks on my monologue, which I had chosen from Ingmar Bergman's *Face to Face,* a dark, complex portrait of a psychiatrist's descent into a nervous breakdown. At seventeen, I found that I liked exploring the dark side of the human psyche. There was something familiar about it. Mr. Toppo seemed stunned by my openness in rehearsal. He said I had a great instrument. Finally, on the day of the contest, I couldn't hold myself back.

"Mr. Toppo . . . I think I'm falling in love with you," I said.

"If this were another time and place, perhaps," he said, correcting papers.

"Mr. Toppo?"

"Yes, Jenny."

"I can't tell if I'm good at acting because I'm in love with you or because I'm just good at acting," I said.

"Tonight is only the beginning for you, Jenny," he said. "Good luck out there."

I was out of my body the night of the Declamation

Contest. The auditorium was filled with an audience in the hundreds, the judges, and most of all my love for what I was doing. I took the stage as Bergman's embattled protagonist wearing a diaphanous nightgown, uninhibited and completely free. I ripped through my monologue, giving it my simplest, most honest interpretation. The crowd went wild. I won. When the head of the American Legion stood up to announce my name as the winner, Valerie and Meredith shouted and whooped in the aisles. Mr. Toppo stood at the fire exit with his arms folded, quietly nodding. Backstage, Mrs. Oberstein, the elegant school speech therapist, approached me weeping, thanking me for my performance. Mrs. Landau, the empress of all English teachers, who had preferred teaching my more studious sisters and had taken much less notice of me, pulled me aside.

"You became a woman tonight," she said, looking into my eyes. I felt humbled and gracious. I shook hands and kissed people congratulating me as Mr. Toppo, my first acting mentor, graciously stepped back into the shadows. I wasn't in love with him anymore, but I loved him.

I think I was born to act. Unfortunately, I was also born to stop myself from acting. For some reason, I didn't trust my love for it. Acting felt too good or something. I just didn't understand how anything in life could come so easily. There had to be a catch.

Almost immediately after my emancipation onstage in the Declamation Contest, self-doubt came a-calling. Self-doubt was a problem I'd inherited in part from my mother and one that I would fight for years. I was fine working at jobs I didn't love. But when it came to the pursuit of my deepest passions, I felt inhibited sometimes and unworthy. My father had been born with a sense of entitlement. He believed he had the right to walk into a restaurant and change its menu. In my attempt to separate myself from him, I think I might have gone too far in the other direction. Sometimes I didn't feel entitled to my dreams at all.

I went on to study acting at New York University, but self-doubt seeped into most every performance and my every opportunity to work. I would become physically sick from stage fright. I'd call Valerie from backstage moments before an entrance, telling her I couldn't go on.

"What's the worst that could happen?" Valerie asked.

"Die," I said, choking on fear.

"You're afraid to live is what," she said. "Just get out there and pretend you don't give a shit." Okay, so she wasn't Stella Adler. But Valerie convinced me to get out onstage and do my job. "Just complete," she said. I managed to make my mark onstage on a few glorious occasions.

Valerie had always fascinated me. She was my older

sister. She had been a parent to Meredith and me. Valerie had never missed a single one of my performances, including dress rehearsals. After college, she was right there loving me through difficult patches, praising my successes. No one believed in me more than Valerie. She believed I saw things first, knew them first—well, you know the drill. But you didn't want to ask Valerie what *she* was working on.

"Crap," she'd say. "That's what." My sister Valerie clearly understood the importance of work. She had worked her ass off from the time she was fifteen. She was never without a job. Hers was one puzzling résumé. Valerie had studied English in college. She wanted to be a writer. But for five years, ten years, fifteen years after graduation, she didn't write.

"I can't write," she'd say. "My writing is like an alien's writing." Okay. I realized I had my work cut out for me. Valerie had been my life's guide, my first one. She put me through the basic training that had solidified my values, my habits, and my work ethic. But when Valerie hit her twenties, boy, did she ever need a kick in the pants from Meredith and me, her own graduating class.

Valerie and I were always creative soul mates. Meredith didn't understand our mind-bending, never-ending quandaries. Meredith figured if you wanted to do something, you did it all day, as simple as that. She had gone to college and immediately to grad-

uate school. She had pursued jobs in fashion merchan-
dising because that's what Meredith wanted. Boom.
Done. Valerie and I, on the other hand, constantly
questioned our motives. We talked endlessly on the
phone and over coffee and into the night about the creative process. Not that we had many creations in
process—we just liked to put our minds to the issues
of art and creativity.

It was thanks to Valerie's patience over the years
that I was eventually able to accept the fact that work
brings disappointments along with success, that work
isn't a bed of donuts. I learned that work was always
going to be a mixed bag, no matter the job. But Valerie
herself wasn't interested in mixed bags. She felt that
unless she wrote like Tennessee Williams, she should
be stripped of the right to write.

"We already have a Tennessee Williams," I told her.
I wanted Valerie to know that we needed one of her,
too. Just because I wasn't Meryl Streep didn't mean I
shouldn't act. Also, if acting was going to give me so
much to think about and *so little to do,* maybe I should
consider changing jobs. I was learning maturity. I was
learning a give-and-take. Valerie taught me that give-
and-take, but she'd forgotten to teach herself. Now I
mentored her. I tried anyway. She wrote five short plays.

"They pretty much suck," said Valerie, handing me
the scripts. They were fine plays. They needed work,
but the grain of goodness was right there on the page.

"Do you think you can work on these?" I asked. Valerie worked on the plays and saw them performed.

"So, what did you think?" I asked, after a roomful of people clapped for her plays.

"I think I need work," she said.

"Yes, isn't that great? There's so much to do," I said. Valerie was starting to know that everything— every painting, kitchen cabinet, chocolate soufflé, could use some improving. The point of the game was to stay in it. You had to be in it to win it. Valerie and I taught each other that taking risks was difficult and necessary.

After college, my friends from the NYU Theater Department started a company called Naked Angels. Out of curiosity, I went over to The Space on Seventeenth Street, the company's new home, and I didn't leave for years. Acting was giving me a tough way to go. I tried working through my fears at Naked Angels by taking a part in the Joseph Heller play *We Bombed in New Haven. We Bombed on Seventeenth Street* was more like it. I wasn't that good in the play. But, truth be told, I wasn't that bad, either. More than anything, acting had just become a source of annoyance and frustration. I made a conscious decision to walk away from it for a while. I could always come back if I wanted to. In the meantime, I figured, I'd be a producer. Valerie said it: I'd always had a knack for seeing the big picture.

Naked Angels was a great place to cut your teeth if you were a fledgling actor, playwright, director, or stage designer. My fellow company members included so many talented artists: Marisa Tomei, Rob Morrow, Kenneth Lonergan, Jon Robin Baitz, Gina Gershon, Nicole Burdette . . . but there was no one running the joint. My friend Merrill and I built up the office from zero. Merrill had some great ideas. He showed me the importance of a dynamic board of directors. He and I were careful to build a board that would give back to the company: raising money, bringing ideas, and donating in-kind services. John Kennedy was on the board. He provided me with many in-kind services. First—let's just put this on the table—the man was insanely elegant and gorgeous. I had just never seen such grace in a human being before. Another Naked Angels board member, Martha McCully—also insanely gorgeous— and I would sit at meetings, bewitched by John. His was an uncommon beauty. John was a mentor—I learned a lot about self-discipline working side by side with him. He was a master at letting things roll off his back. I tried to copy him.

If I may be so bold, I'd say Naked Angels eventually became *the* place to be for emerging artists and audiences. We never advertised our plays, but orchestrated a word of mouth that gave Naked Angels a cache, an air of mystery, a certain underground glamour. Naked Angels became the hottest ticket in town, not only because we were savvy in our "branding" but because we nurtured gifted artists in their formative years. We promoted art in progress—an excellent product, in my opinion.

I remember watching the Academy Awards as a girl and wondering what producers did. I could picture actors and directors and costume designers at work—but it was hard visualizing a producer. This is what I did as a producer: I took productions of plays under my wing. I worked every aspect of productions, from getting corporate backing to working with writers on scripts to advising directors, listening to actors, and selling tickets. If the heat wasn't coming up through the pipes, that was me. The producer was responsible for soup through nuts. If Jacqueline Kennedy Onassis was stopping by the office to talk to me about John and his love for the theater, I had to make myself available. (Talking with Mrs. Kennedy Onassis was one of the great honors of my life.) During the day, I worked hand in hand with the company and the board to ensure that The Space was a nurturing place. At night, I worked the schmooze, dining and dishing and drumming up excitement for Naked Angels. I got people to fall in love with Naked Angels and give us things. Some nights thinking about work, I was too excited to sleep. I was crazy in love with my job. For my five years as producing director, Naked Angels previewed the next generation of talent—my generation.

When it came to my career, I was never a pampered pooch. I was never groomed to run the family business. I had made my own way, so that one day I could offer my son or daughter or niece or nephew the chance to inherit and improve upon what I had built. I was a student in business from the start. Mentors had been a key to my learning, so I sought them out aggressively. I picked up the phone and called Sue, Kathie, Simon, John, Michael, and others whom I'd admired from afar and wanted to learn from and asked if I could meet with them. I was always afraid that the person on the other end of the phone would think, *Who is this little pisher calling me?* But I called anyway. It was never easy picking up the phone. None of it was easy, come to think of it—the nerves, the cold calling, making meetings with strangers—but all of it was necessary.

"I just want to do a good job, Simon," I said, during my job interview with him. I was interviewing for the position of account executive at the public relations firm Baker Winokur Ryder. I didn't really know what public relations was, but after Naked Angels, I just had to start earning a decent wage for myself. "I just want to do a good job," I said again. Simon got a big kick out of my wide-eyed earnestness—he was a bit taken aback by it. I was never too good at business-speak—you know, that buttoned-down way of presenting your case. My strategy was going into an office and speaking my heart. It wasn't necessarily a winning strategy, but it did win me the chance to roll up my sleeves and get started with Simon.

I spent the money as soon as I got it. That was just my way. Making more money, I figured I could spend more on my sisters, my mother, my future husband—wherever he was hiding—and my nieces and nephews. Simon Halls gave me a chance to earn more—so I could share more. I was confident about my prospects. Almost as soon as I started at Baker Winokur Ryder, I hatched my next plan—the big kahuna. I had always wanted to produce movies. I dreamed of bringing high-quality entertainment to millions of people, and there were two people I wanted to work with in making it happen—Valerie and Meredith. With valuable experience under my belt, I hunkered down for hard work in my glorious thirties. I looked forward to a life sentence of hard labor. Then I got sick.

One of my favorite plays was *The Three Sisters* by Anton Chekhov. In one scene the three sisters sit around the samovar, talking about their lives. They are still hurting from the death of their beloved father a year before. Although the sisters are full of dreams, they feel directionless. Then they remember—*the work*. It is a revelation for them, a forgotten treasure. Yes, the sisters are heartbroken. Yes, their lives haven't worked out as planned. But suddenly they are invigorated by the following realization: They still have work to do. It was the same with Valerie, Meredith, and me. When all seemed lost, when Reed walked out my door, and illness prevented me from doing the same, my sisters and I still had *the work*. ALS wasn't our first choice of work, but it was what we were dealt.

There wasn't time to stop and worry about whether our work was pretty or a masterpiece or inspiring. As a bunch of nonscientists, we didn't stop to worry if we were allowed to challenge science and medicine. Fear and self-doubt had become luxuries my sisters and I couldn't afford. We had a lot of work to do, and we didn't have much time. My sisters and I became the Charlie's Angels of ALS.

I was the stay-at-home Angel, working phones from my bed. My ALS was moving into my arms and torso, so going out on the town wasn't an option anymore. It was too dangerous. Even with a custom-made wheelchair, I had trouble holding my body up. One wrong move, one uneven curb, and I would have gone flying off the chair. I couldn't rely on my muscles to keep me safe and upright. Living on my bed for most of the day worked in one respect: I got a lot done. It's not like I could hop up and go out for lunch. My fingers were getting less nimble. It was hard dialing friends just to talk. I worked more than I had ever worked before, because I couldn't get away from it. I used a headset while Lorna dialed for me. For conference calls, Jules, Meredith, and Valerie gathered around my speakerphone. I learned a million ways to say the same thing: The state of ALS was unacceptable. Project A.L.S. was going to change it. Can you help us?

As I romanced corporate America from my bed, Meredith and Valerie worked over the scientists to come up with new, more aggressive approaches to research. These doctors, who seemed nice enough, hadn't managed to come up with medicine for ALS in two hundred years. Why was that, exactly? We knew they could do better—we set out to help them do their best work and hold them accountable. My sisters, Jules, and I had been held accountable in every job we'd ever had. Either we completed a task by the stated deadline or we were fired. We taught scientists about deadlines: I was talking *dead*lines. Project A.L.S. led with cattle prods. I think that the researchers and doctors appreciated our directness.

While I worked at home, Angels Valerie and Meredith hit the road, recruiting the most gifted, creative scientists—many of whom had never thought about ALS before—and molding them into a dream team. Project A.L.S. funded this dream team on the condition that the players work together, share data, meet regularly, and beat deadlines. Traditionally, scientific research was done in isolation—the guy in Podunk worked on his project, the gal in Hodunk worked at her project, and they never met to share their findings or to discuss how their projects might connect to the larger body of ALS research. The traditional work model seemed totally ludicrous to us. Scientists worked as competitors, not collaborators. Crazy! Teams, armies, communities, a houseful of sisters, a country as one—every major championship, war, and consensus that America had won, it had won through some form of togetherness. We founded Project A.L.S. on the same notion—that ALS would be solved not by brilliant individuals working in isolation, but by committed, aggressive teams of researchers working together. It was the American way. It was our way. It was the only way we were going to win this thing.

One of our first breaks came in early 1999, when Valerie got a hot tip about a renegade scientist and neurologist from Children's Hospital at Harvard University. Evan Snyder was using stem cells to make mice that had been genetically engineered to shake and wobble stop shaking and wobbling. Valerie and Meredith went up to Dr. Snyder's lab and pinned him against the wall—kidding. They asked him if he thought that stem cells might also help people who wobble with ALS, or other degenerative brain diseases or injuries. Dr. Snyder said he thought that they could, and a new idea was born—using stem cells to understand and treat ALS.

Over the next two years, Project A.L.S. created a world-leading consortium including stem cell experts, molecular biologists, ALS clinicians, and others to test different kinds of stem cells in laboratory models of ALS. In one set of experiments, Douglas Kerr and John Gearhart of Johns Hopkins University showed that stem cells helped paralyzed rats walk again. A group of scientists led by Hynek Wichterle and Thomas Jessell of Columbia University and the Howard Hughes Medical Institute showed that stem cells could be *nudged* to become brand-new motor neurons, the cells that die in ALS. Both groundbreaking studies were formed, funded, and overseen by Project A.L.S. We knew how to nudge, too. I loved that Dr. Jeff Rothstein was on our team now. The same man who had told me my motor neurons were dying and they'd never be replaced was starting to show that stem cells might one day prove him wrong.

Work allowed me to take out my frustration over the fact that nothing had been done about ALS by doing something. Work was an outlet for my fear, too. My arms got weak so fast. My fingers started curling in. They reminded me of *The Wizard of Oz,* when the witch's feet curl up under Dorothy's house (for me, the scariest part of the movie). Soon I wouldn't be able to feed myself. I had a night nurse now, Karen Jack, who rubbed my feet and listened to my midnight confessions. Dishing with Karen became a ritual that I looked forward to. I noticed that my breathing was becoming ever so labored, which meant that my diaphragm, the flat muscle that expands and contracts the lungs, wasn't working as efficiently. With ALS, the writing was always on the wall. Each day I came across a clue telling me which part of my body was going to be destroyed next.

At the same time my body wiped out, my pride grew mightily. I marveled at Valerie's and Meredith's ability to go out into the world, challenge it, and bring home the kill. They worked with such grace, intelligence, and economy.

"I learned it all from you," Meredith said as she crunched numbers on my bed.

"I learned it all from you," I said.

"And I would be chopped liver," said Valerie, who became director of research for Project A.L.S. Listening to her talk to scientists on the phone made me feel hopeful. It took her about ten minutes to learn their language. She had mentored me; now she was motivating some of the world's greatest scientists to do better.

Build it and they will come. We did and they did. As Project A.L.S. made inroads, magazines and newspapers got interested. *The New York Times* and *People* ran stories about us. Then my friend Patricia Harrington introduced me to Katie Couric. One day, when Valerie and Meredith were down in Washington at a meeting with the Food and Drug Administration, Katie came to my bed. We talked and talked and talked. Outside there was a blizzard. As the snow piled up, Katie and I spent the whole day getting to know each other. I felt as if I'd known her before. No doubt, we would have been best friends as girls. She probably would have been as good if not better than I was at the Hula Hoop. I admired Katie's demand for journalistic excellence— she seemed to be a perfectionist like me. I totally fell in love with her soul. It was profoundly kind and kindred. Not to mention we were on the same page when it came to men. As single women (Katie had lost her beloved husband, Jay Monahan, to colorectal cancer), we both wondered about our chances of finding new love.

Soon after our meeting, Katie reported an in-depth segment about Project A.L.S. on the *Today* show. It elevated us to a whole new level. Our phones rang off the hooks. More corporate sponsorship followed— *InStyle* magazine, Bloomberg—and more researchers signed on. Valerie built a tight-knit research advisory board of universally respected scientists and administrators to guide us to our next level of discovery in the laboratory. Jules, Meredith, and I put together our board of directors, a downright remarkable group of friends, activists, and philanthropists. My sisters and I were on our way. We didn't know if we'd get there in the time of my life, but we swore to get there, to the mountaintop, where hard work, love, and determination foretold medicine for people who were dying.

My work for Project A.L.S. made me feel more entitled, though not in a selfish way. I was just so confident. I felt that I could do anything. I couldn't reach out literally anymore, but I wanted to keep reaching in every other way. Forget fear and self-doubt. If by some miracle I got better, I'd do a lot more acting. I'd ring Reed's doorbell and the doorbells of many men. I'd be uninhibited and free and confident. I pictured myself as a woman in health, running, not walking, toward what I wanted.

Chapter Nine

AFTER TWO YEARS living on Twelfth Street, I started calling my carpet "the food and beverage carpet." People spilled on it all the time. No one knew why. It was a phenomenon. If a friend came in to my room with a Diet Coke, chances are she was going to spill it. Friends would say, "Oh my God, Jen, let me get some paper towels." And I'd say, "Please, please don't worry about it. This is the food and beverage carpet. Everyone's spilling." Even more mysterious . . . my ocean blue carpet appeared to absorb everything from beer to pasta, and it never stained or smelled.

"We should really get Stanley Steemer in here to clean this carpet," Meredith said, after knocking over one of her trademark iced teas.

"I don't think we need it, Mer," I said.

Aside from the food and beverage carpet, my bedroom was unremarkable, except for the photos covering every inch of my walls, bureau, and radiator. The faces of my nieces and nephews made people stop in their tracks—they were *that* beautiful. One of the most mesmerizing was a close-up of Kate, Valerie's daughter, the latest addition. I was never able to hold Kate in my arms by myself. When Valerie brought her home from the hospital, she lay newborn Kate in my lap and put my arms around the baby and held us there. That was about the best we could do.

As my arms and hands became paralyzed, as my body shut down, I was grateful to be able to commune with photos of my friends. Some people look to crosses or the Torah for inspiration. As I got sicker, I looked to photos of my friends. Some were of my friends with me when I was healthy, at parties, at the beach, in the good old days. I couldn't believe how much my body had changed. I had been a much prettier person than I remembered.

My friends showed up in person, too. Old and new friends came to my bed. Before I got sick I was all over New York. Nothing made me happier than throwing on some jeans and catching a movie with Martha and Merrill, or meeting my posse after work at the Odeon, a Tribeca restaurant with great roast chicken and mashed potatoes. Going out with friends wasn't always easy breezy. There was a certain pressure that came along with showing up at all the right places with all the right people—and being *on*. What if *I* wasn't right—what if I was *off*? Many nights I would have much rather stayed home alone with a cake. But the more I challenged myself to get out there socially, the more I began to relax and enjoy myself.

Now I rarely left my bed, which after two years of constant use had become a whining, arthritic queen. Each time my nurses sent it up or down with the clicker it groaned with dissatisfaction. I remembered the early days of ALS, when Meredith and I dressed up my bed with fabulous sheets and comforters. Now we just couldn't be bothered. My nurses used a plain flat sheet to move me around. I had to be shifted constantly. I breathed easier lying on my side. Coughing was easier sitting up. On the millionth count-of-three, Lorna, Karen, or my new nurse, Juliet, would pull my sheet and me toward the closet or toward the window or toward the door or toward the wall, depending on whether I needed to breathe or cough or eat or sleep. They lifted and lowered my arms, legs, and trunk. They adjusted my hands and my head. My nurses were like hands on the deck of a ship in a never-ending storm. My bed and I were the ship that they steered and manipulated.

As I was being lifted, shifted, and rolled, I thought about my summer with Reed two years before. I had been much more mobile then. When Reed had held me that summer, I could hold him back. I had been able to absorb the insulting bumps and bruises that

New York dished out to people in wheelchairs, but I couldn't cut it anymore. I missed my laugh a lot. Without laugh muscles, all I could muster now was a flat, forced "aaaaaa." I hated that sound. It was a real joke killer. A baby monitor was my latest piece of equipment. It became a lifesaver, as my once booming voice and laugh—my friends had always said they knew exactly where I was sitting in a theater—disappeared. The baby monitor was my connection to my nurses in the living room.

The living room, also known as Project A.L.S. World Headquarters, was just beyond my door. During the week, our associate director, Nina Capelli, worked in the office as I worked on my bed in my room with my sliding door closed. First thing in the morning, I would hear Nina out there pleasantly answering the phone, "Project A.L.S," and our executive director Dana Kind, and producer Jonathan Burkhart strategizing for our next event, while Lorna and I were behind closed doors trying to get my head through a turtleneck. My lifestyle was less traditional than ever: I lived where I worked. I ate where I slept. I bathed on my bed. God knows I would have traded it all for a husband and a house with a normal carpet, but that wasn't my fate.

I saw the world from my bed. Lorna got me ready. She would sit me up in my black turtleneck and black cotton pants, cross my legs, and balance my hands on my knees. She'd prop me up all around with bean-filled pillows. I looked like a Buddha or a tepee. Then she'd slide the door open and my friends would come in. I can imagine how nervous people were to see me. They probably didn't know what to expect as time passed. But once my friends came to the bed, they didn't want to leave. I didn't want them to leave, either.

My friends were impressed with the food and beverage carpet. They loved my whole room. They said it was out of time, that it was a time machine. My friends said my room was sanctum sanctorum, a sacred place where they didn't feel judged. They said it was a spiritual spa where they could relax and let it all hang out. As their confessions flowed, my desire to listen to them grew stronger. I wanted to offer help where I could. I wanted to help so much. I had sleepover dates with Simon, four-hour lunches with Katie, business strategy sessions with Sue; all of it seemed out of time, as if my friends and I existed in a parallel place.

Martha McCully walking into my room—there was a gift. My friend Martha looked more beautiful to me with each visit. Martha and I had shared a taste for the best things, always—beautiful people and restaurants, fabulous vacation spots. In health, Martha and I were weight-conscious to a fault. We wanted to lose ten pounds forever. That forever nagging feeling was so far away now. Talking on my bed, Martha and I felt more and more that we were a-okay, and that ten pounds would never separate us again from the lives we wanted. Martha brought over her new boyfriend to meet me. I felt like Judge Judy while they sat there holding hands and answering my pointed questions. I was so proud that Martha was in love, the most empowering feeling, but I wasn't totally sold on the guy. He was a little defensive. Plus, where were the flowers and candy? For Martha and me, romance was always a subject "to be continued." Focusing on how we could improve ourselves for *ourselves,* and not for our potential boyfriends, remained one of our biggest challenges.

I may not have been a whiz when it came to my love life, but friendship I knew. I had a knack for giving my friends dead-on romantic advice. It gave me joy sharing my best feelings about Martha *with* Martha, being Katie's bed spy, letting Caroline wrap me in the pale blue cashmere blanket that she had brought for me from Europe and hearing about her latest date.

I was always a big believer in family values. You'd be, too, if you had a family like mine. Friends were my family. I'd have toasted them right there on my bed: *To my friends—that family of mine* . . . but I couldn't hold a glass anymore. I probably would have spilled on my carpet anyway. After her piece about Project A.L.S. on *Today,* Katie came back to my bed with a new boom box for me and encouraged me to listen to music again. Thanks to Katie, Frank Sinatra was back in my life. In short order, Katie brought me another man, my new Sinatra. Rob Kaplan was Katie's friend, and he quickly became my brother. Rob and I bonded the moment we met. We talked about love, his upbringing in Kansas, and Project A.L.S. I learned the finer points of leadership and philanthropy on the bed with Rob. He and I covered territory in a hurry. Ours was a deep friendship in fast motion. We wanted to get everything in. Rob and I were busy people, but we always had time to check in with each other by phone. He had occasional questions about women. I had eternal questions about men. I was Rob's romance 4–1–1. He was my spiritual 9–1–1. Rob became my Sinatra, my brother, my husband, business mentor, and eternal friend. I don't know what Freud would have said about Rob and me, but I had stopped trying to please Freud a long time ago.

"You're an old fuddy-duddy," Valerie had told me when I was ten. "You're an old lady or something." Some saw a wisdom in my chubby face—a certain age, a knowing. My math teacher came to me for advice. So did kids in my class and their mothers. My own mother had taught me the master class in friendship: If I could help her, I could definitely help others. My mother and I confided in each other throughout her divorce, subsequent remarriage, and boyfriends.

"I don't have *boyfriends,*" my mother sneered.

"Okay, *man*friends," I said.

"I don't have manfriends. Men are fools, every last one of them," she hissed.

"With all due respect, Ma, you're never without one." I believe my mother loved men more than she loved herself—that was the biggest problem. Over coffee with the woman I idolized, I observed the many subtle ways in which brilliant, gifted, exotic women diminished themselves in relation to the world. Men did it, too. I wanted to stop the people I loved from doing this. From a young age, I had tried to save them.

"Who do you think you are, Holden Caulfield?" Valerie would say. "Why don't you mind your own business?" I have always felt that other people's business *was* my business.

When my mother fell head over heels, crazy in love with the man who became her second husband—I called him Number Two—I was forced to bring my A-game. It was really scary. After three dates with Number Two, my mother had already changed her smart wardrobe to all flouncy dresses; she had permed her hair and started talking in uncharacteristically girlish whispers. She was another person. It was like *The Stepford Wives.* Hey, I liked a good makeover as much as the next girl. But this was ridiculous.

"Isn't he an elegant creature?" my mother marvelled as we sat in the car watching Number Two exit the liquor store with a brown bag. "Watch how he *moves,* Jenifer. He's all about economy." He sure was. Number Two was so cheap, he and my mother took over Alison and Valerie's room after they got hitched, without even asking. The guy sure saved on rent.

My mother was definitely in love with Number Two. I was genuinely happy for her. I don't think she'd ever been in love with my father. But the price she paid! My mother gave Number Two the farm. The farm was all of her intelligence, her strengths, and her elegance. She projected it all onto him. *He* was the elegant one. It was hard staying patient with my mother sometimes. I told her she needed to look in the mirror. Then she would see her worth—and that perm had to go. When I was a girl, I had noticed a lot of girls and boys, and women and men, giving away the farm. It was epidemic. A lot of people looked to *the other* instead of looking inside for happiness. It was like me buying a Rolls-Royce or a house in Malibu, expecting that those beautiful things would fill me up, or like Dorothy searching for fulfillment in Oz when her heart was home—inside of her—the whole time.

I advised my mother. I advised my friends. They filled empty spaces for me, too. After my father left, Valerie, Meredith, and I rebuilt our family with friends. We all shared the same ones. We made our house home to them after school. We broke bread with our friends. We went away for weekends with them.

At fifteen, Valerie was de facto head of our growing household. Through living with friends, my sisters and I learned the value of one big, happy family.

It wasn't all rosy. After my father left, the holidays were especially depressing. When I was a girl, my mother had always made such a big production of our Jewish Christmas. I was Eloise at The Plaza. Christmas was my absolute favorite time of the year. I think I believed in Santa until I was thirteen. On Christmas mornings, my sisters and I would rush downstairs to find that the living room had been magically transformed into a winter wonderland with hills of gifts in shiny wrapping. I still looked forward to Christmas, but the tenor of it changed after my father left. My mother definitely wasn't up for magic making. I was worried about her.

Then Donna and Elsa came in. Donna and Elsa were more Valerie's friends, but Meredith and I looked up to them so much. Valerie met Donna on the Harrison Huskies girls' basketball team. Valerie played forward; Donna was their outstanding point guard. Elsa was Donna's best friend, a college student who watched games from the stands with her sunglasses on. Elsa was so cool she could have been Fonzie's sister. Donna and Elsa became Valerie's parents. Elsa picked Valerie up after school in a cool brown Firebird; Donna cooked Italian dinners for her. We all felt safe around Elsa and Donna.

One Christmas Eve during high school I was struck by a sad silence. Our usual friends had gone home to be with their real families for the night, and the house felt cold and hollow. My mother was alone in her room with the door closed. Valerie, Meredith, and I just sat there as the afternoon got darker and darker. Then Elsa and Donna busted through the front door, carrying a huge Christmas tree. We'd never had a Christmas tree before.

"Please, Mommy, can't we have a tree?" I remember asking my mother when I was little.

"Jews don't have trees," she'd say. Well, they did now.

As Donna and Elsa hoisted the tree inside, our house filled with the smell of pine.

"Take a deep breath," I said, filling my chest with rarefied air. Meredith and I roamed around the house just taking it all in. Then we all decorated the tree together, with lights and ornaments that Donna and Elsa had brought. When we were finished, my mother came down the stairs, took one look at our tree, and started to cry.

"How beautiful . . . how beautiful," she kept repeating, as she wept in Donna's and Elsa's arms. For some very lucky people, family is a fixed entity: one loving mother and one loving father supporting their healthy, happy children, and they all live to be 150. But for me, family was friends. It was growing and ever changing—it could always be bigger. Elsa and Donna bringing over the tree was an act of faith that I will never forget—it marked a renewal of my own faith. I ended up feeling very religious that Christmas. Family, in its ever changing shapes and sizes, was my religion of choice.

My friends had helped me to come of age in high school. My friends put Project A.L.S. on the map. As I navigated my third year of ALS on the bed, friends kept coming on board to make our mission a reality. It was my friends' belief that our growing family would wipe ALS from the face of the earth. The world's leading researchers, who worked intensely with Valerie, became our father figures. Corporate leaders—people like Stephanie George of *InStyle* magazine—became sisters and brothers to Meredith as she honed our business plan. I made a new friend in Senator Arlen Specter, United States Senator from Pennsylvania, who invited me on behalf of Project A.L.S. to come to Washington to testify before his and Senator Tom Harkin's Labor, Health and Human Services Subcommittee. Senators Specter and Harkin had coauthored a controversial bill proposing federal funding for stem cell research, and they wanted a panel of knowledgeable Americans to answer the subcommittee's questions and concerns on the matter.

Thanks to Project A.L.S. and others, scientific research had already provided intriguing evidence that stem cells might ultimately save ten million people dying with ALS, Alzheimer's, Parkinson's disease, and life-threatening disorders of the spine and brain like multiple sclerosis and spinal cord injury. We thought that the government should see about saving ten million Americans right away. Project A.L.S. was going to Capitol Hill.

The Amtrak trip to Washington was a blast. Reed flew in from Los Angeles just for the occasion. We reserved a whole train car for the Project A.L.S. entourage. There were Valerie and Meredith, board members, friends, Reed, my nurses, a lot of candy going around, the press, and me rehearsing my remarks. Later that morning, I had the honor of testifying alongside Christopher Reeve, my shining knight in the fight for increased and concerted government support for stem cell and scientific research. In my speech I talked about the American Dream that I had had as a girl growing up. I told the subcommittee that ALS was a national disaster that needed the government's attention immediately. I spoke of Project A.L.S.'s hard-earned laboratory results with stem cells. My goal was to inform the gentlemen and -women of the Senate. I think I succeeded. A few months later, Senator Specter invited me to testify again. This time I spoke with Chris, and more new friends, Mary Tyler

Moore and Michael J. Fox. We had all joined the fight. When it was my turn to speak, I reminded the subcommittee that people blindsided by life-threatening illnesses and injuries had the same American Dream as everyone else. I felt Chris, Mary, and Michael's support as I ended my remarks: *Each day I speak from inside my body, which has now become a prison. I am still here and dreaming of an America that will protect our rights to life, liberty, and the pursuit of happiness for all.* Applause followed. Afterward, Senator Specter thanked me for coming. I told him I hoped to see him again soon.

During the train ride home from my initial subcommittee appearance, as towns flew by, I thought about Project A.L.S. and the progress my friends and I were making. I thought about my friends, the incredible artists who had pledged their ongoing support for Project A.L.S.: Ben Stiller, Katie Couric, Melissa Etheridge, Julianna Margulies, Edie Falco, Caroline Rhea, Sheryl Crow, Rob Morrow, Marisa Tomei, Kristen Johnston, Camryn Manheim, Sarah Jessica Parker, Matthew Broderick, Gina Gershon, Billy Baldwin, Laura San Giacomo, Helen Hunt, and the list goes on and on. I thought about my friends, the thousands of Americans who were sending in generous donations and letters of encouragement. I thought about my friends Katie and Martha, who gave me hope for womankind. I thought about my friends the Wertliebs, the Abramsons, the McGraths, the Decters, and the Kaufmans, families from all over the country fighting with us to save their children from the devastation of ALS. I thought about my friend the courageous young Katherine Moore of Rocky Hill, Tennessee, whose father had died from ALS, and who had asked her friends to donate to Project A.L.S. instead of giving her presents for her tenth birthday. I looked forward to receiving Katherine's thoughtful cards. Maybe one would be waiting for me when I got home. The train kept going. I had a lot to look forward to—reaction to our first trip to the Senate, working on the next Project A.L.S. public service campaign, and my sleepover. Simon and I were supposed to have a sleepover that night back on the bed. Simon gave great dish.

I could feel us—my sisters, friends, and I were a bullet train speeding toward the answers to unanswerable questions. Scientists were unearthing stunning facts about stem cells, cells that were somehow attracted to areas of injury, migrated to those areas, and fixed what was broken there. What a miracle, the miracle of life. It occurred to me that the people I loved were like those cells. Me, too. We were attracted to areas of injury. We migrated to those areas. We did what we had to do for each other. Project A.L.S. was moving fast and efficiently. It was my dream company, a train that wouldn't be stopped. Could stem cells or any of the other potential therapies that Project

A.L.S. researchers were working on come in time for me?

Sometimes I would dream about getting better. There I'd be sitting around a huge family table with thousands of friends celebrating. We'd pass around roast turkey, mashed potatoes, and platters of perfect chocolate cake. We'd eat the meal that made America strong.

"Please pass the potatoes, Senator Specter," I'd say to the gentleman to my right.

"Passing you the potatoes would be my distinct pleasure, Miss Estess," Senator Specter would reply, as our dinner went on until dawn.

Once when I woke up from the dream, I noticed that my breathing had become even more labored. I was working too hard for each breath, straining my neck muscles to help me. My neurologist, Dr. Rowland, came for a house call. Sitting on the bed, he confirmed that my breathing had been affected—my diaphragm muscle and my chest muscles had grown weak. He prescribed a bi-pap, a truly unattractive ventilator that would force air into my lungs and suck it out through my nose, force it in and suck it out—in an unending cycle of assisted breathing. When the bi-pap was delivered to my door, Valerie, Meredith, and I cried.

Karen helped me put the mask on. The bi-pap mask was like a second, even bigger nose. It was a gawky plastic triangle that formed an airtight seal against my face. It wasn't a good look for me. A huge hose connected me and my mask to the breathing machine on my nightstand. Basically, I was now wearing a vacuum cleaner to stay alive. The bi-pap scared me. Even more than paralysis, the bi-pap represented a point of no return. Deep inside I knew that the medicine Project A.L.S. was fighting for probably wouldn't come in time for me, but that my friends and I had to keep working. We had children to fight for.

Valerie slept next to me my first night using the bi-pap. It took us a long, long time, but eventually Karen came in with blankets and we got some sleep. The sun, Valerie, and I rose the next morning after my first successful night of using a machine to breathe. The bi-pap was a setback, but not an insurmountable one, as the next day reminded me.

The day after my first night with a ventilator was a banner day for Project A.L.S. Valerie came in excited about a phone call that she had just received from Fred Gage, a researcher at the Salk Institute in La Jolla, California, who was working with Project A.L.S. on stem cells. Dr. Gage told Valerie about a new discovery in his lab. It wasn't stem cells, but a new *gene therapy* that he thought might be effective in ALS. Did Project A.L.S. want to fund a pilot experiment? As Valerie shared the good news with our research advisors, Meredith, Jules, and I locked in a $100,000 corporate sponsor for our next big event in Los Angeles. It was a great day, but Project A.L.S. needed to wrap up early, at about four o'clock. Lorna, Karen, and I needed to get me washed and dressed for Katie, who was coming to my bed that night with Warren Beatty. I fell in love with Warren Beatty when he fell in love with Natalie Wood in *Splendor in the Grass* on the Million-Dollar Movie. I wondered what Warren was going to say about my mask, or if he would acknowledge it at all. He would probably say something funny about it, and comforting and helpful. I was so nervous to meet him. But you had to have faith in the man. I looked forward to making a new friend.

Chapter Ten

I LOVED LORNA more than life. She was my arms and legs, but she was totally clueless when it came to my hair.

"Just do a comb-over," I said, sitting and waiting on my bed as Lorna attempted a last-minute blow-dry.

"I *am* doing it," she said. But she wasn't, folks, not even close. My dryer came with attachments, which should have made her job easier, but Lorna struggled. She cast the blow-dryer in the general direction of my skull and missed—again. She might as well have been fishing for sea bass. I couldn't move at all to help Lorna help me. It was just plain crazy. This game had been going on for an hour. I was already late for my plane.

My plane and I were taking off for a luxurious six-day vacation at the Dorado Hotel in San Juan, Puerto Rico. Meredith and Peter were coming, too. Oh, and so was Reed. I'd invited him and he'd said yes. We hadn't seen each other in a year. I heard Reed drop his bags in the living room while Lorna and I focused on getting ready. I was extremely nervous to see Reed and for him to see me with the mask. Thankfully, my breathing was decent enough so that I didn't have to wear it for most of the day. I looked forward to some real face time with Reed on the beach.

It took a village just to get me out the door. While Lorna worked the hair, Karen's perfect bun spun out like a pinwheel. She was rushing around, packing a hundred suitcases filled with the bi-pap and its back-up, my volume ventilator (which gave me little puffs of forced air when I didn't quite need the sustained support of the bi-pap), fifty feet of plastic tubing, extra wheelchair parts, a dozen bean-filled pillows, and my vacation wardrobe. Nothing was harder than packing clothes for Puerto Rico. My fashion choices had become limited to what I call pull-ups—basically, pants without form, zippers, or buttons. Pull-ups were modified sweatpants and, although I was never a sweatpants kind of girl, I'd set out to find the chicest pull-ups out there. Karen stacked them and packed them. I'd also bought a couple of pastel cotton tops to match, just in case a certain someone in San Juan wanted to go under my shirt for any reason.

As the precious moments to takeoff ticked away, I barked orders from the bed. I was the Scarlett O'Hara of ALS. I liked things just so. "Don't forget the ambu-bag," I reminded Karen. The ambu-bag was what Julianna Margulies had in mind when she ran down the hall shouting "Bag her!" on *ER*. It was a collapsible plastic bottle that people could use to force air into my lungs in case of an emergency—an electrical outage, for example. I had two ambu-bags, one pink and one purple.

"Ambu-bags, packed and ready—*yesterday,*" said Karen, glaring at me. She was so prideful.

"Extra mask for the bi-pap?" I asked, ticking off must-haves.

"Extra mask, check-*m,*" said Karen.

"I think you forgot the Annick Goutal," I said. I wanted to bring along my favorite moisturizer, Annick Goutal. I loved the way it smelled. I thought that Reed might like it, too.

"Annick Goutal packed *yesterday,*" said Karen. "Correction—*last week-m.*"

"Maybe *you* want to dry my hair then?" I asked Karen. I was intrigued by the lilt in Karen's speech. Being from Trinidad and Tobago she added sweet little *m* garnishes to words sometimes. Late at night, as Karen and I talked about life, death-*m,* and my chances of marrying Jon Stewart, I found her lilt comforting, like a song. At moments like these, with my plane revving up for my first vacation in six years, I found the lilt completely irritating.

"If the lady thinks her hair is important above all else-*m,* I shall drop what I'm doing and fix the lady's hair," said Karen. When it came to witty banter, the Algonquin Round Table had nothing on Karen and me. We tossed it around the infield pretty good. But repartee was a luxury that neither of us could afford at the moment. I had to get to Teterboro Airport in New Jersey or miss my flight to Puerto Rico. Meredith and Peter called. They'd been waiting for us at the airport since breakfast.

"I don't know what you're worried about," said Valerie, who had stopped by my bed with coffee and a blueberry muffin to say bon voyage. Valerie had built great momentum with our team of scientists pursuing gene therapy. An announcement was due any day. To Valerie, a vacation at the beach meant nothing compared to the possibility she'd receive news of further progress in the lab.

"It's a private plane," Valerie reminded me, giving me sips of hot coffee from Jessie's, my new favorite deli. "*They* wait for *you.*" Silly me, forgetting. That plane wasn't leaving without me. It wasn't *moving* until I dried my hair. That plane was *my* plane, a shiny Gulfstream IV, the ultimate in luxury.

My existence had become a surreal mix of loss, pain, accomplishment, and, now, ultimate luxury. As Project A.L.S. caught on as a movement, generous people came out of the woodwork to give my sisters and me support and advice, and to pave my working days with comfort. Thanks to Katie Couric, and to pieces in *The New York Times, People, Science, The New York Observer, Nature, InStyle, Forbes,* and *The Wall Street Journal* that chronicled the strides we were making in research and in fund-raising, Project A.L.S. was receiving national attention. As a result, scientists and philanthropists approached us with ideas. My sisters and I were busier than we had ever been in our lives. And, frankly, I became a bit of a celebrity. My hard work was paying off. I was living the life that I dreamed of as a girl: other people packing my bags, a handsome man waiting for me in the living room, private planes and limousines. No autographs, please.

Believe me, I was perfectly happy traveling commercial, that is, until about a year and a half into ALS, when Simon and I took a horrifying Continental Airlines flight from New York to Los Angeles for a Project A.L.S. fund-raiser. We had the worst time. It was devastating, really, seeing service-oriented professionals treat people in wheelchairs like animals. The flight crew told Simon and me that the FAA didn't allow standard wheelchairs on airplanes. Fair enough, but in order to board, they said, Simon had to transfer me to a standard issue . . . it wasn't a chair, really, but a rickety toy wagon. It was fine for a doll. Simon and I had a feeling it would break any second. As soon as we loaded in, he was hauling me down the aisle like a crazed shopper. I felt like the groceries. When the FAA banned standard wheelchairs from commercial flights, you'd think that maybe it would have created a comfortable, humane alternative. The flight staff was rude to Simon and me for the entire flight. These people seemed so miserable in their jobs. We got a lot of those annoyed "special needs" glares from flight attendants whispering in the galley. After we landed, the pilot tried to squeeze by me in the aisle. But Simon and I were having trouble getting me back on the toy wagon.

"What's the holdup here?" the pilot demanded of a flight attendant. He didn't even have the courtesy to address me directly. The flight attendant rolled her eyes, while Simon tried desperately to balance me.

"I can't wait for *this*," the pilot said, meaning me. Maybe he was late for a meeting with the FAA. Finally, he kicked my wagon and stepped right over me. Simon and I were shaken to our core by the experience. When Meredith and Valerie saw our faces after landing at LAX, they thought that something terrible had happened. It took me a few hours to stop shaking. Simon and I needed a vacation just from the flight.

The next time I had to be in Los Angeles for work, I decided to phone in from my bed. The prospect of flying again was too humiliating. Then Chris and Dana Reeve offered me a ride to Los Angeles in a private plane. Chris flew all the time for work. When

Dana called to offer me a lift, I started to cry. Their gesture was so incredibly generous. If not for the Reeves, I would never have seen L.A. again. Through Chris and Dana, I met my future travel mates, Bobby, Robert, Andreas, and Cynthia, three strong, handsome firefighters and an excellent nurse, who specialized in helping Chris travel the world. Thanks to the Reeves, I built my very own entourage.

I never flew commercial again. Project A.L.S. board member Brad Grey, who had lost his grandfather and mentor Sam Levin to ALS, made sure I flew safely from then on. Brad and Richard Santulli, the charitable chairman of NetJets, purveyor of the finest private aircraft in the world, donated Gulfstream jets to Project A.L.S. when I needed to go somewhere. Mr. Santulli, a man I'd never met, an angel, gave me my wings. From then on, I flew high and proud and safely.

Private airplanes were only part of my fun. There were diamonds, huge rocks that the jeweler Harry Winston gave me on loan to wear to Project A.L.S. benefits. The earrings came with their own armed guard. I did the red carpet in my Harry Winstons. Simon pushed me alongside my better-known friends Ben Stiller, Brooke Shields, Helen Hunt, Scott Wolf, and Richard Kind. We made our way down red carpets together to speak with journalists wanting to know more about Project A.L.S.

Once our whirlwind tour started, it didn't end. Project A.L.S. was named *Vanity Fair* magazine's "it" charity. I sat for a photo session with the renowned photographer Brigitte Lacombe. Charlie Rose interviewed two of our scientists, Valerie, and me on his TV show. I chatted with George Clooney and Sheryl Crow in green rooms. *Glamour* magazine awarded me Woman of the Year. Restaurateur and chef Bobby Flay came by to cook dinner for me and twelve of my best friends. When Lorna wasn't available, the John Barrett Salon of Bergdorf Goodman provided me with the full range of complimentary beauty services bedside: Nicole cut and blow-dried my hair. Rosa gave me manicures. Mercedes did eyebrows and makeup. Thomas did my color, navigating obstacles posed by the bulky bi-pap and the fact that my neck was so weak it couldn't support my head. Thomas was a magician, gentle, sweet, and talented. The John Barrett team made sure that my hair remained my best asset and that I always looked my best. My bed became a celebrity landmark. Tired and weary from pacing the Hollywood Walk of Fame, celebrities came to my bed just to say hello.

My sisters were hot tamales, as well. Valerie and Meredith appeared in public and on TV. Clothing designers offered to dress them. My sisters and I appeared on *Entertainment Tonight* and *Access Hollywood* in Calvin Klein and Salvatore Ferragamo.

When in L.A., Ricky Benjamin, driver to the stars and the owner of a sleek, wheelchair-friendly van, took me and mine wherever we wanted to go—into the Hollywood Hills, out to a beachside restaurant in Santa Monica, the Bel-Air Hotel, please. It was dizzying. The champagne wishes and caviar dreams that I had always had for my sisters and me were finally coming true. And I was dying.

If you want a job done right, call a firefighter. Bobby and Robert carried me onto the plane at Teterboro as if it were nothing. Reed put me on his lap. I asked him to help me on with my new Chanel sunglasses, a present from Meredith for the trip. Then he held me tight as we sank down into our plush leather bucket seat for takeoff. Reed's arms around me, his legs wrapped around mine steadying me for flight—well, it definitely beat a seat belt. We fit together so well. Taxiing down the runway I thought, *How can this guy not be in love with me?* I looked at Meredith and Peter. They were so great-looking, so at home on the Gulfstream IV, and so in love with each other. The Hulberts always appeared windswept—like they were coming *back* from a vacation. I felt grateful that my sisters and I were tasting luxury, maybe not under optimal circumstances, but together in our lifetimes. I smiled at Meredith. She smiled at me. After the pilot and flight attendant wished us a good flight, we cued up Frank Sinatra on the CD player. The Gulfstream engine roared like a jungle cat, and we were number one for takeoff. As Frankie sang us up, up, up into the bluest sky, I thought that it all happens so fast, ultimately. The day starts and you can't imagine how you'll get through it—then you're through it.

Red rose petals were there at my feet when we landed. My mother's friend Linda Singer, a travel agent, made sure that my room at the Dorado was appointed with fragrant red petals, bottles of wine, and a view of the water. As the first order of business, everyone—Reed, Peter, Meredith, Lorna, Cynthia, Robert, and Bobby—carried me on a lounge chair, just like Cleopatra, down to the water. On our way to the water we said hi to the hotel staff, who were already setting up for our private beach barbecue that night. They told us to expect a singular evening, a mariachi band at sunset and plenty of horses, my favorite creatures. Everyone set me down at the edge of the sand. Then Reed transferred me into the water. He carried me out until the water was up to our shoulders. Warm waves broke around us. Reed held me deep in the ocean all afternoon. It was the most romantic moment of my life.

In the water with Reed I could move again. There wasn't gravity where we were. I was free. I looked toward the shore. My entourage stood watching us.

Reed swung me around. I looked out at the ocean. It was endless. My life stretched both ways, I realized, to the shore, where I was going to have a barbecue, and toward the other end of the ocean, where my future was. Reed and I held each other in the water between the shore and infinity. There wasn't much for us to say. We just looked at each other. Then it was time to move on.

Later, before dinner, Reed tried to get the two of us into a hammock. That wasn't happening. As he lowered us down, we flipped over and I hit the deck. I felt totally humiliated. I mean, I was a grown woman lying there, unable to move at all. It was very Humpty Dumpty. My ALS had progressed to the point where even Reed didn't know if he could get me up from the ground. He shouted for Lorna. Then he stepped back to assess the situation.

"Jen," he asked, "is there anything you can do about the diet?"

"Reed," I said, "you have just crossed a line that I don't think you'll come back from."

Just then we caught sight of Lorna strolling over with the ambu-bag. She sure was taking her sweet time. I don't know what had gotten into Lorna, the sea air, sheer exhaustion from a morning of blow-drying, maybe, but there she was with the ambu-bag tucked into her arm like a purse, soaking up the sights, conversing with the birds. When Reed and I saw Lorna coming down the lane, we looked at each other and we started to laugh, tears mixed with sweat. Then we were hysterical, laughing and inconsolable. Lorna walked along just smelling the flowers while Reed and I laughed all night.

Most people get skeleton-thin from ALS. Naturally, I was the first person in the two-hundred-year history of the disease to gain weight. My neurologist, Dr. Rowland, who had seen more cases of ALS than any living person, claimed he'd never witnessed anything like it.

"Can you go on a diet?" Dr. Rowland asked as he sat on my bed during a house call.

"You want me to go on a diet?" The indignities, the mortification, the humiliation never stopped. "I have a better idea, Bud. Why don't you give me some medicine to help me breathe?"

"Let's see what you and your sisters come up with," he said. "I have my fingers crossed." Dr. Rowland—my own doctor—was relying on Project A.L.S. to come up with medicine for ALS. How crazy was that? I have to admit, it was gratifying as well. Bud Rowland was truly impressed with the research progress that Project A.L.S. was making. As for the weight gain, the truth is, I wasn't eating that much.

"Are you sure, Jenifer?" asked Meredith, who understood my tendency to pack it away in private.

"I swear," I swore. It's not like I could just roll into the kitchen and grab a box of cookies. If anything, ALS brought my stormy love affair with food to an end. Food and I fell in love when I was a baby girl. Our house could have been burning down. Give me a Twinkie, I was happy. I wasn't inhibited around food. If I wanted something, I ate it. I was free. When Kaka came to New York for the first time to visit us as grown-up girls, I prepared her a surprise platter of cut-up Twinkies and attractive wedges of Hostess Cupcakes. I couldn't think of a better way to welcome my babysitter from Rock Island. Food warmed and comforted me. It smelled good, looked good; it satisfied every time.

Then when I hit thirteen, my relationship with food turned illicit. It became my secret lover. I snuck it. I felt embarrassed for wanting it. As I grew, so to speak, I felt further and further from my body ideal, also known as the Harrison High School cheerleaders. Realistically, I probably had ten or fifteen pounds to lose, but the girl I saw in the mirror was way bigger. I dieted and dieted. I failed and failed. I wasn't alone. Every girl I knew wanted to change her shape, even the Harrison High School cheerleaders. Every girl dieted. Every girl failed.

We girls couldn't win for losing. Dieting seemed rigged to me, like pro wrestling. Still, I couldn't take myself out of the game. As a single healthy woman in New York, I spent many nights at home alone feeling "not quite right" when I could have been out there. I tried taking Valerie's advice and accepting my body for what it was. But sustained self-criticism, which girls seem to learn as willingly as boys learn the fundamentals of baseball, came more naturally.

Several years into ALS, I wasn't even eating real meals anymore. The truth is, I could barely swallow. When ALS told my muscles to let go, they did as they were told, systematically, every last one of them, including those I used to chew and swallow food. My favorite things to eat—turkey on a roll, roasted chicken, Caesar salad—were too dangerous for me to try, so I said good-bye to them. For the first time in my life I didn't look forward to eating—I feared it. I was afraid of choking. Lorna, Karen, and Juliet cut up my food and fed me like a baby. Eventually they ran everything through a blender three times. Meredith and Valerie brought over their own liquid creations for me to try—cream of cream of cream of broccoli soup, gravy with a dollop of mashed potatoes. Nothing went down easy. My days of taking food by mouth were numbered. Yet, incredibly, I gained weight.

I called myself Puff Jenny—P. Jiddy to the inner

circle. As I lost muscles, I lost muscle tone. As I lost muscle tone, I began to look like another person. Unfortunately, that person wasn't especially slender. She was puffy, really puffy. I was never a small girl, but ALS cut me down and blew up my ass. It was a shame. I'd peaked physically before I got sick. I was thirty-five at the time, a little late in the game maybe, but I was coming to a new understanding of my body. Thanks to working out and eating right, I'd never felt more beautiful. ALS was my tough luck: I wasn't eating and I gained weight ... I was wearing the Queen's diamonds on my ears, but I could hardly hold my head up to support them ... I was running a multimillion-dollar company devoted to wiping out a disease that had already destroyed my body, piece by piece. My plate was full and I couldn't eat.

Puerto Rico proved that although I wasn't at my best physically, I could still feel beautiful. Reed had something to do with that, I think. But beauty, as in looking my best, had always been of the utmost importance. Best foot forward—best smile, best hair, and best face, no matter what. I worked to present my best self to the world, always with a little lipstick. I discovered my own look and went full tilt in that direction. As a girl, I accepted that there were movie stars whom I didn't and could never look like. There were certain women, however—Cher, Barbra Streisand—whose looks seemed totally achievable. I liked Cher because I looked like her. I really loved Barbra Streisand. In every photo, film, or song, she seemed to be saying: *Just because I have a big nose, don't tell me I can't have everything I want.* I liked her subtext. Just because I wasn't Lana Turner didn't mean I should jump off a cliff. So I worked it. I started by copying Cher, and I kind of jumped off from there. I grew up knowing that *my style* was terrific and beautiful and the only one that counted. I knew it on an intellectual level, anyway. In reality, doing the day was incredibly challenging, no matter what I wore. Doing the day was my life's work. It was hard work.

When I got ALS, I craved beauty. I filled up my senses with it. More things were beautiful to me. My palette expanded—along with my figure—when I got sick. To me, the sight of working legs was beautiful. A cheeseburger deluxe was beautiful. Meredith brushing Jane's hair into a ponytail was beautiful. I still admired the undeniable beauty of, say, a Michelle Pfeiffer. It's just that my scope was so much bigger now. My capacity to take it all in—Martha's eyes, Willis's hands, Valerie's face when she promised that everything was going to be okay—was limitless. Was I *beautiful* rolling down the red carpet in a wheelchair all puffy with no husband or children, and no foreseeable future? I guess so. I guess I was beautiful, in a way. I had learned to take it all in. That's not to say I'd ruled out plastic surgery. As God is my witness, I vowed that if I ever got better I'd haul it in for a total body lift. Just pull the whole thing up and over and get out the scissors. Until then and after that I would cherish every beautiful moment: *Just because I have a big nose and a World War II mask in this wheelchair, don't tell me I can't have everything I want.*

Did Reed dig my look in Puerto Rico? Was he attracted to me for ten seconds? I'm gonna go out on a limb and say yes, but I'll never know for sure. Nothing happened between us at the beach in San Juan, except for everything. We didn't sleep. We talked all day and night for six days. Reed rubbed my shoulders. He lay down next to me on the bed. He put his forehead against mine and we laughed. The sound of the checkout notice sliding under the door of my hotel room at four in the morning signaled the end.

The moment my Gulfstream IV hit the New Jersey runway, Reed bolted for L.A. It was like the worst part of *Cinderella*. We hit the ground and my private plane turned into a filthy wheelchair van . . . my entourage turned into nurses and firefighters who had to get home to their own families . . . Meredith and Peter turned into parents talking reassuringly into their cell phones to their kids, who'd missed them terribly . . . and Reed, my prince, turned into a guy who couldn't wait to get home to walk his dog. I guess that made me Cinderella, wheelchair strapped in, trying to keep her balance during a bumpy van ride home to Manhattan.

We'd all had a beautiful time in Puerto Rico, a great vacation. As I was loaded out of the van and onto my bed on Twelfth Street, I was filled with sensations of Puerto Rico: Reed and me in the hammock; him helping me touch a white horse that walked up to us on the beach; Lorna strolling along with the ambubag; being in the water with Reed, Meredith and Peter watching us from the shore. Then the sensations went away. By the time Karen and I settled in for my welcome-home foot massage, I couldn't feel Puerto Rico anymore. It was weird how fast moments turned into memories.

No life of beauty and glamour is complete without a movie being made about it. After we returned from Puerto Rico, I heard that the documentary filmmaker and HBO honcho Sheila Nevins was interested in coming to the bed. I knew Sheila to be a big deal. She had a trunkful of Academy Awards. She was one of the first women to make it big as an entertainment executive. Sheila Nevins was known for speaking her mind.

Sheila came to my bed with Sara Bernstein, her colleague at HBO. She told Valerie, Meredith, and me that she'd heard a lot about Project A.L.S. *She's me,* I thought as Sheila walked to the bed, this woman who was living the life I wanted. She was a great business-woman, funny, self-deprecating, creative, so powerful. We sat with Sheila and Sara for a while, not really knowing why they'd come. After spending an hour together, Sheila said she wanted to do a movie about us, a documentary for HBO. She asked if she and her crew could come to my apartment in two weeks and film my sisters and me right on the bed. In three months, Sheila and HBO put the finishing touches on *Three Sisters: Searching for a Cure,* a forty-minute film that captured the essence of Project A.L.S. Brad Grey had just formed Plan B Films, which produced *Three Sisters.*

At last, my big-screen debut. It wasn't glamorous. There I am in the movie with my bi-pap cranking and my Hannibal Lecter mask. I look pretty ravaged up there. "Oh, well," I said to Willis, as we watched a rough, rough cut.

"You're the prettiest woman on earth, Jen," he said.

My movie debut felt like my swan song. Late at night, when my sisters went home, I began feeling a restlessness that was hard to describe. For six years of ALS, I could always lean on whatever function I had left. When my legs became paralyzed, I leaned on my arms. When my neck was paralyzed, I leaned on my trunk. I loved my lips and mouth. Now they were going. I was having trouble forming words. Now I had nothing left to lean on, except for Valerie and Meredith, the loves of my life.

Valerie reported to me deep into the night by e-mail about gene therapy, her work with scientists and the NIH and the FDA, and now our first move to human trial. We were getting closer to a shot for me, she promised. She urged me to hang in there. All I could think was that the upper right side of my lip was going.

Meredith called me one morning after taking the kids to school.

"No one understands what I'm saying anymore," I told her.

"You sound clear as a bell to me," she said.

"Katie, Martha, Caroline—I say something and everyone says *What? What did you say?*" I said.

"Wait a second. I think I just heard the doorbell," said Meredith. I knew there was no doorbell ringing.

"You don't understand what I'm saying, do you, Merry?" I said. More and more, when we spoke on the phone, Valerie and Meredith suddenly had to get doorbells ringing or pots burning on the stove or save children from falling on knives. My sisters created these smoke screens because they couldn't quite bring themselves to tell me the truth—that more and more they didn't understand what I was saying. My lips and mouth were getting weaker. I couldn't wrap them around my words. Not being able to sit on the bed talking with Valerie and Meredith—that was my life. It had always been my life. ALS was taking my speech, my last remaining treasure. ALS had shaken me down to my last penny. I tried to be strong.

Why me? You've asked that question, I'm sure. I have. My sisters have. Why us? Why did a fatal disease with no medicine break up our miraculous love and cut it short? I don't know. All I know is that everyone has a *why me.* Look at Christie Brinkley. You wouldn't think she has a *why me,* but I bet she does. Look at your parents and friends. Look at your children. Look in the mirror. Everyone faces a challenge—or not, as they so choose. Everyone has a *why me.* I got a pretty bad one. But the key for me and my sisters had always been looking at our *why me* straight on and getting to work, getting to love, in the time we had left.

"I still think we're gonna get out of this," said Meredith, as we sat on the bed, the bi-pap cycling air in and out, sounding like waves in a mechanical ocean. This was our millionth "I still think we're gonna get out of this" pep talk. Meredith always kicked it off, followed by Valerie's saying yes, we'd definitely get out of it, followed by my saying I hoped we'd get out of it. That was the script, but this millionth time, everyone forgot their lines.

"I do," said Meredith. "I think we'll get out of it, but we really have to move it along."

193

"Hmmm," I said.

"We've gotta get out of this," said Valerie.

"I think there's still a chance," said Meredith.

"You know," I said, "even if we don't get out of this, we're still getting out of it." I knew I was right. My sisters knew I was right. Maybe science wasn't going to catch up with me. Maybe it was, but it probably wasn't. All I knew was that Project A.L.S. was going to fight and push and work and love until ALS was gone. This disease was going down.

"Bring it on," I said, as Lorna brought me my last cup of coffee on earth on the bed. A few months after I got back from Puerto Rico, I officially declared my swallowing shot. Lorna tipped the cup to my mouth, and the coffee from Jessie's Deli went down. The hot coffee warmed me inside out. Life was just so beautiful.

Chapter Eleven

WHEN I WAS in high school, August was about inhaling, going to the beach with Meredith, and exhaling. That was the rhythm of our days. Every day in August, Meredith and I drove to Sherwood Island in Connecticut to work on our tans between the peak hours of noon and two. Windows down, our hair blew wild. I remember the sun on my face. I remember the sun on Meredith's face as she drove. Meredith always drove. She said I was a horrible driver. Fine with me—I wanted my own chauffeur someday anyway; so did she, for that matter. There was no doubt about it. One day we were going to live in huge houses side by side with our own chauffeurs. Driving with Meredith, deep breaths, the reassurance of the Connecticut tides—it was all very August.

Then August changed. After six and a half years of being sick, I watched the summer grow dark from my window. August became the dark, stormy heath of reckoning where Shakespeare's characters ranted and raved about betrayal and lost children. At first the heath was pretty quiet, as in "all's quiet on the western heath." Then the wind kicked up. From my bed I watched the summer wind blow with a vengeance. Was I the only one to notice? The wind had a personality all of a sudden. It wanted me dead.

Then King Lear, make that Valerie, marched in.

"I wanna kill someone. I just wanna wipe the idiotic looks off people's faces." Spoken like the director of scientific research for Project A.L.S. Valerie paced back and forth in front of the bed.

"Lorna," I said.

"Coming," said Lorna, who came quicker from the living room these days. Lorna was on high alert in August.

"We need to go out and down with the mask," I said. Lorna pulled the mask away from my face and shifted it downward. Still not right.

"Out and down, Lorna," I repeated. Lorna, a home health aide who had become the most skilled ALS caregiver on the face of the planet, tried and failed again to reposition the mask on my face. I couldn't get a decent breath in August. Lorna and I spent hours at a time just trying to get the mask to sit properly. Valerie paced, fuming at the world, Lorna, and me.

"I'm the one you want to kill," I said to Valerie as

Lorna tightened the Velcro straps that held the mask in place. "I'm the one who ruined your life."

"Why do you have to be so selfish?" Valerie said. "Why does everything have to revolve around you? I have my own life, Jenifer. I have my own problems that have nothing whatsoever to do with you."

"That's why I think you should go home and be with your children," I said. The sicker I got, the harder Valerie and Meredith worked. They worked in the living room, on the bed. They never went home.

"We're this close to medicine and you want me to go home?" she said. Valerie raged in August. It was too bad. Things couldn't have been more promising from the research side. For one thing, it was official: Dr. Gage's gene therapy helped ALS mice to live over one-third longer than untreated ALS mice. These stunning findings were about to be published in the prestigious journal *Science* and announced all over the news. It was the best therapeutic result seen in the history of the disease. According to Valerie's calculations, the gene therapy human trial would begin in a little over a year. She demonstrated where I'd be getting my shots. They were going to inject my neck and my legs and my arms and my chest.

"They better hurry up," I said.

"Just don't you worry," said Valerie, as if she knew something I didn't. I was so proud of her. Valerie had put the scientists together. She had mothered them, exacting best efforts from them. Gene therapy was only the beginning. Stem cells continued to show great therapeutic promise. Project A.L.S. researchers were also zeroing in on "disease pathways," or why ALS occurred in the first place. On account of Project A.L.S., the research community was working together as a family—as the family that would beat ALS. If August was dark and disturbing from my window, the landscape of ALS had never appeared sunnier.

Valerie fell at my feet and cried. She said she'd been doing a lot of that lately, feeling angry, then sad. She raged, then mourned, and she didn't know why. I knew why.

Meredith came in. Let's call her Viola, Lady Macbeth, and Juliet—all of the women of Shakespeare plus the sonnets—wrapped up into one majestic twenty-first-century mama. For six years, Meredith had searched the world for meaning and money for research. She built Project A.L.S. from "an Ikea desk and two milk crates"—as the actor Richard Kind had once said about us—into a $20 million company. She had drafted thousands of Americans into the unpopular war against brain disease. I was so proud of her. Meredith, too, was in a foul mood.

"Is this *it* for you and work?" she asked me, glaring. "Just tell me because I need to know. We have three events coming up. If I *can't* count on you I need to know *now*."

"Suction, Lorna," I said. In August, Lorna stood by my bed like a soldier. My swallowing muscles had grown dangerously weak. We used a machine to suction my so-called secretions, or saliva, because swallowing—just regular everyday swallowing—made me choke. Lorna inserted the plastic suction tube into my mouth.

"Just tell me who to call, Merry," I said over the whirring of the machine, "and I'll call."

"That's what you said last week," said Meredith. I wanted to keep working from the bed but, truth be told, I usually didn't have the energy. In all my forty years, I'd never let anyone down on the job, but here we were. Who knew that an honest day's work was one of life's great luxuries? Meredith was fit to be tied in August. She wasn't sleeping and she didn't know why. I knew why.

I got pneumonia. Pneumonia is to ALS what fire is to the Scarecrow. It came on in an instant, and because I couldn't move, breathe, cough, or clear my throat or lungs, the infection settled in my lungs and spread fast. My lungs filled with fluid. It's funny saying this, but besides the ALS I was actually a pretty healthy person. I couldn't remember the last time I had had a fever. But I was burning hot. Nadine, an excellent registered nurse, or RN, was on duty that day. I couldn't afford to be without an RN anymore. My situation called for the heavy artillery, major RNs like Juliet Hercules, Nadine Donohue, Maureen Carlo, veterans of the wars. These chicks didn't mess around. Along with Karen and Lorna, they threw me onto my side, sat me up, pounded my chest and back, gave me Heimlich maneuvers. They dripped sweat daily to keep my systems cleared. They knew my body better than a husband. In rare moments of respite they heard my confessions. I told them how I feared for Valerie's and Meredith's future and for the future of their children, my children, without me. I confided my deepest emotions to these women I barely knew. I obsessed with thoughts of Valerie and Meredith in a world without me. *Will they be okay without me? Will they be okay?* My nurses listened. They told me I wasn't going anywhere and that I didn't have to worry about such things. In wartime my nurses and I spent each second fighting together for the next.

When my temperature hit 102 degrees, Nadine called 911. St. Vincent's Hospital was located conveniently right across the street. Nadine, Valerie, and the paramedics put me on a stretcher and ran me and my bi-pap right over to the St. Vincent's emergency room, where an X-ray of my chest revealed a left lung black with fluid. I choked and burned with fever. Dale Ryan, a nurse in the ER, made it right. Dale set me up.

She got an IV line in me—no small task, because I had extremely hard-to-find veins—and kept me hydrated and nourished. Nurse Ryan had pounded a few chests in her time. She talked to me in a kind voice and stroked my hair. Dr. Linda Kirshenbaum—or Dr. K., as my sisters and I called her—an expert in emergency medicine, took me up to the critical care unit. Dale and Dr. K. became instant family. I stayed in the CCU at St. Vincent's for almost a week until I responded to antibiotics and stabilized. I was the youngest person there. Valerie and Meredith lived in the waiting area of the CCU for that week. They didn't leave my side.

Cameras were rolling in earnest on the latest movie in my head, *The Beds of August,* a new comedy-drama about a woman so sick she goes from bed to bed to bed, all over the city. That very night, only a few hours home from the hospital, I "threw a plug," a Shakespearean term that my nurse Maureen used to describe the sudden inability to clear mucus. Mucus obstructed my airway while I was watching TV, and I lost consciousness immediately. Karen called 911.

This time I was totally out of it. The paramedics couldn't find a pulse on me. They put me on the floor and worked to bring me back. I don't remember much—the sense of gentle men's voices and Karen calling Valerie on my phone, telling her to hurry over. Later, Valerie told me it had looked like a nativity scene when she got there. It was four in the morning.

My room was lit by a lamp, she said. Paramedics worked around me on the floor quietly, lovingly, expertly. Karen stood over them with her hands clasped. Valerie knelt at my feet.

"Got a pulse," said one of the paramedics after a while.

"I love you, Jenifer," said Valerie. "I love you." I loved her so much. I heard Valerie, but I couldn't reach her. I didn't see a white light or a tunnel. All I felt was a wanting to get back to my sister, a reaching, the same reaching I'd always felt when I was near her and Meredith. I reached as I always had—to get back, start over, do better.

"You can't leave anyway," Valerie said. "Do you hear me? You're gonna be on Katie in an hour." At Valerie's mention of the *Today* show, on which the results of our gene therapy work were to be announced that very morning, I opened one eye. I was back. In the end death was no match for my chance to appear on national television.

"Jenifer," Valerie said, holding me.

"I'm here," I said, opening my eyes. And back we went to the ER at St. Vincent's. My bed there was still warm. Dr. K. was none too pleased to see me again. She felt that at this rate I was asking for big trouble. She wanted to perform a tracheotomy, immediately. She wanted one of her colleagues to cut a hole in my neck and attach a ventilator to the hole. Arguably, having "the trach," as they call it in ALS circles, would make my breathing and the act of suctioning a little easier. But after having given the matter much thought over the years, I had already decided against the trach. As it was, I had adapted so much in so many ways to being sick. Living with a trach and all that that meant—the constant need for suction, a nurse by my side every second of every day, probable loss of my already waning ability to speak and eat—wasn't for me. Dr. K. felt we needed to move on it right away.

Valerie called her team at Johns Hopkins. The Hopkins doctors, led by Dr. Jeff Rothstein, had evolved into the leading clinical team in the country. They were amazing that day. Dr. Charlie Weiner, associate director of medicine at Hopkins, who had had extensive experience helping ALS patients to breathe, took the next Amtrak north to New York to assess me. I had never even met Charlie, and there he was by my side. Charlie told Dr. K. he thought that I could go for years more on the bi-pap. In fact, he said, he'd never seen a patient use a bi-pap for so long and look so good.

I was feeling cocky. I had narrowly escaped the trach. Still, because I had aspirated or choked the night before, Charlie and Dr. K. agreed that I needed to have a feeding tube surgically inserted into my stomach as soon as possible. At this point, food going down the wrong way would mean instant death. They shipped me uptown to Columbia Presbyterian for the procedure.

The most uncomfortable bed of August was the one at Columbia Presbyterian, where I had my feeding tube inserted. The staff was slightly off during my stay—a lot of people entering without knocking.

"You know ALS doesn't affect the hearing," I said to one resident who recited my vital signs to me very s-l-o-w-l-y and very LOUDLY. "I understand what you're saying," I reiterated. I wanted him to know that ALS didn't affect my cognition, either. I also wanted to give Columbia the benefit of the doubt. I loved Columbia. Project A.L.S. had directed some nice cash to research at the university; my neurologist, Dr. Rowland, was a Columbia man; three of the five treasured research advisors to Project A.L.S. resided at Columbia, including Gerry Fischbach, an elegant researcher, advocate, and now dean of the Columbia Medical School. It was August, after all—maybe the neurology unit's A Team was on vacation.

One young neurologist said he needed to take a blood gas—a painful blood test that measures the level of oxygen in the blood—right away. Earlier that afternoon I had asked his supervisor if instead of the blood gas I might get a good night's rest. The supervisor thought that rest was a great idea and that I could just as well have my blood drawn the next day. Late that night the young neurologist snuck into my room, as determined to take my blood as I was powerless to move. He stuck my wrist over and over. He couldn't find my artery. My wrist was bloody and bruised the next morning.

No matter how hard you fight to maintain your dignity in the foxhole, you can expect moments of humiliation and disappointment. There's no avoiding them. These moments are built in to the life-and-death experience. I didn't know if that young neurologist meant to one-up me or his boss—and I didn't care. I was sure that the millions of people sick and dying from untreatable brain diseases in fine hospitals all over the country didn't care, either. Putting up with the humiliations, these unfortunate moments made of man's inhumanity to man, would be so much easier for us to bear—if we just had some medicine.

When you're in the foxhole you have to thank the stars for people like Daniel Brodie, a young doctor who I believe represents the future of medicine. Dr. Brodie, a pulmonology fellow, came to my bed at Columbia not knowing me but curious to meet me. Daniel was so kind. We talked for hours about breathing and my chances for survival. Amazingly, I still had the strength to appreciate a good-looking doctor. Life without romance isn't worth pursuing. I looked at Daniel Brodie knowing that his life would be richly romantic, as mine had been. He had a light in his eyes. He had a passion for work that I recognized. My romantic imagination was still a comfort to me, even that August in the foxhole. I had always worked to keep romance alive in some form. When I didn't have true love in my life, I got by with fantasies, memories, and crushes. They were all part of my workout until the real thing came along. Visits from Daniel Brodie kept me sharp in August. He entered my romantic imagination and, as a result, I felt prepared. I was ready for anything.

My bed had served as a temple, a stage, a place where I learned to see the world. The Beds of August—whether in the ER at St. Vincent's, in the CCU, on the neurology floor at Columbia Presbyterian, in ambulances, or at home—were foxholes. In August I hunkered down in my bed and held on as the bombs flew above me. There was no margin of error in the foxhole—one wrong move and I was a goner. Luckily, the wisdom of the foxhole, my most basic survival instincts, kicked in. They had always been there in reserve. I believed that they lived in everyone. *Live now,* I said to myself, *now and now and now.*

I talked myself through one second at a time in August and praised myself for every effort: A nurse came toward me with an ambu-bag when my bi-pap went out. *You can do this,* I thought, and I did. I put all of my energy into working with the nurse and the ambu-bag until the bi-pap was up and running again.

Willis was excited for our date to watch a Johnny Depp movie on the bed, but I didn't want him to see me struggling. I wanted to cancel our plans for the sleep-over. *I must do this,* I thought, and Willis and I lay next to each other watching movies all night. My nurse Maureen came toward me with a huge plastic syringe to give me my first feeding through the new plastic tube in my stomach. *This I can't do,* I thought. *I just can't do this.* I took a beat, a private moment. Was there an upside to my taking baby formula through my stomach? *Maybe these cans of crap will make me strong again.* "All right, bring on the dog food," I said, and Maureen injected a putrid, enriched formula into my brand-new stomach tube. I felt a cold sensation in my stomach. I never ate another meal. Rather I had "feed-ings" four times a day. I was like an animal at the zoo. My whole life I'd counted on food for everything from genuine pleasure to avoidance to celebrating with friends. Food gave me a major something to do. When my breathing went, I leaned on my ability to swallow food and drinks. When my ability to swallow went . . . I saw the sign up ahead: Beginning of the End.

When do you wave the white flag? As sick as I was, I held on to a thread of the belief that I might get better. I think that that's just the way of the human heart. The heart's desire is to be repaired. The heart beats in the name of repair from birth until the end. I longed to ben-efit from the breadth of knowledge, the resources and technology, the great promise and wealth of the age I lived in, of this new century. Was I a fool to believe that all good things might converge in time to save me? I wasn't a fool. I just loved my life. I wasn't a fool. I was a dreamer. I also happened to be realistic. I knew that I might die soon.

The first order of business was to make sure that if death came no one would try to jump in there with me, especially Valerie and Meredith. Obsessive thoughts of death had begun to color my days and nights. I was adamant about not sharing these thoughts with my sisters, the children, Scott and Peter, Katie, Simon, Rob, my friends, or my mother. The fear of death spreads fast in the foxhole. Fear breeds panic and chaos. I decided that showing my fear was no way for me to go on— even if I was going out. I learned that I could carry my fears with dignity. I could bear more than I ever thought. That was a revelation. The people I loved had their own pain. My pain was mine. My sisters were having a hard enough time. They were so angry.

"Love is the answer," I said to Valerie during one of her homicidal rants.

"Who are you, Mahatma Gandhi?" she screamed.

"Was Mahatma the man or the woman?" I asked. I never could keep those Gandhis straight. So accomplished, that family.

"Just leave me alone," said Valerie. But I didn't want to leave her alone. She didn't want to leave me alone, either. For all of our lives, Valerie, Meredith, and I never wanted to leave one another alone. After three trips to the hospital in August, when I was finally back at home, my sisters and I had the chance to sit on the bed and assess the big picture. With a lovely feeding tube inserted safely in my stomach and no further sign of infection, Valerie and Meredith seemed to think we had actually bought some time in August. I wished they were right.

"I hope you're right," I said.

"I'm right," said Valerie.

"Merry?" Meredith was awfully quiet.

"Hmm?" she said.

"Do you think we bought ourselves some time?" I asked.

"I guess. Yeah," Meredith said. But it was clear to me from her tone and the cloud of concern that had settled over us that we didn't know how much. My sisters and I couldn't look at one another. Their anger was giving way to sadness and a sense of defeat we weren't ready to acknowledge. We sat on the bed, each of us crying and looking away.

The big blackout of 2003 hit the next afternoon. My two generators combined delivered only five hours of backup electricity for my bi-pap. So when the lights went out, I went back to St. Vincent's. It was like old home week for me over in the ER, which was jammed with people looking for a place to rest their feet during the blackout. There wasn't a bed to be had when we arrived. Then Nurse Dale Ryan appeared. She said she'd been expecting me from the moment New York lost light.

"I knew you were coming, Jen," Dale said, leaning on my old, faithful ER stretcher she'd marked with a Day-Glo Post-it: RESERVED FOR JENIFER ESTESS. Being in the hospital during the blackout wasn't great for my body. The constant back-and-forth to hospitals in August had taken a major toll.

At the end of the day at the end of August, I worried. When I settled into sleep, I worried in my dreams. I dreamed about flying. That part was good. I dreamed I was flying up strong and free in the dark. My hair blew in the wind. Then I heard the sounds of children. The sounds awoke me with a start. I woke up worrying about the children. I looked for a sign, some assurance that—with or without me—the children would live in happiness and health. I knew that nature didn't grant such assurances. Nature was harsh. Only the fittest survived, it said. The occasional baby bird or lion cub or llama fell through the cracks, got eaten or abandoned because nature dictated it. But I thought it should be different for the children. Freeing the children from a future of disease and heartbreak—we ought to do that, by whatever means necessary. What separated humans from animals was our ability to teach nature a thing or two.

I never had children of my own. That was my greatest dream unrealized. It was my one and only personal tragedy. But in a way I always felt the love that a mother feels. I knew the power of my love and of my listening to help children grow and change. I understood the power of the words *I know you can do it* to go a really long way. I knew that with a little encouragement—true parenting—the children in my life could feel empowered to go out there, teach nature a thing or two, and change the world.

My beautiful, amazing children: Jake, Willis, Jane, James, Kate. As I turned the page from August to the winter of my life, I looked for a sign that they would be all right. My children had the best parents in the world. Meredith and Peter and Scott and Valerie would keep up the good work because their love for their children was just so huge. I wanted to tell my nieces and nephews a little something, too. I wanted them to know I wasn't scared. I wanted them to know that even if I died they would be okay.

The children would always be a-okay. I knew this for a fact because I saw them being born. Jake was the first baby. Meredith and Peter conceived Jake on my bed in my apartment on Seventy-first Street. (I was out with friends that night.) Nine months later, on March 10, Meredith's water broke on my same bed. Meredith, Peter, and I took a cab to New York University Hospital early the next morning in the snow and cold. I was always a lucky third wheel when it came to the children. I was always there at the birth. I stood by Meredith while she was in heavy labor. She was working her contractions along to a tape that Valerie had made of our favorite songs from high school. The boom box blasted and Meredith pushed. I think it was Carly Simon's "Embrace Me You Child" that put her over the top. Meredith pushed one last time and Jake was born on March 11 at 1:59 A.M. Jake was a skinny thing. He looked like a wise old man. Peter stood there in his scrubs, weeping, "It's a boy. It's a boy." The whole family came to see the first baby under the warming light of his baby bed. Jake looked like a grandpa sunbathing in Miami. Fittingly, we ordered up corned beef and knishes from Sarge's Deli and partied in the waiting room for a day and a half. Being there at the birth taught me that there was nothing to be scared of either in coming into the world or leaving it.

There had been so many births. I watched Jake grow into a strapping young man. Willis was born, my Hubbell on earth. Jane came, my spitting image, a beautiful, strong girl who put others first. Kate ran in. She was a little Jodie Foster and reminded me so much of Valerie. Then there was James, an artist in the making. James had been tentative around me. At five, he had only ever known me as a sick person. He was especially scared of the bi-pap mask. I knew how he felt. As a kid, I was scared of people who looked very ill. One night James was adamant about telling me something in private. Meredith, Peter, and the others cleared the room, and James climbed onto my bed and into my lap. James had never come onto the bed before. He had never touched me. He put his face to my ear.

"Jen Jen," he whispered, "I'm not scared of the mask anymore. I'm not scared." And he held me for a moment, climbed down, and went home. James had the heart of an artist all right. He moved right through his fear. They say that people don't change. That's hogwash as far as I was concerned. James changed. My sisters and I had changed through the years. We had become more open as women, more savvy as business-people, a little softer around the edges. Scientists changed. They were motivated by a new urgency to figure out ALS. Just like James, I would continue making changes. I knew that if I ever got better I sure would make at least one radical change. I'd be a lot more physical. There would be a line of men around the block waiting to have liaisons with me. Watching people change, changing my own life—that was the main attraction for me.

I started to ramble—kind of like this—after

August. I started thinking about things in the abstract, which was totally unlike me. I pictured worst-case scenarios; I entertained vague visions of brighter futures—exactly whose futures they were, I didn't know. Spending a lot of time in the foxhole left me a little "general" in my thinking. I engaged in mental walkabouts. They bothered me. I knew myself. I had to commit myself to a project, something concrete, or else I'd go nuts, so I planned a combined birthday party for Willis, who had turned ten, and Jane, just nine. Lorna dressed my place with streamers and balloons. We made gift bags for everyone. According to my strict instructions, Lorna bought and wrapped almost a million presents for Willis and Jane. I ordered everyone's favorite food. Everything was in place for the big blowout.

The morning of the party I woke up early. I felt the old excitement of Christmas. I couldn't wait for my family to come that night and for the children to open their presents. Everyone waited in the living room while Lorna sat me up. Then she flung open the doors. Everyone came to the bed and we had a great time. Willis really liked the fifty-seven video games I bought him. I'm sure Jane liked her American Girl dolls. I bought her the one that she wanted, a pretty pioneer. I bought the accessories that every pioneer needed, sold separately: utensils for eating hearty meals by the fire, boots for the long trek, and a bed for resting at the end of days filled with discovery. It was the complete pioneer's package. It was a great birthday party. Lorna got ready to go home.

"When will I see you again?" I asked her.

"Tuesday morning," said Lorna.

"That's so far away," I said.

"Tuesday's close, Jenifer," she said. "It's real close." My family hung out for a while, then Karen breezed in fashionably late for her night shift.

"Everyone needs to bundle up-*m,*" she said. "It's a cold night." The passage of time is different in the foxhole. Somehow, just as Valerie's and Meredith's anger gave way to sadness, August had given way to December. I didn't remember much about the months in between. The children put on their warm coats after a great party, climbed one by one onto my bed, and I kissed them good-bye. They walked into the cold night. I never saw them again.

Chapter Twelve

I DIED ON DECEMBER 16, two days after the birthday party. It was early in the morning, a little after five. I was deep asleep and dreaming my usual. I don't know what medical event occurred. I stopped breathing is all, my heart stopped beating, and I was on my way. One second I was dreaming, the next second I was traveling.

I'm on my way, as Paul Simon says. I don't know where I'm going. Maybe to heaven or straight into the hearts of the people I love or into lettuce fields or carrot patches or cut flowers. Everyone has a guess on the matter of where we go when we die. All I know is that I'm rising. That's a good sign, don't you think? As far as general directions one wants to be heading in are concerned, up is definitely my first choice. So far it's been dark the whole way. I'm moving through a deep navy blue ocean dark that isn't scary. At this point, anything seems possible. Changes in hues, colors, or the lightness—there's no way for me to predict what's going to happen. I'm sure only of the rising. There's no more pain. I am moving again. My ALS is totally gone, which makes perfect sense. ALS can survive only if it's sucking the life out of a living, breathing human being. As of this rising, it's probably entering the nerve cells of another unsuspecting sister, brother, mother, or father. ALS isn't picky—it's an equal opportunity disease. But quite frankly now, I am pure joy. I am the joy of movement. I know that sounds like an aerobics class, but it's true. I am joy rising.

People said I looked really good dead. They said I looked the way I did before I got sick. After I died, Lorna put on my lipstick of choice, "Pearl" by Mac; she brushed my hair and put me in a black turtleneck and my favorite pants. I was a babe in that box. Friends stood over me in the hospital morgue and in my viewing room at Riverside Memorial Chapel. They loved seeing me without the Hannibal Lecter mask. I had a really pretty face. I loved my body. I'd forgotten.

"Beautiful Jenifer," said Lorna, crying as she touched my face. "You're in the arms of Jesus now." Truth be told, the cradling image kind of works for me. I find the image of being rocked in someone's arms or in the branches of a tree comforting. It gives me something to look forward to. I haven't passed any robed figures or men with beards on this ocean blue highway. I haven't seen women in gowns. No obvious angels. That's not to say I won't. I'm just moving through the dark alone now. We'll see what we see.

My last night alive was pretty usual: formula through my feeding tube for dinner at eight, a couple of hours watching TV, phone calls with Valerie and Meredith, and a foot massage. Christmas was coming. The same night of the birthday party, Valerie, Meredith, and the kids had brought up a tree and decorated it outside my room. I don't know why, but I wasn't quite ready to look at the tree. That night, for the time being, I watched reflections from its lights on my wall. My home health aides Basilia and Rosanne, who were filling in for my regular nurses, helped me off to sleep somewhere between three and four in the morning. The night was typical; the day before hadn't been.

That day, Monday, was the last time I saw Meredith, my Meredith, the daylight. We sat on the bed, working. One of our board members had been planning a power breakfast to honor Project A.L.S. Meredith and I considered the scenario. We discussed the details of the annual Project A.L.S. holiday party, which always took place in the general vicinity of my bed. Then Meredith and I checked in with *General Hospital*.

Meredith stayed later than usual. She normally

took a five-something train home, but Peter was coaching Jane's basketball team that night, then taking the kids out to dinner, so Meredith and I had a few hours to hang out. My baby sister looked tired on the bed, but statuesque—always statuesque, even at her worst. I looked just horrible. My energy was at an all-time low. I could feel my airways—the intricate paths through which oxygen flows, nourishing our bodies—growing smaller by the day. My infrastructure was shrinking and caving in on itself.

"Sometimes I'm scared," I said, "that we just fade to black. That it's just lights out at the end."

"I don't think so," said Meredith.

"What do you think?" I asked.

"I don't know, but I don't think we fade to black. I mean *after all this*?"

"What are you gonna have for dinner?" I asked her. I lived vicariously through Valerie's and Meredith's eating.

"Whatever," Meredith said. She was crying. She looked away.

"You look really beautiful, Mer," I said. "You really have that body to beat all." Although Meredith was weary, she looked just great. She had lost about ten pounds on the South Beach Diet, not that she needed to.

"I can't go on," said Meredith.

"You will," I said. "It's Valerie I'm worried about.

She's gotta get to the gym." I wanted to reach out for Meredith and hold her and tell her I knew she could get through anything. She'd already been through anything *and* everything. It was kind of odd—as close as we were, my sisters and I never did much touching. Not a lot of hugging and kissing and cradling going on. It was a tradition that had been passed through the chilly bloodlines of our family. As babies and as girls, my sisters and I learned to hold ourselves. We were self-held kids. But you should have seen us with our kids. We shattered the no-hold tradition—and then some. We held our kids whenever we got the chance. I know that if I had gotten healthy, I'd have held them all again. The children would probably have been graduating from high school by that time, but I could see myself picking up my grown nieces and nephews and swinging them around. My sisters wouldn't stand a chance—I'd jump all over them for joy. I'd walk on out to Santa Monica and kiss Reed . . . go twelve rounds with a couple of neurologists I have in mind. I'd never stop moving.

A palpable sadness had settled over the Project A.L.S. camp that Monday, the day before I died. A couple hours after Meredith left the bed for the last time, she called to ask me if I got joy from anything anymore. She said she needed to know. I told her that joy on earth was hard for me to come by recently.

"Does seeing the kids make you happy?" she asked.

"I get joy from seeing them, Mer, but I'm losing my energy to love them in the way that I need to."

"I don't believe that," said Meredith. She didn't believe that the Love Girl was running out of steam. But it took strength to love—really love someone—and in recent days I'd felt that energy changing. Loving on the level that Valerie, Meredith, and I loved throughout our lives takes so much generosity. Loving isn't passive. I think that people feel slighted most of the time. They don't want to give love out to others—they don't want to put out the effort—because they didn't get love themselves. It takes a real effort to turn hurt feelings around. It takes real courage to put your love out there. I longed to put my love on the bed, on this earth, with all of the people I loved in the flesh, but I was being called away. My last conversation with Meredith wasn't our most satisfying. I talked to Meredith about my deteriorating speech, which had made it hard for me to form words like deteriorating. Meredith and I tried to imagine sitting together on the bed not being able to talk to each other. Not being able to shop together, eat together, talk—neither of us could picture it, the not talking. I worried about not being able to take care of her anymore. Who would take my place? Meredith and I said good-bye at around eleven.

I had said good-bye to Valerie the day before, on Sunday. She was in the living room, working on this book. I'd slept all day. She stopped writing at about five to come in and see me. She knocked and slid back the door.

"Hey," she said.

"Hey," I said. "Can you believe how much I sleep?"

"Sleep is a good thing. Sometimes it's the best thing," she said, sitting on the bed. Sleep wasn't the best thing. The best thing was feeling Valerie writing on the other side of my bedroom door. She had worked hard that day. She looked like she could use a break, so we turned on Lifetime. Valerie and I watched a made-for-TV movie starring Meredith Baxter and Swoosie Kurtz until night. We loved TV movies. In this one, Swoosie's daughter was having an affair with the husband of her mother's best friend, played by Meredith Baxter. The husband was so unappealing! Valerie and I couldn't figure out why anyone would want to throw it overboard for him. We talked about our book during commercials.

"I'm so proud of the writing," I said. "I'm so proud of you."

"There's nothing to be proud of," Valerie said. No matter what I said to Valerie lately she couldn't take it in. She was temporarily made of stone—completely unable to absorb a compliment. She seemed determined to stay in this stony state until I got healthy again. She wasn't going to budge until the miracle came, until I got up and danced. I think Valerie saw it as her job to make me better. Until that day came, nothing else would matter. I kept trying to tell Valerie that the celebration was now—our forty years together.

"I love what you've written so far," I said. "You're such a good writer."

"I just listen to your voice on the tapes," she said. "Stop overblowing things."

"Okeydokey," I said as Meredith Baxter hauled off and slapped Swoosie right across the face in a shopping center parking lot. When Swoosie reeled back from the blow and banged into a parked car, Valerie and I laughed until we couldn't breathe. That was maybe about two seconds for me—but you know what I mean. Valerie and I loved acting and actors and movies. All acting; all singing; all dancing—bring it on forever. I remembered when Valerie was going to write movies and I was going to produce and act in them. Valerie, Meredith, and I were going to have our own film production company. That would have been great, I thought, but no greater than this—sitting on the bed with Valerie watching Lifetime.

Here's the thing with this rising: My memories are fueling the ride. My memories are providing the rocket fuel. It turns out I can't go up—unless I go back. The more I see my life as it was, the more I rise. The memories are coming fast and furious: watching Meredith and Peter kiss during our first picnic at West Point; holding two-year-old Willis as he shook with delight after Aldo the horse ate a carrot from his hand;

dancing in my apartment on Seventy-first Street before work; braiding Jane's hair; eating a blueberry muffin at my desk at Naked Angels; changing Jake's diaper; getting kisses and kisses from Kate; holding hands with my boyfriend Michael as we walked through the high school breezeway; watching James take his first steps; joking with Scott at the dinner table while Valerie served up chicken and rice; shopping for fake nails at Polk's; taking my bows with the cast of *Men in White,* a play at NYU; eating corn on the cob with Simon in Shelter Island; throwing a clay pot on the kick wheel at Buck's Rock Work Camp; feeling my body against Reed's in the ocean—the ocean, the ocean; running with my sisters as girls in the surf at Playland Beach; wondering in awe at the mystery of my mother's beauty; holding a cup of hot coffee.

I made my own way in life. I had my own style. We all make our own ways and create our own styles. Yes, I wish that I had had more time to hone that style, to tweak it and love it completely just because it was mine, but I didn't. I am thinking and I'm sure, even if life deals us the unimaginable, the absolute ugliest, most intimidating set of circumstances, we can cut a road through it. My sisters and I built a road. We built a road and grew up to be loving, caring, hardworking people, in spite of the odds. My friends and family and I built a road. Project A.L.S. will continue to search until it finds medicine to help people who are dying cruel and inhuman deaths. There are so many roads for us to build that we can and must build. The building is the miracle. As we build, as we work, the ugliest of circumstances will start looking a little less ugly, then less ugly, then they'll look decent bordering on mildly attractive. One day, the road we build will end in a destination. We'll celebrate our fine work together until which time we must go it alone.

I see Meredith now. She's in her kitchen. She is taking a container of sliced cantaloupe out of the refrigerator. She puts the cantaloupe and some bananas on the counter, where Jane and James are sitting and eating breakfast. Jake comes in. He is doing his homework at the last minute. His mother is mad about the homework. She tells him to take a banana. James puts an entire strawberry into his mouth. Here comes Peter, Big Poppa. He's wearing a crisp white shirt for work. He's carrying a tie to put on in the car. He's on the run. The whole family is looking forward to the workmen coming today. Soon the Hulberts will have an addition built on to their house. It will have a playroom, a family room, and a new bedroom for Jake, who is really coming into his own. I have never seen love like this— the yelling and eating and getting ready. After Peter and the kids leave, Meredith will spend the rest of the morning crying on her bed. Then she'll stop crying and take a train into the city. She will buy a large iced tea with one Sweet'n Low and take it up to the office, on Twelfth Street, where she will work for Project A.L.S. until night. Before she goes home on the train, she will drop off her favorite pictures of me at the frame shop. When she gets home she'll tell everyone about the pictures of me that will be coming into the house. Then everyone will go to sleep. Meredith will call Valerie about a hundred times during the day. This is after they've spent the entire day working together at the office.

I see Valerie now. She is almost ready to wrap Christmas presents. She's in my room on Twelfth Street. It's late at night on Christmas Eve. It's one in the morning. Valerie will wrap presents for Willis and Kate at my house because she doesn't want to get caught doing it at her house. Kate believes in Santa Claus. This is probably the last year that Willis will believe, but he still believes. Valerie has come straight from Riverside Memorial Chapel, where she picked up my ashes at about nine o'clock. The man at Riverside gave her a shopping bag with a cherrywood box inside. Valerie took the bag back to the car, lifted the box out of the bag, and put it in the passenger seat. She put the seat belt around the box, then she and I went for one last ride around the city. We drove by the tree at Rockefeller Center, and Naked Angels, which is now a thrift shop, and my old apartment on Seventy-first Street. Valerie wept and drove. She rolled down the windows and screamed at New York.

Then she stopped weeping. She parked the car, came up to my place, and put Annie Lennox on my boom box. Now she is starting to wrap. She'll finish in time to surprise Scott and the kids with presents and breakfast in the morning. It's beginning to look a lot like Christmas. Valerie will call Meredith from my phone in the middle of the night. They'll talk. They'll see each other Christmas afternoon. Meredith is making dinner for everyone in Harrison.

We go on. The gentle, three-headed monster Valerie-Jenifer-Meredith will continue to roam the earth. That's what my sisters and I do. We love. We work. We roam. I'm not in the phone loop anymore, but I am here, rising, free, moving, sending love. Everything is going to be okay. There are no boundaries for me now. This is the next world. It is a world of action—rising—and no equal and opposite reaction, at least so far. There is one, unchallenged motion here—up. At the moment, my love is free to rise and seek and stretch out. I like it. It reminds me of the way I felt when I was in the water with Reed, when I felt my love for life stretching out across the infinite ocean.

I don't know what's next for me, if there is a next. If there is, I'd be grateful for a skating rink of some kind. I like this upward motion, but I still have an urge to glide on ice. I could do it now. I could do it again now that I'm free. The ice was always so beautiful in my life. My mother would dress my sisters and me alike in yellow jackets and blue stretch pants; then she'd send us out. As the afternoons wore on, we yellow jackets would meet in the middle of the rink and form a smaller circle of our own. We'd hold on to one another, skating in a circle until the night came. Our yellow jackets were the brightest thing in the dark. When it was closing time at Ebersol Rink, my sisters and I would all just fall down dizzy onto our backs on the ice. I'd look up at the stars and take a deep breath. Oh my, the stars. Oh my. I wanted to touch them and knew that someday, in some way, I would. So here I am. I'd be grateful for a skating rink. I hope there's a snack bar. Meantime, I can say about death what I knew about life: It's not about letting go, but reaching.

Afterword

BY VALERIE ESTESS

MY GUIDE, the love of my life, my sister Jenifer died on December 16, 2003, then Meredith and I finished this book. Our hearts were shattered but we completed the job. Jenifer always taught me that starting a job was one thing—and admirable—but that following through and completing—well, that's where the bravery is. Ultimately, it didn't matter if the end product was magnificent or mediocre or critically acclaimed. What mattered, Jenifer told me, was the work itself, from beginning to middle to end. So I delivered this manuscript covered with tears to our abiding publishers a couple of weeks ago.

I hope that this book serves up a small inspiring portion of Jenifer's life to you, the reader. Jenifer wasn't wealthy or a supermodel or a pampered pooch. She was a working girl who put on her best face, fought for the life she dreamed of having, and dedicated her last years to fighting the sorry state of brain disease research. Not a shabby résumé. Not her first choice by any stretch, but Jenifer's story shows that sometimes, your Plan B can be okay, better than okay—miraculous. There's gold for us along the way if we can open our eyes enough to see it. The gold is in the getting there, in the holding on, in the reaching. That was Jenifer's experience. Maybe it's yours, too.

Meredith, Project A.L.S., and I continue the fight against ALS and its relatives, Parkinson's, Alzheimer's, and Huntington's diseases. It would be downright un-American of us to quit now. We will keep working from our love for Jenifer and our respect for the millions of adults and children who are being cut down needlessly by these scourges. Project A.L.S. and others are helping scientists approach research in a whole new way. Scientists are working as teammates now—as a dedicated family—so we should be putting effective medicine into place soon.

I always used to whine to Jenifer that the world seemed divided into two groups: the haves and the have-nots. When Jenifer was diagnosed with ALS at the age of thirty-five, I cried that my sisters and I were have-nots. As I railed and stomped my feet, Jenifer just sat on her bed, regal, suggesting that I might want to take a closer look at my own life. As far as Jenifer was concerned, anyone who shared the love that she, Meredith, and I had shared was a have. For Jenifer, having it all was a simple, exquisite recipe, like the one for Kaka's brownies. Combine love, work, compassion, and you will some day, in some way, get to the mountaintop. Making the climb is the ultimate honor and privilege, I now know. I love Jenifer for teaching me that and everything else.

Acknowledgments

My sisters and I acknowledge the extraordinary efforts of Harriet Abramson, Jace Alexander, Jane Alexander, Jennifer Aniston, Debbon Ayer, Hank Azaria, Jon Robin Baitz, William Baldwin, Willow Bay, Vicki and Marc Beckerman, Kathie Berlin, Michael Berman, Cynthia Bernardie, Sara Bernstein, Basilia Billups, David Blaine, Joe Blake, Tessa Blake, Michael Boatman, Michael Bolton, Barry Bostwick, Sofia Bragat, Matthew Broderick, Daniel Brodie, Andrea Brown, Robert H. Brown Jr., Nicole Burdette, Jonathan Burkhart, Rob Burnett, Bobby Canavalle, Nina Capelli, Maureen Carlo, Gail Carson, Tom Cavanaugh, Arnie Civins, Robert Clarke, George Clooney, Lorna Cofield, Maddie Corman, Katie Couric, Sheryl Crow, Carson Daly, Ronnie Davis, Alice and Phillip Decter, Darci DeMatteo, Diana DeRosa, Matt Dillon, Nadine Donahue, Kathi Doolan, Caryle Duffy, Karen Duffy, Paul Eckstein, Ron Eldard, Cornelia Erpf, Alison Estess,

Marilyn Estess, Melissa Etheridge, Edie Falco, Gerald D. Fischbach, Steven Fisher, Brenda Friend, Michael J. Fox, Robert Fumarelli, Fred H. Gage, Matthew Gallagher, James Gandolfini, Janeane Garofalo, Kathleen Gates, John Gearhart, Stephanie George, Gina Gershon, Thomas Gibson, David Marshall Grant, Clark Gregg, Brad Grey, Jill Grey, Harry Grossman, Marlene Haffner, Simon Halls, Lorraine Hamilton, Donna Hanover, Mariska Hargitay, Patricia Harrington, Peter Hedges, Joanna Heimbold, John and Peggy Henry, Juliet Hercules, Gloria and Howard Hirsch, David Hoffenberg, Julianne Hoffenberg, Juliette Hohnen, Joy Huang, Peter J. Hulbert, Bonnie Hunt, Helen Hunt, Kevin Huvane, Robert Iger, Karen Jack, Myra and Allen Jacobson, David L. Jaffe, Andrew Jarecki, Nancy Jarecki, Thomas Jessell, Kristen Johnston, Jane Kaczmarek, Robert S. Kaplan, Brian Kaspar, Carol and Gerald Kaufman, Daniel Kellison, Jimmy Kimmel, Dana and Richard Kind, Greg Kinnear, Linda Kirschenbaum, Jill Knee, Jane Krakowski, Peter Krause, Regina Kulik, Brigitte Lacombe, Jonathan LaPook, Laura Lavelle, Charla Lawhon, Sharon Lawrence, Sue Leibman, Robert Levine, Jaqueline Lividini, Kenneth Lonergan, Bryan Lourd, Joseph Lovett, Richard Lovett, Kyle MacLachlan, Mitchell G. Mandell, Pam Manela and John LaFemina, Camryn Manheim, Julianna Margulies, Jesse L. Martin, Sandy Martin, Michael Mastro, Adam Max, Diane Max, Chi McBride, Martha McCully, Ashley McDermott, Jeffrey

McDermott, The McGraths, Valerie McLarty, The
Meads, Memory, Jack Merrill, Cori Miller, Dana Miller,
Penelope Ann Miller, Katherine Moore, Julie and Rob
Moran, Rob Morrow, Geoffrey Nauffts, Sheila Nevins,
Fernanda Niven, Philip Noguchi, David O'Connor, Jim
Oelschlager, Cheri Oteri, Pippin Parker, Sarah Jessica
Parker, Luke Perry, Brad Pitt, Michael Price, Jason
Priestley, Frank Pugliese, Tim Ransom, Dana and
Christopher Reeve, Caroline Rhea, Ron Rifkin, Scott
Robbins, Janine Rose, Jeffrey D. Rothstein, Lewis P.
Rowland, Alan Ruck, Paul Rudd, Reed Rudy, Dale
Ryan, Laura SanGiacomo, Richard Santulli, Lou
Saporito, Kim Schefler-Rodriguez, Annabella Sciorra,
Frederic Seegal, Molly Shannon, Edward Sherin,
Brooke Shields, Linda G. Singer, Evan Snyder, Vincent
Spano, Fisher Stevens, Jon Stewart, Ben Stiller, Michael
Sweedler, D. B. Sweeney, Pamela and Laurence Tarica,
Jamie Tarses, Christine Taylor, Carol Thompson, Maura
Tierney, Marisa Tomei, Nancy Travis, Blair
Underwood, Asnal Valcin, Jamie Walsh, Jennifer Ward,
Juliet Weber, Steven Weber, Marion Weil, Titus
Welliver, Tom Werner, Linda and the Wertliebs,
Bradley White, Debbie Wilpon, Fred Wilpon, Richard
Wilpon, Cyd Wilson, Scott Wolf, Richard Wood, and
the thousands across the country who have given so gen-
erously of their time and efforts on behalf of finding a cure.

I especially wish to recognize Judith Curr for her
vision, and my editor, Tracy Behar, for her singular
guidance in writing this book.

ABOUT THIS GUIDE

The suggested questions are intended to help your reading group find new and interesting angles and topics for discussion of *Tales from the Bed*. We hope that these ideas will enrich your conversation and increase your enjoyment of the book.

Many fine books from Washington Square Press feature Readers Club Guides. For a complete listing, or to read the Guides online, visit http://www.BookClubReader.com

Questions and Topics for Discussion

1) *Tales from the Bed* allows the reader to get to know Jenifer Estess and follow her throughout the various emotions she experiences before and after being diagnosed with ALS. Do you identify with Jenifer? What are the aspects of her personality that you relate to and why?

2) Jenifer recounts her various experiences with doctors and medical professionals after being initially diagnosed. Do you think her experiences are unique? Discuss the role of the physician and other medical professionals in cases involving life-debilitating or terminal illness, such as ALS. What should be

expected from health professionals on both a personal and professional level?

3) Do you think running Project A.L.S. had an impact on Jenifer's health? Discuss the role of work in maintaining a sense of well-being.

4) Discuss how Jenifer relates her childhood experiences with her experiences after being diagnosed with ALS. What are some of the lessons she draws from those experiences?

5) Jenifer employs several metaphors and similes throughout the memoir. Explain how phrases such as "The doctors invited me to a square dance" and "Piece by piece, my morning fell to the sidewalk like leaves" help tell her story. How do these literary devices help personalize the story and enhance Jenifer's personality?

6) Jenifer provides an in-depth view of her close relationships with Valerie and Meredith. Describe each of their roles in their shared family history and how those roles were applied to the logistics of running Project A.L.S., as well as their support system throughout Jenifer's illness.

7) Explore Jenifer and Reed's relationship. How does the theme of romantic love figure into how Jenifer

views her own illness? What does Reed symbolize to Jenifer? To the reader?

8) The theme of family is present throughout the book. Though the sisterhood shared by Valerie, Jenifer, and Meredith is thoroughly examined, there are other family members Jenifer writes about. How have these family members impacted Jenifer's life? How do her parents, other siblings, and nieces and nephews affect her outlook on life, illness, and death?

9) In recent years, A.L.S. has come to the forefront in media outlets and the scientific research community. Prior to reading *Tales from the Bed,* were you familiar with A.L.S. or Project ALS? Discuss the impact Project A.L.S. has had on the research, and the role that stem-cell therapy may have in the future.

10) The final chapter of the book is unique. How did you feel reading it? Do you think reading the last chapter, written from Jenifer's point of view, offers some closure to her story?

Wings

of
Morning

Kathleen Morgan

These Highland Hills
Book 2

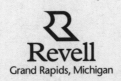

Revell
Grand Rapids, Michigan

Published by Fleming H. Revell
a division of Baker Publishing Group
P.O. Box 6287, Grand Rapids, MI 49516-6287

Second printing, May 2007

Printed in the United States of America

Library of Congress Cataloging-in-Publication Data
Morgan, Kathleen, 1950–
    Wings of morning / Kathleen Morgan.
        p.   cm. — (These highland hills ; bk. 2)
        ISBN 10: 0-8007-5964-8 (pbk.)
        ISBN 978-0-8007-5964-3 (pbk.)
        1. Scotland—History—16th century—Fiction. 2. Highlands (Scotland)—Fiction. I. Title.
    PS3563.O8647W56 2006
    813'.54—dc22   2005019747

This book is dedicated to Kelli Standish,
a great champion of Christian fiction.
Your deep and unstinting love for
God and the ministry of Christian fiction
is so very much appreciated, my friend.
Thank you from the bottom of my heart.

I

STRATHYRE HOUSE, CENTRAL SCOTTISH HIGHLANDS, JUNE 1566

All was in readiness.

The bedchamber was spotless, the linens so recently washed the faint scent of sunshine and fresh air clung to them still. The stout oak bedstead had been hand-rubbed with oil until it gleamed. The stone floors were scrubbed and laid with newly cut, summer-sweet marsh rushes.

Beeswax candles, impaled on tall, iron stakes, flickered and burned on either side of the bed. A fire smoldered in the hearth, adding its own warmth and light to mute the chill darkness of stone-damp castle and dreary summer night.

Still, seventeen-year-old Regan Drummond shivered, clasping her arms protectively about her night-rail-clad body. Gooseflesh tightened her fair skin. The thin, lawn fabric was, after all, not meant for warmth but enticement. Regan could only hope, after tonight, her wedding night, she'd be able to put away the ridiculously impractical gown forever.

But not just yet. Tonight, no matter how senseless all the bedtime ceremony seemed, she'd grit her teeth, keep her opinions to herself, and do her duty. Aye, do her duty, and not give dear Roddy cause to question her devotion to him. Already he was in such a state of agitation over their impending coupling, Regan had all but forced him into the arms of his inebriated younger brother and other male wedding guests.

"Give me a time to prepare myself," she had urged her new husband. "A cup or two of wine won't harm a braw lad like ye," she then added, motioning Roddy away. "Indeed, it'll ease the night to come for the both of us."

Misgiving in his warm brown eyes, Roddy had reluctantly joined the party of revelers, leaving Regan to her maidservants and the bedtime preparations. If the truth be told, she was in no hurry for the marital consummation. If the truth be told, she was as frightened and unsure of what this night held as he.

With a sense of foreboding, Regan walked to the big, four-poster bed, climbed in beneath the cool, linen sheets, and pulled the down comforter up to her chin. The sound of raucous male voices echoed down the long, stone corridor, voices thick with drunkenness and loud with crude songs. She shivered. It was the wedding party, at last delivering Roddy to his bride.

It was only for a night, Regan reminded herself, and only for a short while at that. Roddy would manage his husbandly duties, then fall asleep beside her. On the morrow, they'd rise, share breakfast, and fall back into the comfortable routine and relationship they had always known before.

Aye, Reagan thought. It was only for a night—well, the worst of it, leastwise. It was also, in the total scheme of their lives, a very small part indeed.

The singing and shouts grew louder. The remarks came again, crude and ribald. Hot blood warmed Regan's cheeks. The boors. The vulgar, insufferable boors!

Then they were at the door, kicking it open and spilling into the bridal bedchamber like a horde of Viking marauders. Hair disheveled, shirts wine-stained and half hanging from their kilts, the group of twenty or so clansmen, led by Roddy's younger brother, Walter, slid to an abrupt halt at the sight of her. Roddy, carried aloft by the other revelers, looked up from his perch and blinked in surprise.

It took only a moment, however, for his surprise to transform into a drunken leer. "Och, there ye are, my bonny bride," he managed to slur. "Ready and waiting for yer man to make ye a woman, are ye?"

At that, Roddy's companions roared in laughter and resumed their unsteady trek toward the bed. Regan watched them approach, their grinning passenger held overhead like some precious cargo, her desire to dive beneath the covers warring with the impulse to leap from bed and pummel the lot of them. Only her fierce Highland pride held her where she was. That, and the hurt Roddy's insensitive acquiescence to this ridiculous performance stirred in her.

She had begged him not to allow the traditional activities that always culminated in drunken men milling about, making bawdy comments in the marital bedchamber. And he had given his word that no such escapades would mar their wedding night. Yet here he was, as inebriated and lewd as the rest, joining in with the most unseemly—and traitorous—enthusiasm.

But there was no time to dwell on his hurtful betrayal. The MacLaren men halted at the foot of the big bed. With suddenly the greatest of care, they lowered their laird and deposited him there. Apparently oblivious to Regan's murderous glare, Roddy immediately rose to all fours and crawled up to meet her.

"A wee kiss for yer husband," he growled, his liquor-bleary gaze roving over her. "Show me how badly ye want me, lass."

Regan steadily traded glances with him. "First, send them on their way," she said, her voice low but taut with fury. "What's between us, if indeed there's aught to be salvaged this night, isn't for the sight of others."

As if trying to fathom the meaning beneath her words, her husband blinked stupidly. A light of comprehension flared, signaling that a shred or two of sense still remained. He nodded slowly, then, half turning, looked behind him.

"Away with ye," he snarled. "I've better things to do than celebrate with the likes of ye."

"But ye haven't even crawled between the covers!" one of Roddy's compatriots shouted. "And we've yet to verify ye're properly bedded."

Roddy turned back to Regan. She could see the liquor beginning to regain its foothold, the uncertainty rise. "Send them away," she whispered. "Please."

"She said ye must leave," he muttered thickly, never taking his gaze off her.

"And since when does a wife tell her husband what he can and cannot do?" a voice rose from somewhere beyond the foot of the bed.

"Aye, bridle the filly before she takes the bit, and she's forever out of control," another man yelled. "Teach her to obey now, or ye'll never tame her!"

"And ye'd know that better than most, eh, Fergus!" yet another added, and they all laughed.

At that, something hardened, went dark and shuttered in Roddy's eyes. Despair rippled through her. She had lost what little influence she may have had over him. Or, leastwise, this night anyway.

The laughs and suggestive comments rose again, until Regan felt smothered in their dreadful, demeaning cacophony. She shut her eyes, attempting to block it all out. And then Roddy leaned close, took her chin in one hand, and slammed his mouth down on hers.

His kiss was rough and awkward. The taste of wine, the odor of smoke and sweat, was on him. Nausea roiled in her gut.

Suddenly, Regan couldn't breathe. Panic seized her. She struck out frantically.

Roddy tumbled backward, falling off the end of the bed. For a fleeting moment, his companions fell silent, then roared all louder in laughter. It snapped the last thread of maidenly modesty and decorum Regan possessed.

With a cry of rage, she leaped from bed and grabbed one of the tall, iron candlesticks. Pulling the beeswax taper free, she tossed it aside. Then, swinging the candle stake's pointed end in a wide arc before her, Regan advanced on the clansmen.

"Out of here, I say," she screamed. "Get out before I run ye through with this!"

The sight of an enraged, night-rail-clad woman must have finally been enough to sober the assembled men, at least temporarily. They fell silent; their mouths dropped open, and they stared. She knew, though, she must press her advantage while she still could. The candle stake held before her like some battle spear, Regan advanced on them.

"Get out, ye leering, liquor-besotted swine," she all but shrieked. "Out! Out of my bedchamber!"

She punctuated her demand with a sudden lunge forward with her lethally pointed weapon. With an indignant gasp, the men parted before her. Another sharp thrust, and they began to crowd backward toward the still-open door.

Like she would with a flock of sheep, Regan slowly but surely herded them out the way they had come. When the last man stepped back over the threshold, she finally set aside her weapon. Taking the door, she slammed it shut and bolted it.

There were a few defiant shouts and muttered curses, but from the footsteps now echoing down the corridor, it was evident all the revelry had at last ebbed from Roddy's clansmen. Soon, silence reigned once more. It took a time for Regan's anger to cool and her heart to resume a more placid beat. At last, though, the candle stake in hand, she turned back to the bed.

Roddy was sitting on the floor where he had fallen, a crooked smile on his lips. Though most times that boyishly endearing look was enough to erase any lingering anger or exasperation Regan might still harbor against her dearest friend, this night there seemed nothing behind that smile. Nothing, leastwise, that could come close to justifying what had almost happened.

"Are ye planning to impale me on that wee spike, lass?" her now apparently contrite new husband inquired. "It wouldn't sit well with the clan, ye know, killing the bridegroom on his wedding night."

"Yet almost ravishing me before half the men of the clan would?"

He gave what looked to be a half-apologetic shrug. "Well, mayhap I let things get a wee bit out of hand . . ."

Regan gave a disdainful snort. "A *wee* bit?"

Roddy heaved a weary sigh. "Fine, it got far too much out of hand. And I'm sorry, lass. Verra sorry."

All the fight drained from her in one big rush. "Ye . . . ye promised, R-Roddy." Despite her best efforts to contain it, her voice quavered. "And ye knew how badly I didn't want such a degrading spectacle on our wedding night. Yet ye . . . Och, how *could* ye go against yer word?"

"Lass, lass." He shoved to his feet, swayed unsteadily, and had to grab for one of the bedposts to keep from toppling over. Once more, a sheepish grin split his handsome face. "Let me make it up to ye. Come here. Come to me, for I fear I'll surely fall and crack my skull if I try to walk verra far."

She knew what would happen if she went to him. Yet, despite what had just transpired, despite the lingering pain at his vow breaking, Regan knew she couldn't avoid the inevitable forever. And at least the bedchamber door was now firmly bolted against any intruders . . .

"I'm not thinking ye deserve aught from me this night," she muttered, even as she made her way back across the room, "but if ye give me yer solemn vow ye'll never do that again—"

Just as soon as she came within arms' length, Roddy grabbed her and pulled her to him. "Wheesht, lass," he said to silence her. "I promise. It'll never happen again."

With that, he lowered his head toward her. At first the kiss was gentle, even tentative, but as Regan moved close and yielded to him, his mouth slanted harder and more insistently. He crushed her lips with an increasingly savage intensity. His hands began to rove over her, touching places no man had ever touched before.

She wrenched her mouth away. "Roddy . . . please. Ye're hurting me!"

He lifted passion-glazed eyes to her. "Wheesht," he mumbled, his voice gone hoarse and frighteningly unfamiliar. "Ye've had yer apology. It's time ye give me what I've been wanting for years now. It's time ye begin acting the obedient wife."

Whirling around, Roddy forced her up against the foot of the bed. Regan fought to keep her balance, but her husband's greater weight and strength inexorably bore her back until they both fell onto the bed. And then his hands were tugging at her night rail, wrenching the delicate fabric until it tore.

The sound of the ripping cloth sent Roddy past the point of reason. He threw himself atop her, his fingers entwining in her hair to twist the long locks painfully in his hands.

"Roddy," Regan cried. "Stop! Ye're going too fast!"

Her husband—the gentle man she thought she had married— was no more. A madness the like of which she had never seen before came over him. Terror filled Regan. Panic rose to nearly strangle her. Instinctively, she fought back, pounding at him, striking his head and face, all the while screaming for him to stop.

And then, he did. He went limp and slumped over her. At first, all Regan could do was struggle to catch her breath. Gradually, though, as her heart eased its pounding and the room ceased its crazed twirling, Regan realized he hadn't stopped of his own volition. Roddy had either succumbed to the vast amounts of wine he had surely imbibed this eve, or she had inadvertently knocked him out in her terror-stricken thrashing.

She shoved him off her and, for a long moment, lay there beside him. Then, rolling away, Regan slid from bed.

His face relaxed once more, Roddy looked again like the friend she had grown up with all these years. He looked familiar, comforting, kind—nothing like the madman of a few minutes ago. But it didn't matter anymore. She had seen a side of Roderick MacLaren she didn't like. Didn't like at all.

Regan glanced down at her nightrail. Nausea welled. Suddenly she couldn't bear to be in the same room with the stranger who was now her husband. She shrugged from the ruined garment, hurriedly dressed, then ran from the room.

✝

"The alarm's been raised, m'lord. Reivers have attacked Shenlarich and taken the cattle."

Not another village, Iain Campbell thought late that evening, *and that only a fortnight since the last attack.* Though he loved the Highlands dearly, there were times when he grew mightily weary of all the lawlessness, plundering, and blackmail that were such an integral part of the Highland way of life. He had suffered enough at the hands of power-maddened, narrow-visioned men. All he wanted was to live in peace.

But apparently the fulfillment of that particular wish wasn't in the offing anytime soon. With a sigh, the laird of Balloch Castle and tanist to his cousin and clan chief, Niall Campbell, glanced up from his spot in the chapel pew. "And have ye word, as well, Charlie, as to which clan's doing the thieving?" he asked.

"It's likely the MacLarens, m'lord." Charles Campbell's mouth lifted in an apologetic grin. "I'm sorry to be disturbing ye at prayers, and this well into the eve and all, but if we're to have a chance of catching them . . ."

Iain closed his prayer book, set it aside, and leaned back in the pew. "Dinna fash yerself. Clan honor won't permit such a humiliation. Best we see to the task forthwith."

"Shall I call out the lads to ready themselves then?"

Though understanding for his reluctance burned in his captain's eyes, Iain knew his men would leap at the chance to avenge the thievery. They'd be eager for a late night's rousing ride, thirsty for retribution against a band of other clansmen likely out for naught more than a bit of excitement and a few cattle to prove the mettle of their manhood. Still, the crofters who had lost their beasts were poor folk and could hardly spare even one less animal. Even more importantly, they were Campbells and looked to him, as their laird, for a reckoning.

"Was any crofter seriously injured or killed?"

Momentarily, Charlie's weathered brow furrowed in thought. "Nay. Daniel, the smithy, was banged upside his head, and old Angus got a foot stomped on by a passing horse, but no one was much in the mood to defy armed men. Most just stood back and watched."

Things might not go quite as peaceably for the MacLarens, Iain well knew. Once his men's blood was stirred to recapture their cattle, the possibility was strong that lives might be lost. MacLaren lives, as well as the lives of his own men.

Iain grimaced. He'd had enough of fighting and death in the past two years to last him a lifetime. He'd had enough of treachery and misguided Highland honor. Yet few seemed to share his sentiments. Few Highlanders, at any rate.

"Well," he said, rising, "though we didn't start this absurd custom of reiving, we've no other choice but to end yet another instance of it." He shook his head. "As if Roddy MacLaren and his clan are on the verge of starvation, now that he's gone and wed that Drummond heiress."

"Mayhap he intends to present the cattle to his wee bride as a wedding gift." Charlie chuckled. "The MacLarens are themselves, after all, poor as church mice. And a man, even a poor one, has his pride."

Iain gave a snort of disgust. "So a stolen bridal gift is better than no gift at all, is it? Nay. I don't see it that way, and never will, Charlie."

The older man stepped aside for Iain to slip from the pew and head down the aisle of the ancient, stone chapel. "Nay, m'lord," he softly called after him. "But then, ye're not like most men, are ye? And thanks be to God that ye aren't. Aye, thanks be to God!"

✟

"R-Regan? Regan, are ye all right? Regan, wake up!"

Cold, stiff, and miserable, Regan awoke in the pale light of dawn to a sweet, childish voice. For a fleeting instant, disorientation, as thick as the morning mists hanging heavy on the air, swirled about her. Then, as she tried to stretch her drawn-up legs—and found she couldn't—remembrance returned.

She was in the garden, crammed between the high stone wall and the yew bushes that formed a backdrop for the fountain with its crumbling statue of an archer. Her gown and woolen cloak were damp with dew. Her toes, clad as they were in a pair of thin leather slippers, were numb.

"Regan?"

She looked up and, through the parted branches, saw Molly. Roddy and Walter's little sister gazed back at her with frightened eyes. Regan's heart went out to the seven-year-old. Likely she had heard the noisy celebration last night. And, just as likely, she had been awakened in the wee hours to Roddy roaring about like some wounded lion. No wonder the bairn was confused and afraid.

"I'm fine, lassie." She attempted a reassuring smile. "I was just playing a game with Roddy and Walter, that's all."

Molly's pert little nose wrinkled in puzzlement. "But Roddy's not even here, nor is Walter. So why are ye still hiding?"

Good question. "Och, well, I suppose I dozed off while I was waiting. But now there's no reason to hide anymore, is there?"

"Nay, there isn't."

With a sigh, Regan rolled to the side and crawled from her hiding place. It was past time she face the world again, whatever time it actually was. Fortunately, no one was about in the garden, and the mists effectively blanketed her from view of the tower windows.

As she climbed to her feet, however, a chill breeze swept through

14

the little, enclosed courtyard, sending needles of ice to pierce her sodden garments. Regan shivered and wrapped her arms about her. If she wasn't careful, she'd surely catch the ague from the past night's sorry refuge in the garden.

Served her right, she supposed, for running out on Roddy last eve. Not that he had long remained in his drunken stupor. Scarcely a half hour later her husband had roused and taken to storming though Strathyre House, shouting her name and demanding she join him posthaste. For his efforts, Roddy had stirred anew his still-inebriated clansmen, who had then proceeded to add to the pandemonium.

Not that any of the blustering and threats had pried her from her secret bower. Regan was no fool. Roddy was a man changed when under the influence of liquor. A man whom she had only recently discovered she neither liked nor trusted. Or, leastwise, didn't like or trust when he drank. No matter how he bellowed and pleaded, she had refused to face him again last night.

One betrayal in her life was far more than she could bear. She'd not risk her heart again.

At the irony in that thought, Regan's lips lifted in what she imagined was a parody of a smile. Roddy's abandoned promises last night had been an unexpectedly savage wounding. It might indeed take a long time to heal, if it ever did. But she hadn't really been thinking of his shameful behavior. She had been remembering an even more troubling, long past ordeal.

Odds were, though, that Roddy and his clansmen would return soon. After a time of searching the tower house, her husband had given up his efforts to find her. He and his men had ridden off, apparently in pursuit of the nearest tavern. She only hoped the drunken lot had managed not to fall from their horses and been trampled in the doing. That's all she needed. A hungover *and* injured husband.

"Er, shouldn't we be going inside?" Molly asked just then. "It's verra chilly out, ye know."

Regan glanced down at the little girl. With a mop of long, blond curls, big, blue eyes, and the sweetest smile, Molly was the sister Regan had never had. She had been born late in Roddy and Walter's father's second marriage, and her birth had killed her mother. Regan, with the help of the servants, had essentially raised her.

"Aye, ye're right as always, lassie," she replied. "It *is* verra chilly out."

Taking Molly's hand in hers, Regan skirted the flower beds that angled out from the fountain, then headed down the flagstone path between the two, long rows of herbs and vegetables leading to the ground-floor entry. Slipping inside, she made her way to the turnpike stair leading up to the first floor, which opened immediately onto a large kitchen. Cook and her two helpers were already hard at work, preparing what Regan realized, with a start, was the noon meal.

"And what've ye been about," the older, pleasantly plump woman demanded as she caught sight of her, "to be slinking into my kitchen like this?" She shot Molly then Regan a quick, assessing glance before returning her attention to the bread dough she was kneading. "Ye look a drenched cat, ye do, Regan MacLaren. Best ye hie yerself up to yer bedchamber and have Isabel draw ye a nice, hot bath. Meanwhile, I'll prepare ye a wee bit of breakfast to tide ye over, and have it sent up. The young lord has yet to return. Ye've still time to prepare yerself, not to mention gather yer wits about ye."

Regan could feel the warmth flood her cheeks. She looked down at Molly. "Why don't ye go over and see if Sally has any sweets left from last eve's meal?"

The little girl seemed to like that idea and scampered off. Once she reached Sally's side, she tugged on the woman's apron.

"And why would I be needing to gather my wits about me?" Regan asked then, sidling up to Cook even as she faced the humiliating realization that her and Roddy's marital spat was indeed known by all.

"Why else than to show that man of yers the proper way of

things?" Cook gave a hoarse laugh. "He acted the craven boor last eve, and well ye know it. Ye mustn't let him off lightly. Not if ye've even an ounce of pride in ye, at any rate."

Cook meant well. Indeed, over the years living at Strathyre House she had been the closest thing to a mother that Regan had had. In the end, though, she was now a MacLaren. Her first loyalty must ultimately be to Strathyre's laird.

"I've my pride," Regan muttered. "But I'll deal with my husband in my own time and way, thank ye verra much."

The expression on the other woman's face fell. "Och, I beg pardon, m'lady. I didn't mean aught by my comments. Of course ye must deal with the young lord as ye see fit."

She had bruised Cook's feelings. Compunction filled Regan. "Och, I didn't mean aught by my unkind comments! I value yer advice, truly I do. It's just that . . . well, I've a lot to think on before Roddy returns."

"Aye, that ye do." Cook smiled in sympathy. "And it'll all go better after ye've had a bite to eat and a nice, hot bath." She made a shooing motion with her flour-dusted hands. "So off with ye now. Just as soon as ye hie yerself to yer room, I'll send up my two lasses with the buckets of water."

Regan's mouth quirked in gratitude. "Thank ye. I don't know what—"

A cry went out from high overhead. It was the sentry walking guard on the tower house parapet. Regan and Cook's gazes met. It was surely Roddy and his men, headed home at last from their night's escapades.

Now that the moment was upon her, Regan wasn't so certain she was up to facing her husband. Perhaps it was best to take to her chambers for a time, then find Roddy in a less public moment. But that smacked of some beaten dog slinking away to hide, and she had nothing to hide or be ashamed of.

She squared her shoulders and lifted her chin. "The time for gathering my wits, I see, has passed. I must go and greet my husband."

Understanding flared in Cook's eyes. "Aye, m'lady, ye must. Naught else would be fitting, would it?"

"Nay, it wouldn't." Regan hesitated, her glance alighting on Molly now seated at the table, her face smeared with strawberry jam from one of the tarts she was eating. "Best Molly stay down here. Until I've had a chance to speak with Roddy."

Cook nodded. "Aye, best she does. We'll keep an eye on the lass, we will."

"My thanks." With that, she turned and left the kitchen.

Though Regan's intent to have it out with her husband had sounded confident back in the kitchen, as she made her way to the stairs, then up another flight to the Great Hall where she intended to await the men, fresh doubts assailed her. How should she receive Roddy? What should she say, or should she say aught at all? Might it not be best just to let him do all the talking?

One thing was certain. He must understand, and understand thoroughly, that his behavior last eve was reprehensible and wouldn't be tolerated ever again. He must, or there was no hope of salvaging their marriage.

She removed her cloak and laid it on a bench as she passed into the Great Hall. Her gown was still damp, but no one would likely notice in the excitement of the homecoming. There wasn't aught to be done about her hair, but then, the dampness only made the thick mass of chestnut locks even wavier, and Roddy was well used to that. Regan doubted he'd note aught amiss in her appearance.

Drawing up before the hearth fire, she first took a seat in one of the high-backed, carved wooden chairs placed there. Finally, however, when it began to seem Roddy and the others were taking an interminable amount of time to come inside, she stood and began to make her way across the wide expanse of rush-covered floor. Before she could traverse even half of the room, however, the MacLarens walked in.

Regan jerked to a halt. Between the double file of clansmen, they carried what looked to be a length of tautly stretched plaid. For an instant, she stared at them in puzzlement. In the yet gloomy day, it was difficult to make out what they carried between them. Then, as the men drew nearer, Regan saw a body lying on the plaid.

She noted now that many of them were bloodied, their shirts torn, and some wore bandages. Fear stabbed through her. What had they been about last eve?

Her glance searched them more closely now, seeking but one face in the mass of men approaching her. Walter, his face twisted in anguish, strode along at the side of one of the men carrying an end of the plaid. Regan's hand went to her throat. Nowhere did she see Roddy.

And then she knew. They carried Roddy!

With a strangled cry, she ran to them, shoving her way past the men, crowding up to stand beside her husband. The men halted, and she could finally see what had been hidden before. Roddy lay there, pale and unmoving. She reached out, touched his cheek. It was cold.

"How?" Regan forced out the word. "How did this happen?" No one replied.

"How?" she repeated on a thread of hysteria. "How?"

"He wanted to prove himself to ye," Walter said at long last, moving to her side. "He wanted to make amends by giving ye a fitting bridal gift. So we went on a wee ride into Campbell lands to lift a few fat cattle."

She turned a horrified gaze to Roddy's younger brother. "Ye . . . ye went reiving? On my wedding night?"

"It wasn't my idea, lass," Walter said. "I tried to talk Roddy out of it. Ye can ask any of these lads here. They'll vouch for me, they will."

"What happened?" Regan dragged in a shuddering breath. She gestured to the lifeless form of her husband. "How did *this* happen?"

"The Campbells weren't in a verra forgiving mood when they caught up with us. We found ourselves fighting for our lives. Finally, Roddy cried out to the Campbells that we yielded. That seemed to satisfy them, once we had thrown down all our weapons. I thought then that we might actually live through this, especially when the Campbell leader next ordered us to depart. Things got a bit confused then, in the darkness and all, and I lost track of Roddy. Soon thereafter, a shot rang out.

"The clouds momentarily parted and, in the moonlight, I saw Roddy fall. I wheeled about just in time to catch a flash of a silver pistol in the hand of the man who had just fired it. Fired a bullet into my brother's back." His mouth contorted in hatred. "The cowardly, cold-blooded knave!"

Time stilled. Blood pounded through Regan's skull until she thought she'd scream. All the while, though, a chill calm spread through her. Roddy was dead, and the man who had murdered him still lived.

"Who?" she gritted out the demand. "Who killed Roddy?"

"The laird of Balloch Castle, no less," Walter hissed. "None other than Iain Campbell himself."

2

It's strange what kinds of thoughts enter yer head when ye least expect them, Regan mused three days later as she watched the final shovelfuls of dirt tumble down onto Roddy's casket. Rather than dwell on the morbid scene of glum MacLaren clansmen or the still wailing *bean-tuiream*—professional mourning woman who had followed the coffin to the kirk graveyard—Regan chose instead to consider her current options. Mayhap it was just her way of distancing herself so she might cling fast to the tattered remnants of her control. Or mayhap she truly was, in the end, as cold-blooded and hard of heart as Roddy sometimes accused her of being.

One way or another, Regan knew she had to maintain her sanity, had to survive. That resolve hadn't changed but only evolved over the years from a childish, unthinking instinct to one of now-conscious intent. With Roddy gone, however, the only question remaining was should she continue on here or attempt once again to return to her own clan? Unfortunately, the decision was no simpler than it had ever been.

Walter had already made it clear that her place was here, that in everything but birth she was now a MacLaren. And there was some truth in the fact that Strathyre House, whether she had ever wished it so or not, had long ago become her home.

She had been only five when her parents had brought her here to stay with one of her mother's cousins, a dour-faced, imposing woman who was by then Roddy and Walter's stepmother. But only for a few months, her parents had assured her, while they journeyed to Edinburgh to attend the widowed queen, Mary of Guise's, appointment ceremony as Governor of Scotland to rule in the place of her young daughter, Mary, until she came of age. Though that day had been over twelve years ago, Regan recalled it yet as if it had been yesterday.

She had begged her parents until she was hoarse, then screamed and wept until her voice was gone, pleading with them to reconsider and take her with them. But they had remained adamant, promising to return just as soon as they could. Their departure had sent Regan to her bed for nearly a week, in which she refused to eat or be consoled. Indeed, what could be said that would justify such desertion? It was a wounding the likes of which she hoped never to experience again.

But experience it she had, but three months later, when word came that both of her parents had died of typhus. All good intentions aside, they had never returned for her. They had never even set out on the road back home, having died in some miserable, louse-infested lodging in Edinburgh.

This time, Regan was inconsolable. Though but a child, she knew the truth of what had happened. Her beloved father and mother were gone, headed for a distant place she could never reach in this life. They had left her behind. They had rejected her. They didn't love her.

But neither had Regan found much comfort or love from her two caretakers. Roderick senior had been too busy trying to provide for his family to spare the grieving five-year-old much time. And his wife, for some reason still unknown to Regan, found a strangely sadistic pleasure in taunting her at every turn, accusing her of driving her parents away and, in the process, inadvertently causing their deaths. The cruel words, however, didn't long suffice. And then the beatings began.

Not that Clan Drummond, her father's people, appeared to bear her any true sort of love either. Though at the time of her parents' untimely demise Regan had been too young even to think about returning to her ancestral home, much less even care to do so, factions had soon risen within the peevish Drummond clan over who should or shouldn't assume the now-vacant clan chieftainship. And, with several uncles to contend with—all of whom, for one reason or another, felt their claim was the most legitimate—no one had given much thought to a wee girl child's own, even more valid, claim. No one had lifted any hue and cry, for that matter, that she should even be returned from the temporary—and presumably far safer—care of the MacLarens.

In her heart of hearts, despite the brutality of Roddy and Walter's stepmother, Regan knew she had always been far safer at Strathyre than in her own lands. It was why, over the years, she hadn't ever seriously broached the matter of returning home. And it was why she gave it only passing consideration now, as she stood at Roddy's grave, contemplating what path her life should next take.

She was now a MacLaren and would live her life as one, until the day came when some other man would take her as his wife. She wasn't a fool. Her only value lay in whatever future suitors saw in her. After all, having squandered the one opportunity to become impregnated with Roddy's heir, Regan knew Walter would now inherit Strathyre and its lands.

He could never wed her himself, though, *if* he even desired to do so. Highlanders were an independent lot and frequently ignored the laws and social strictures of their cousins to the far south. The taking of one's widowed sister-in-law in marriage, however, wasn't one custom easily discarded. Especially not when the Kirk itself also frowned on such a practice.

For that reason alone, Regan had little worry Walter would ever consider her as a possible wife. Unfortunately, he also lacked the funds to put together sufficient dowry to entice any other potential husbands. Only her claim to the Drummond fortune would offer any hope for future suitors. *If* they were of a mind to go to war with her uncles over it.

In the distance, thunder rumbled. Regan lifted her gaze to the pewter gray skies. Rain was in the offing, as it frequently was this time of year. Best they hie themselves home while they still could, or soon be trudging through a torrential downpour and the resulting mud.

Not that Strathyre offered any promise of respite, Regan thought as the gathering finally began to disperse. Even on the sunniest of days, it was still a damp, dreary, rundown place. Once the seat of a mighty clan, Strathyre, perched on the shores of Loch Voil, was a superbly defensible tower house that had, in the last century, been additionally fortified with two additional conically capped turrets on opposite corners from the already existing gabled watchtowers.

As she headed up the hill toward the old stone dwelling, Regan's gaze lifted. A four-story, square tower topped by an attic and a garret story beneath its steeply pitched roof, the building's seven-foot-thick walls had withstood numerous assaults in the three hundred years of its existence. Made of local stone, the dark gray house was a sophisticated balance of intricacy and symmetry. It was also, however, a dwelling of few comforts or amenities.

The ground floor, which held storage cellars, a small armory, and two prison cells, was dark and dank, its only illumination three narrow, vertical, defensive loopholes. A turnpike stair led to an L-shaped first floor, which housed the kitchen, several more storage rooms, and a general workroom. It at least, though, had three windows and a garderobe. The Great Hall on the second floor, plastered and painted with rapidly fading scenes, was even more brightly lit, with windows in each wall, two with stone seats, a fine fireplace, and garderobes at both ends of the south wall.

On the third floor, in addition to the two, large bedchambers with fireplaces, was another, smaller bedroom in one of the turrets that had always been Regan's. Or, leastwise, she thought sadly, her room until her wedding night, when she had gone to join Roddy in the largest of the two main bedchambers. Access to the lower stories of the turrets—which additionally held garderobes—was also available from the third floor.

The fourth story was the attic. Besides offering entry to the upper stories of the turrets, in inclement weather the attic was used to hang the wash from ropes strung from the rafters. It had also been, throughout the days of her girlhood, a favorite place for her to play.

At the memory, Regan's lips curved in a sad little smile. Many the times she had escaped up there to hide from the wrath of Roddy and Walter's ill-tempered stepmother. Perhaps the woman had been dull-witted enough never to suspect the attic as a hiding place. More likely, though, with her ever-increasing corpulence, she lacked the energy to climb the additional flights of stairs on the twisting, circular turnpike.

One way or another, the attic had become Regan's haven. From its imposing height, she could peer out the windows on each wall and see for miles in every direction. Sometimes, when the weather was particularly miserable, Roddy and Walter would even deign to entertain her childish pleas to play with her. Together, they'd create all sorts of scenarios, of knights and ladies, of heroes and dragons, and sometimes, though not as often, of saints and martyrs.

High up in the lofty heights of the attic, for a short while Regan was temporarily able to set aside the raw wound of her grief, the ever-present doubts and questions about her role in her mother and father's deaths, the waking nightmare that had become her life. In those blessed, highly imaginative moments, she could almost believe her parents were yet on their way home. She could almost believe that they'd soon be reconciled as the loving, happy family they had once been, and all the misery and fear would disappear as if it had never, ever happened.

Those fleetingly happy times with the two brothers, however, had soon faded. Roddy's interests rapidly turned to more carnal ones, and he began spending what seemed both day and night pursuing every maiden in sight. And Walter, but two years younger, wasn't long in joining him.

By that time, wee Molly had been born, and Regan soon had her care to preoccupy her. So Regan watched the two brothers' escapades in curiosity, then shook her head in bemusement, secretly grateful they continued to view her as naught more than their little foster sister.

The day came, though, when all that changed.

"R-Regan!" a male voice, unsteady most likely from the exertion of running up the steeply winding hill to Strathyre House, rose from several feet behind her. "Hold up, l-lass. I need to speak with ye."

It was Walter. She heaved an inward sigh. Notwithstanding that she didn't always get along with Roddy's self-absorbed, eternally calculating younger brother, she was in no mood right now to talk. All Regan wanted to do was retire to her little turret bedchamber, be alone with her thoughts—and especially her regrets—and shed some more tears.

Still, Walter was grieving too. Perhaps he but wished for a few words of comfort, for assurance that all would someday be right again with the world. Problem was, Regan wasn't convinced of that herself.

Nonetheless, she halted and turned to await his arrival. Walter soon drew up at her side.

His dark brown eyes skimmed her slender form and, as always, Regan couldn't help but wonder what direction his thoughts were taking. She soon discarded that consideration. No one could ever really be certain what Walter was thinking. To dwell on it was a pointless waste of time.

He was as tall as his brother had been, but instead of Roddy's sturdily muscled form, Walter was thin and wiry. His hair was brown, but a drab shade, with none of the glinting highlights of Roddy's wavy mane. And there was nothing of singular appeal about his face. He was neither handsome nor ugly. The best and worst that could be said of Walter MacLaren was that he was . . . average.

"Aye?" Regan met his impenetrable gaze with an open, steady one of her own. "What is it?"

He stepped around to her side and took her by the arm. "As I said, lass. I need to speak with ye—in private. Come," he said, tugging now on her arm. "I'm thinking the library would be best."

Irritation at his suddenly high-handed manner surged through her. Did he think, now that Roddy was gone and he was laird of Strathyre, that he could begin ordering her about? But then, perhaps Walter, who had always stood in Roddy's shadow, was but unfamiliar with being in a position of authority. She shouldn't misjudge him so quickly.

"As ye wish." She fell into step beside him.

It wasn't long before they reached the big tower house and climbed the stairs to the third-floor library. Tucked in one corner off the Great Hall, it was a cozy, if windowless, room, lined with two half shelves of books, a long, high-backed oak settle, and two plainly fashioned wooden benches.

The room always had a musty, closed-in smell, but Regan didn't care. Few people frequented the little library, save for a private conversation or meeting, and so she generally—and quite happily—had the place all to herself.

She entered, and Walter followed, closing the door behind them. Regan walked to the settle, took her seat on one end of its wooden expanse, and quickly smoothed a fold of her most elegant gown, its severe lines of gray wool adorned with but a bit of lace at the edge of the high-collared neck and ends of the long sleeves. It was, at the very least, five or more years out of date compared to the current fashions at Queen Mary's court. Fine dresses these days, though, came dearly for the now almost penniless Clan MacLaren. Not that it mattered much to her. She had long ago learned to content herself with the everyday dress of a simple clanswoman.

Only the silver cross, rich with openwork scrolls and flourishes, that she wore constantly about her neck reliably alluded to her higher standing in the Scots' nobility. At the cross's center was a tiny hinged compartment for keeping a written prayer close to the heart. It was a parting gift from her mother, and though the script on the enclosed scrap of yellowed parchment was now faded with age, Regan kept it still. As she'd likely do until the end of her days, she imagined, her fingers touching it fleetingly before falling once more to her lap.

She cocked her head at Walter, who hadn't yet exited his spot by the door. "Well, what is it? Ye've never been one to mince words before, so what's holding ye back now?"

He inhaled a deep breath. "Now that Roddy's been prayed over and buried, we need to talk about what to do about the man who murdered him."

Regan went still. Och, holy saints and martyrs! What would going after Iain Campbell accomplish now at any rate? Roddy was dead, and no amount of talk of revenge or reliving that fateful night would bring him back.

But mayhap Walter needed to speak of this. And mayhap, in the speaking, it would ease a bit of his pain.

He had always kept his feelings close, not sharing much of his heart with anyone. Indeed, she was perhaps the only person who had ever been privy to any of Walter's thoughts, and even that was a rare happening. But she saw the look that had haunted his eyes since Roddy had first been brought home, already cold and lifeless. It was there still, gnawing at him like some relentless beast that refused to release its fallen prey. In his own way, Walter had likely loved his older brother far more deeply than Regan—and perhaps even Roddy—had ever realized.

"Aye?" she prodded when he chose not to continue with his unsettling pronouncement. "And what of it? Roddy's dead. What more is there to say?"

"It's one thing to die fighting yer enemy face-to-face. There's some honor on both sides in that." Walter paused and glanced away yet again. "But when yer enemy chooses to spare yer life and sends ye on yer way, only to then backshoot . . ."

For a long moment, Regan just stared at him. She knew now where Walter was going with this. Roddy's murder was grounds for a feud. No Scotsman worthy of calling himself a Highlander would deny there wasn't just cause to call out the clan. But to go up against the mighty Campbells . . .

"Aye, ye're right." Regan expelled a long, slow breath. "At the verra least, Iain Campbell must be brought to justice."

Walter gave a harsh, high-pitched laugh. "And who'd dare bring the Campbell clan's tanist to justice? He's cousin and dear friend to the clan chief, and once even saved his life." He shook his head with a savage vehemence. "Nay, we'd get no support from anyone in accusing one of the Campbell nobility. The queen dotes on those two, she does."

Regan knew Walter spoke true. As if Mary's favor in itself didn't squelch any hope of legal justice, Niall and Iain Campbell were both powerful lairds in their own right, owned highly fortified castles, and could commandeer hundreds of men with but a few days' notice. And if the MacLarens declared a feud, clan loyalty would then require the entire Campbell clan join with their two clansmen.

"Aye, we've no hope of bringing Iain Campbell to legal justice," she finally replied. "Yet, in all honor, we're bound to do *something* to avenge Roddy's murder. And murder it is, now that we know how he truly died."

A grim smile tugged at the corners of Walter's thin lips. "There are many forms of justice, some legal and some not. But the final result's the same."

As if a chill breeze had found its way into the room, Regan shivered. "What are ye suggesting?"

He chose that moment to walk over to stand before her. Presentiment brushed Regan before skittering away to cower in some dark corner of the room. She looked up and met his suddenly piercing gaze.

"Iain Campbell must suffer the same fate as Roddy. It's only fair, wouldn't ye say?"

"Aye," she replied warily. "But because he's a cold-blooded murderer doesn't mean we have to become one in the doing."

"Och, lass, lass!" With an exasperated sound, he took a seat beside her on the settle. "It's not murder. It's justice! The only difference is, instead of taking him to the High Court in Edinburgh for trial and hanging, we'll instead be his judge and executioner. And only because there's no other way *to* bring him to justice."

She eyed him with misgiving, even as a part of her agreed with him. Iain Campbell, because he *was* a Campbell, would indeed likely get away with his cowardly attack on Roddy. And a part of her dearly desired revenge. But it wasn't just because Roddy had died. It was also because she felt she had played a part in his death. If she hadn't rejected him, run and hid where he couldn't find her . . .

Somehow, the act seemed nearly one and the same with whatever she had done long ago to drive away her parents.

As if summoned by her memories, Roddy's voice came to Regan, still unsteady from the copious amounts of liquor he had imbibed that night, plaintively calling for her. Calling for her like some wounded child—like a child she had once been—confused and hurt because he had been left alone, and he couldn't quite comprehend why. If only . . . if only . . .

Tears welled at the recollection. With a savage effort, she choked them back and forced herself to return to the matter at hand.

"What ye propose is verra dangerous," she said. "Even if ye were to succeed, ye could be discovered. And then the Campbells would descend on us like a plague of locusts. All honor aside, is it worth the risk to the clan?"

"It is to me. And it's not just for Roddy, ye know. It's for ye too."

"Me?"

"Aye, sweet lass." As he spoke, Walter lifted a hand and, with his fingertip, tenderly stroked her cheek. "I know ye well, I do.

Yer heart's aching for Roddy, but it aches as well over yer guilt in sending him out that night."

It was as if his finger had suddenly turned to flame. Regan jerked away. "I-I don't know what ye're talking about!"

"Aye, but ye do, lass," he said, his voice deepening to the thickest honey. "I know what ye did. I heard my brother staggering through the house, calling for ye. He loved ye, he did, and he thought ye'd abandoned him."

She turned away from him then. *Please, don't say that. Please, don't make me remember . . .*

"It wasn't like that," Regan whispered, wrapping her arms about her. "I just . . . just wanted to give him time for the whiskey to leave him. He wasn't himself that night. I don't know why, but he just wasn't my Roddy."

Hands settled gently on her shoulders. "Wheesht, lass. I know. I only said what I did because I wanted ye to understand why this is so important to me. I wouldn't do this for any other reason. I'm not a bloodthirsty man. But I also won't stand by and see what matters most to me ruined."

A great weariness crushed down on her. She didn't know how to sort through this terrible mess anymore. What, indeed, *was* the right thing to do, and what was wrong? Where was there any fairness in any of it?

"Do what ye think is right," Regan said at long last. "Whatever happens, it's only just."

"Aye," Walter murmured, a strange, oddly triumphant note in his voice. "It's only just."

✠

The attack on Iain Campbell took a time in coming. Walter wasn't fool enough to ride up to Balloch Castle and demand a battle to the death with the Campbell chief's finest warrior. His particular gifts lay in less physical pursuits than sword practice and sweat. Which was well as it should be. As the days, then weeks, passed,

Regan had a gradual change of heart and began to hope he'd not hold fast to their plan.

Finally, Walter's spies returned with news that the Campbell tanist would depart in two days' time for a short visit to the nearby town of Fortingall. Walter immediately moved to gather his men for the long-planned ambush.

By midday, they were armed and ready to depart. Watching them mount up from the front door of Strathyre House, Regan was filled anew with misgiving. Too many times to count in the past weeks, she had reconsidered her acquiescence to Walter's bloodthirsty plan. If anything went wrong with this undertaking, after all, it wouldn't bode well for Clan MacLaren.

He must have seen the uncertain expression on her face. After a few final words to his captain of the guard, Walter strode over.

"A wee kiss for the departing hero?" he asked, taking her by the shoulders.

"Aye," she murmured distractedly and allowed him to press his lips to her cheek. When he finally pulled away, however, Regan met his dark gaze. "Are ye certain this is the best of all solutions? The more I think on this plan of yers, the more uneasy I feel. Mayhap we should—"

"Wheesht, lass." He pressed a gloved finger to her lips. "It's natural for ye to have yer doubts and fears. It's the way of women. That's why it falls to men to be the doers of the braw deeds. Once we make up our minds, we don't waste time wondering if it's the right decision. We take action."

Stung by his belittling appraisal of her reservations, Regan opened her mouth to speak her mind. Then she thought better of it. What, indeed, did she know of men's ways when it came to things of this nature? The only weapon she had ever learned to use was a bodice knife, and that but in self-defense. She truly didn't have any better solution for what to do about Iain Campbell.

Regan pulled his hand away. "Then at least promise me ye'll

abort this plan if it appears there's any chance of failure. There'll be other opportunities. Don't risk yerself needlessly."

"Och, and is that concern I hear?" he asked, a broad grin splitting his face. "One would almost imagine ye'd feelings for me."

There was something behind that lightly given statement that troubled Regan. A fleeting expression of eager expectation, of primal hunger? Whatever it was, the look was so quickly hidden that she questioned what she had really seen.

"Ye're my brother and the only one, besides wee Molly, who's left now of my true family," she chose to reply instead. Lifting on tiptoe, Regan gave him one final hug, then released him and stepped back. "What would Molly and I do if we lost ye too?"

"Well, that'll never be." He grinned. "I'd crawl back on my hands and knees, I would, to return to a bonny lass such as ye."

Walter paused to don his blue bonnet and adjust it until the large, soft, woolen cap sat somewhat sideways on his head. As the new laird of Strathyre House and its lands, and hence a gentleman of the nobility, he now proudly wore one eagle feather on his bonnet. Indeed, it gave even plain-faced Walter a certain flair that he had never possessed before.

Regan knew he had long desired that feather, which, until a few weeks ago, had been the sole prerogative of his brother. But no more, she reminded herself as she watched him turn and swagger off to mount his horse. Naught was as it had once been. Naught would ever be the same again.

In those minutes that next passed, Regan's emotions ranged far and wide. Then, with a shout, the men reined their horses around and rode away. The wind picked up and, as if a shroud had passed over the sun, clouds darkened the sky. She shivered, as much from the sudden chill as from the unreasoning fear that washed over her.

"Ye're wrong to let him go," a gravelly voice rose from over her shoulder.

She wheeled about and found Father Henry standing there. The bald, old priest, his threadbare, black robes fluttering about his ankles in the rising wind, stared calmly back at her. Guilt flooded her.

"Ye know Walter well enough to know he'll do what he wants." Regan brushed a lock of dark cinnamon-colored hair from her eyes. "And justice must be done."

"Aye, justice," the elderly priest said. "But whose justice does Walter truly go out to mete? His or the Lord's? The murderer shall surely be put to death, but mayhap not in the time or manner ye now imagine. And it may not even be the man ye imagine."

He turned then to leave. Regan reached out and grabbed his arm.

"What do ye mean?" she asked, her voice going taut with apprehension. "And what have I to do with it?"

Father Henry looked deep into her eyes. "Lassie, ye stand on a threshold this day. Whatever ye do or do not do, ye can never turn back. I only pray that ye choose the true path. The path that, in the end, will lead ye where ye've always been meant to go."

"And where exactly would that path lead me?" she demanded hoarsely, her heart hammering, her palms going damp.

With the gentlest of touches, the priest pried her fingers from his arm. "Wherever ye wish, dear child. To yer healing and happiness, if only ye've the courage to face and survive the journey. If only ye discover who ye've always been meant to be."

3

Mathilda Campbell, hands on her hips, glared over at her son. "Well, ye've the luck of a charmed man, ye do, and once more have managed to escape the matrimonial snares I've laid for ye. Thanks to this foul weather, there'll be no visiting Lord Fleming and his family this day. And, since they're hoping to set out for Edinburgh on the morrow . . ."

"Och, don't go on so, Mither." With a wry twitch of his lips, Iain turned from the deep, stone-cut window overlooking Balloch's inner courtyard and his view of the rain sluicing down from the leaden skies. "If the truth be told, when have I once refused to meet any of the bonny lasses ye've chosen for me? Can I help it if, this time, the capricious Highland weather—which ye've allowed to cancel yer plans for the trip to Fortingall, not I—prevents my willing participation? Or that Lord and Lady Fleming choose to race through this part of the Highlands, with barely a pause in their journey?"

"Nay, ye're a good son, ye are," Mathilda Campbell replied, then shook her head and sighed. "Meeting someone's a far, far cry from courting, though, and nearly a lifetime away from marriage. And correct me if I've misstated the situation, but ye'll be a score and eight in another two weeks and have yet to take a wife. Why, oh why, won't ye have pity on yer poor mither and make her a grandmither?"

"And would that be with or without the services of a wife?" He shot her a grin, then walked to the small table beside the hearth in his mother's bedchamber. A pottery pitcher of sweetened, mulled cider and two cups stood there. "Care for a wee sip?" Iain asked, holding the pitcher aloft.

"Nay." His mother shook her head once more. "I'm so restless and frustrated I fear naught will satisfy me this day. I'd so looked forward to that visit—and not just for ye to meet Fleming's two marriageable daughters. After all those years in Edinburgh, I confess I still miss the stimulation of court life."

Iain made a sympathetic sound and proceeded to pour himself a cup of cider. After nearly ten years at Court, his high-spirited, gregarious mother must indeed find it difficult to adapt to the far quieter, commonplace life of a rural estate as was Balloch's. Not to mention that the castle, which she had first come to as the new wife of its laird, Duncan Campbell, likely still held many painful memories.

His father, after all, had been a distant, coldhearted, self-serving man. A man who bore no loyalty to family, be it to his older brother, who had been clan chief, nor his nephew, whom he had plotted against for years to prevent from him ever assuming the clan chieftainship, nor even his wife and son, whom he had used to his own ends as well.

But that had all ended with Duncan Campbell's death now almost two years ago. Well, all but the lingering pain and anger, at any rate, which Iain struggled with still, as he knew did his mother. Though her strong religious faith never permitted her to sever her marital vows, she had finally put a physical distance between herself and her philandering husband by moving to Edinburgh to serve the then-regent, Mary of Guise. After the queen mother's death in 1560, Mathilda had remained on in Edinburgh until the daughter, named Mary as well, arrived from France to take up the throne of Scotland.

By the end of 1565, however, Mathilda had finally had her fill of all the political intrigue and machinations of the Scottish court, not to mention the increasingly unpleasant presence of Queen Mary's alcoholic and adulterous second husband, Henry, Lord Darnley. Indeed, she had eagerly accepted Iain's invitation to return home to Balloch.

Nonetheless, though it was apparent his mother was glad to be rid of the less savory aspects of court life, Iain knew she struggled still, even after six months, to find enough here to entertain her. It was likely why she had taken to playing matchmaker with such zeal.

"Mayhap we can pay Niall and Anne a wee visit," he said by way of consolation. "Indeed, it's been nearly a half year since I was last at Kilchurn. Niall will begin to view me as a shoddy tanist if I don't soon make an appearance there."

"Truly?" His mother wheeled around and hurried over to join him. "We can pay Niall and Anne a visit? When? And for how long might we stay?"

Iain took a deep swallow of his cider, then lowered the cup and smiled. "Och, at least a month, so as I can assist Niall with any pressing issues he'll be needing my help with. One way or another, we have to return home before the harvesting begins."

"It'll be time enough, it will." Mathilda smiled in happy anticipation. "And mayhap Anne will have a few eligible lasses in mind for ye to meet while we're there. I'm certain she wants to see ye happily wed as dearly as I do."

"Aye, mayhap she will," Iain murmured, then took another sip of his cider.

His thoughts flew to Niall's beautiful, silver-eyed and auburn-haired wife. He had been in love with her himself and, along with Niall's suspicions that Iain was involved in the treachery that swirled around him at the time, Iain's friendship with Anne had caused a serious and almost fatal rift between them. But Anne's love for Niall had never faltered. Even Iain finally had to face the inescapable fact that Anne would never be his.

It was one of the reasons he had kept his distance from Kilchurn for nearly a year after his father's death, in as much to allow his wounded heart to heal as to permit Niall the time he needed to solidify his position as the new Campbell clan chief, without *his* presence to muddy the waters. It was the least he could do after all the trouble he had caused his cousin, however inadvertently. For Niall *and* for himself.

Problem was, though Iain had finally come to terms with his unrequited love for Anne Campbell, he still compared every woman he met to her—and all had been found lacking. Despite his mother's untiring efforts to the contrary the past several years—for she had worked as tirelessly in absentia as she had in person—Iain was beginning to wonder if he'd ever find a woman to equal Anne. And he wouldn't wed unless he did.

"There's a woman out there for ye, son," Mathilda's voice came of a sudden, drawing Iain back to the present. "A woman who'll be yer soul mate until the end of yer days. A woman chosen just for ye by the dear Lord above."

"Aye, I'm sure there is," he said softly. "It's one of my most frequent requests of the Lord, it is. I but hope to have the good sense to recognize her when the Lord finally does bring her to me."

Iain set down his cup and walked back to the window. *If He ever does*, he silently added, staring once more at the rain pouring from the skies.

✝

Regan rode hard and fast, following the trail left by Walter and his men until the rain came and washed it away. Then, when she was finally drenched through to her skin, the winds picked up, chilling her clear to her bones. The meager sunlight soon faded as the day drew on to dusk. She was finally forced to slow her mount to a walk or risk the animal stumbling on the now mud-slick cow track.

Darkness fell. Clouds scudded across the moon, blocking its light more often than not. After a time, Regan began to wonder if she were even on the path anymore, or headed in the correct direction. Her teeth chattered, her fingers and toes grew numb, and she alternately cursed Walter for his foolish plan and herself for thinking she'd had a chance of catching up with him, much less stopping him.

For a time, the wind lessened. Moonlight managed to thrust past the clouds, and she thought she might yet find her way up the northwestern side of Loch Tay along the route Walter had told her he and his men would take. And then thunder rumbled, the wind quickened once more, and the rain came again. This time, though, lightning accompanied it.

At first, the bolts of light danced several miles south of her. But not for long. As she entered yet another stretch of forest, the thunder lumbered ever closer, until the air fairly sizzled with repeated, jagged flashes. Her horse alternated rearing in terror and threatening to race off with her. It was time to take shelter, but where?

The trees offered no haven, yet she was just as vulnerable out in the open. What she needed was to find a cave or rocky over-hang under which to hide. As the trees once more thinned, Regan searched the surrounding hills now looming before her. Then, blessedly, a burst of lightning illuminated the terrain, and there, up a gently sloping hillside, was a dark opening in a large jumble of boulders. An opening at least large enough for her, if not also for her horse.

She reined her mount to the left and urged it up the hill. Around her, as if the storm had decided to unleash at last the full force of its fury, lightning struck. The air crackled. An ear-splitting explosion engulfed her.

Her horse squealed in terror, reared, and, in the slippery grass, lost its footing. Regan scrambled up on the animal's neck, throwing her weight forward in a futile attempt to add counterbalance and keep the horse from toppling over. Almost overhead now, lightning exploded again. The animal shrieked, lurched to one side, and fell.

The last thing Regan remembered was trying to leap free, but her foot caught in the stirrup. Then her head struck hard, and everything went black.

✠

Iain closed the ledger, set down his quill pen, and, with a sigh, leaned back in his chair. The rain that had begun yesterday had continued off and on through most of the night, culminating in a horrific storm before finally ceasing. In its wake, however, the moisture-saturated air had given rise at dawn to heavy fog. Even now, nearly midday, though the sun and bits of blue sky were at last peeking through the dense vapors, mist still lay heavy in the low spots, swirling and churning like steam rising off some witch's brew.

It was past time, Iain supposed, that he ride out and meet with his farmers about the status of the grain fields. Then he needed to check on the progress of those drainage ditches, not to mention he had yet to get in much sword practice this week.

Balloch Castle's laird shoved from his chair. There were always responsibilities to keep a man occupied. Responsibilities he had assumed at an early age, thanks to his father's decided lack of interest in Balloch and its lands. But then, Duncan Campbell had always had bigger fish to fry and no time for the simple cares of a country laird, much less those of a husband and father.

Iain, on the other hand, was quite content living at Balloch and working hard to improve its lands and the lot of his people. Life was difficult enough in the Highlands, a vast amount of the ground either rocky and ill-suited for farming or consumed by inland sea lochs, marshes, and peat bogs. Still, there was much that could be done if one but took the time, studied the land, and patiently coaxed out its fullest potential. Much like the care required to please a wife and raise a son.

His mouth twisted in grim irony. His father had been blessed early in life with a wonderful, loving wife and excellent mother for his son, and he had all but tossed her aside after a few short years. And *he*, who wanted with all his heart to find such a woman, had yet to do so.

Not that the women weren't there for him. He just couldn't seem to discover the soul mate he sought in the bevy of eager but largely empty-headed beauties who came his way. He was yet a man in his prime, though, and his mother and Anne frequently assured him there was still hope.

In the meanwhile, naught was accomplished in mournful thoughts or pointless worrying. There was work to be done, and lots of it. He had best—

A fist rapped smartly at his door.

"Aye?" Iain called.

"It's Charlie, m'lord. There's a problem downstairs. Seems one of the crofters was out chasing down a runaway cow and came upon this woman . . ."

Frowning in puzzlement, Iain strode immediately to the door. "Aye?" he asked when he had opened it to confront the older man. "And what of this woman? Is she dead or injured?"

"Och, aye. She's injured, and no mistake. Angus found her lying beside her horse, who was grazing quite peacefully. The lass's foot was still caught in a stirrup." Charlie stepped aside and motioned for him to go ahead of him. "Angus thinks she was dragged a goodly distance, and she looks in a verra bad way."

"And where is this woman now?"

"In the Great Hall, m'lord."

"Fetch my mither," Iain said. "In the meanwhile, I'll go down to see the lass."

Charlie nodded. "Aye, m'lord." He then turned on his heel and strode away.

These things happened from time to time, Iain knew. A herdsman was trampled, a maid was kicked while milking a cow, or a rider either fell from his horse or suffered some similar accident. As he hurried down the corridor and then the broad sweep of stairs leading to the second floor and the Great Hall, Iain chastised himself for not asking Charlie who the woman was and if her family had been notified. But no matter. He knew every clansman and woman who lived on Balloch's lands. Once he saw her, he'd soon ascertain her identity.

She was lying on a shabby blanket atop one of the trestle tables in the Hall. A small group had gathered around her, their voices low and solemn. They quickly parted, however, when Iain drew near.

A quick appraisal was all he needed to ascertain this woman was indeed in a bad way. Her hair was long and colored a deep chestnut shot with red. It was also tangled, smeared with bits of leaves and a generous coating of mud. Dried blood from a few deep cuts and some nasty abrasions had mingled in several spots with the mud, leaves, and hair.

Her skin was fair and had taken on a pallid cast, in stark contrast to her blue lips. Her nose was short and pert, and appeared the only place on her face not bruised and swollen. The ankle that had likely been caught in the stirrup was canted oddly, and Iain felt certain it was broken. Her long woolen cloak was dirty and torn, as was the gown she wore beneath it.

And he didn't recognize anything—from her features to her clothing—about her.

From the head of the stairs, Iain heard his mother, accompanied by one of her maidservants, heading their way. He looked about him.

"Gather up the blanket ends and let's take her upstairs. Gently now," he was quick to caution when the four burly men proceeded to jerk the woman up rather roughly from the table. "She may be as badly injured within as she is on the outside. We don't need to make matters worse."

Mathilda was at his side before they were halfway back across the Great Hall. "Whatever happened to the poor lassie?" she asked, drawing up to walk beside the girl.

"Seems she was injured in being dragged by her horse. I'd hazard a guess she was caught out in that storm last night, and her horse spooked."

As they entered the entry area and better light, Iain cast a sharper look at the woman. She was indeed a lass, he now realized, no more than twenty. Her frame was slender, and she wasn't overly tall. Her clothing, he now realized, wasn't elegant but was well made. She wasn't likely a crofter's wife, or even a servant.

His glance met his mother's. Mathilda arched a questioning brow. Iain shook his head.

"I don't recognize her."

"Well, she *is* rather a mess at present. Mayhap when we get her cleaned up, and she wakens . . ."

If she wakened, Iain thought grimly, sparing the mysterious woman yet another considering glance. She had a large purpling knot on the left side of her head, her clothing was drenched, and her color wasn't good at all. Chances were strong the woman might well die before they ever discovered her identity.

✠

From a place far removed, the woman woke to an irritating buzzing sound. She grimaced, turned away, and was immediately rewarded with a sharp pain in the side of her head. She turned her head quickly in the opposite direction, and the throbbing, that she now realized had always been there, intensified until she thought her skull would burst.

A moan rose from deep within her and was caught and strangled in the raw, dry depths of her throat. She licked her lips and found them cracked. She swallowed and realized she was parched.

"W-water . . ."

The word escaped as a harsh croak, startling her. That didn't sound like her—or did it? She suddenly realized she didn't know. Indeed, she didn't know aught, not where she was or what had happened.

"H-help! Help me!" she gasped.

She tried to open her eyes but couldn't. They felt too full, too heavy. Was she blind?

She moved her legs and found her right ankle immobilized in something stiff and hard.

Panic seized her. She tried to push to a sitting position, found her strength insufficient for the task, and flopped back like some helpless babe. A scream clawed its way upward, fighting to break free.

"Wheesht, lass," a voice came of a sudden from the blackness encompassing her. "It's all right. *Ye're* all right. Ye must just give yer poor body time to heal."

From somewhere to her right, she heard something being dipped in water, then rung out. A cool cloth touched her forehead, then was gently stroked down the side of her face. Heavenly, she thought. Och, but it felt heavenly!

"What . . . what happened?" she whispered. "Am I blind . . . and why does my head throb so?"

"Och, lass, lass," the voice, a woman's voice, came again. "Of course ye're not blind. It's just that yer wee face is so bruised and swollen that yer eyes cannot open. And, besides a broken ankle, ye've a huge knot on the side of yer head where we think ye must've struck hard when yer horse ran away with ye. But in time, the swelling will abate and all will be well again."

The woman sounded kind, motherly even. Somehow, that realization brought on a surge of tears. She felt them slip from her eyes and trickle down her cheeks.

"Now, none of that," the older woman crooned, wiping away the tears with the damp cloth. "Ye're safe here, among friends."

A hand slid beneath her head, and she felt herself lifted slightly from the bed.

"Take a sip of this. It's something our healer prepared for ye to ease yer pain."

A cup was pressed to her lips, and a cool liquid flowed into her mouth. She swallowed it down without even tasting it, desperately needing the wetness it provided, if not also the promised pain relief. All too soon, though, the cup was pulled away.

"M-more," she cried, reaching out blindly to find and grasp the cup. "I'm s-so thirsty!"

"Aye, I'd imagine ye are, lass. But give that swallow or two a few minutes to see how it rests in yer stomach. Then I'll give ye more."

As the woman spoke, she ever so carefully lowered her back to rest on the bed. For a while, all was silent. Then the woman spoke again.

"Yer name, lass. If ye'd but tell us who ye be, we could send for yer family. They'd surely be a comfort to ye at such a time."

Her name . . . Aye, that made sense. Her family would come, and they'd know what to do.

She opened her mouth to speak her name when a terrifying realization struck her. It was indeed worse than she had first imagined. Her mind was blank. She had no memory of a name or a family or even of a past life. It was as if she had never lived.

"I . . . I don't know!" The cry was wrenched from the depths of her being. "I don't know my name. I don't know who my family is. And when I try to remember, everything's black!"

She reached out, grasping at empty air, seeking to latch on to something—anything—solid and sure. Hands captured hers, held them tight. The human contact seemed the only anchor left her, securing her to the tattered remnants of her rapidly shredding sanity. So she clung to this unknown, unseen woman with all her might and sobbed until she finally slipped back into exhausted, blessed oblivion.

✝

"We've a wee problem, lad."

Brush in hand, Iain turned from his horse. It was early evening, and he had just returned a few minutes ago from his ride out to the drainage ditches. As was his way, he had immediately seen to the care of his horse.

"We do, eh? And what's the problem this time, Mither? Have vermin been found in the food stores again? Or is someone sneaking down to the cellar to tap off a few more pitcherfuls of wine?"

Mathilda gave a snort of disdain. "As if I couldn't handle such minor difficulties on my own! Nay, it's the wee lass. She finally awoke about an hour ago." She sighed. "Her poor face is so bruised and swollen now she cannot even open her eyes. At first, she imagined she was blind."

Iain's heart filled with compassion. "But that problem will surely abate in time. What matters is do ye think she'll live?"

"Aye, if all goes well and she doesn't catch a chill from being out all night in the rain, the chances are good. She doesn't appear to have suffered any internal injuries." Mathilda paused. "That isn't the problem I was speaking of, though. The lass has lost her memory. She recalls naught—not who she is or where she came from."

He grimaced. "Now that *does* pose a difficulty. In time she may well regain her memory—and we can easily care for her here until that occurs—but, in the meanwhile, her family will be frantic, not knowing where she is. Not to mention we haven't any idea what to call her."

"I've found something on her that might give us a wee clue in that regard."

His mother extended her closed hand and turned it palm up toward him. In it was a nearly two-inch-long, embellished silver cross on a silver chain. At its center, where the crosspiece met the upright bar, Iain could make out a tiny hinged compartment. He carefully flipped it open to find a scrap of folded parchment in its depths.

"I removed that while we were bathing her," his mother continued. "Most other times, I'd never have pried into what might well be a private matter, but once I knew she'd no memory, I thought this one time to take a wee liberty in hopes it might tell us something about her."

He glanced up. "So ye've taken out the parchment and read it?"

"Aye. On it was written 'Dear Lord Jesus, be ever near my beloved daughter Regan.'"

Iain frowned. "And do ye think that's her name then? Regan?"

Mathilda shrugged. "It seems as likely as any. Though she's young, she's old enough to be a mither. But why would she be wearing such a prayer, rather than giving it to her own daughter to wear? And the parchment seems well aged, so I'd wager it was written for her when she was but a child."

"But there was no surname? Nothing else we could use to at least attach her to some neighboring clan?"

"So ye're convinced, are ye, she's not a Campbell?"

He shrugged. "Nay, just that she's not ours. And several clans border us, ye know. She could just as easily be a Menzies, Murray, Moncreiffe, or Stewart. And that's assuming she hasn't come from farther south. Then she could be a Drummond or MacLaren even."

"It seems unlikely a lone woman would be traveling *that* far afield, especially on a night like last."

"Aye," Iain said, "verra unlikely without some verra serious reasons. Nonetheless, we've enough other clans close by to make this a difficult undertaking."

"Well, there's no rush in sending out riders to query those clans. It's enough we've some sort of name that might possibly be hers. And, if the use of it doesn't jog her memory, leastwise we'll now have something to call her." Mathilda put out her hand again. He laid the cross and its chain back in her palm. "It's best I was returning to check on the lass. And to return her cross to her."

Iain nodded. "Aye, best that ye do. It may bring her comfort during these first, trying days. Mayhap we should also ask Father John to pay her a visit."

"That might be well advised." She cocked her head. "And what of ye, lad? As laird of Balloch, it's fitting ye also greet and welcome her to yer home."

He had suspected that request was coming. And it *was* fitting he greet and welcome all guests to their home. Still, Iain was strangely reluctant to do so.

There was something unsettling about the lass. He had sensed it the instant he had laid eyes upon her, and he didn't know from whence the feeling came. Mayhap it was just the first shock at seeing the wretched state she was in. Yet over the years he had encountered people in far worse condition, and though sight of their pitiful forms had touched his heart, they hadn't disturbed him as deeply as she had.

It was the only reason Iain could find to justify his hesitation at seeing her again. Not that his ever-practical mother would accept such a weak excuse. For the time being, however, Iain wished to keep his true motives private.

"There's time enough to visit when she's feeling better," he replied at last. "Allow her at least to get her sight back before she's subjected to additional strangers in her bedchamber. Especially men."

Mathilda eyed him curiously for an instant, then nodded. "Aye, likely ye're right. For a time more at least, she's better off with quiet, soft-spoken women about her, rather than a big lout like ye stomping in, smelling of horse and sweat, and bellowing to the high heavens."

Though he hardly imagined himself a big lout who bellowed to the high heavens, Iain let the majority of his mother's less than flattering assessments pass. "Och, and surely I don't smell that bad, do I?" he asked with a grin.

She laughed then. "Och, nay, lad. Right now, ye smell *far* worse."

4

Late the next afternoon, Walter and his men arrived back at Strathyre House. Thanks to the heavy rains and last night's ferocious storm, the cow tracks had turned to quagmires and the rivers they'd had to ford on the return trip had become swift and treacherous. What should've been half a day's journey evolved into nearly an entire day.

He was soaked to the skin, cold, ravenous, and in the foulest of moods. And he didn't like the thought of having to inform Regan that all his fine plans to avenge Roddy had miserably failed. Even worse than losing a fight, there had been no fight at all. It was hardly the most auspicious way to impress Regan, much less commence his own courtship of her.

But was it his fault that conceited Campbell popinjay was so fussy about the weather? One would almost imagine him born in the Lowlands, rather than a true Highlander, to let a bit of rain forestall his plans.

Well, there was naught to be done for it, Walter consoled himself as he tossed his horse's reins to the stableman and strode into Strathyre. Leastwise, not once his men, who hadn't been overly pleased about reentering Campbell lands in the first place, soon began making noises about returning home. It wasn't as if he could ambush Iain Campbell all by himself.

For all his prissy good looks, Balloch's laird was a formidable warrior. Walter fingered the ragged scar on his chin. He had Campbell to thank for that, and all over some peasant wench he had taken a liking to, now six years past. He had been eighteen at the time, and Iain Campbell but a few years older. Both had accompanied their fathers to a gathering of clan chiefs and their lairds at Kilchurn Castle. Walter had found it the most impressive massing of Highland nobility he had ever seen.

He had also met a particularly bonny lass who was equally as impressive, as impressive as he had imagined she viewed him to be. Yet when he had finally enticed her to leave the others and walk with him into the forest, Walter soon found his advances most forcefully rejected. Mayhap he *had* let his anger at her teasing ways get the best of him, but she was only a peasant lass, after all.

Her screams, however, must have alerted others. One moment he was holding the lass close, silencing her with what he thought was a commanding, manly kiss, and the next he was wrenched back and thrown to the ground. When he finally cleared the scattering of stars dancing before him, Walter looked up to see Iain Campbell standing there.

With a roar, he launched himself at the other man. The battle, unfortunately, was shamefully brief. And then, like some strutting peacock, Campbell offered his arm to the lass and strode off, leaving him lying there with a broken nose, split lip, and gashed chin.

To this day, Walter's teeth clenched and his hands fisted whenever he recalled that humiliating incident. He had learned from his mistake, though. In dealing with more physically proficient men like Iain Campbell, one turned to using one's head instead of one's brawn. And, when it came to cleverness and cunning, Walter was certain he was now the match and more of that particular Campbell. He'd had plenty of time over the years, after all, to learn and practice those skills close to home.

All he needed was the right place and opportunity, and he'd have his revenge. A revenge that had grown apace with each and every recollection of what Iain Campbell had done to him, and with each and every time he saw his scar and his permanently misshapen nose. A revenge that combined very nicely with his other plans, plans he had already set into motion and had now but to bring to their sweetest fruition.

For the first time, as he paused inside the second-floor entry and glanced into the Great Hall, Walter noticed how dark and cold the house seemed. No fire burned in the huge hearth. No candles had been lit, and it was nigh onto dusk.

He frowned. Regan never let the servants neglect their duties. Something was amiss.

Striding into the Great Hall, Walter found no one about. He took the stairs and descended to the kitchen. A pot of something rich and savory bubbled on the hearth. A loaf of bread lay on the worktable, covered with a cloth. But there was no one there save Cook, who dozed on a chair in the corner.

"What's happened here?" he demanded, roughly grabbing the woman and jerking her awake. "Why's there no fire in the Great Hall, or any servants but ye in attendance?

Cook gave a squeak of surprise and leaped up, sending her chair tumbling over. "Och, by the bones of St. Columba!" She blinked in surprise, apparently finally recognizing him. "I-I don't know, m'lord. Mayhap the other servants thought that, since ye and Regan were both gone, there was no need to hang about. But I, not certain when either of ye'd return, felt it necessary to keep something hot and nourishing ready for ye. Not to mention, there was still wee Molly to feed and all."

For an instant, Walter thought he had heard wrong. Regan was gone?

His grip tightened on Cook's arm. "What do ye mean, Regan's gone?"

"Why, she rode out not long after ye, m'lord. We didn't know what to think, but she apparently said naught to the servants, for I questioned them all."

"And she's not back yet?"

The woman's eyes grew wide. "Nay, m'lord."

"And her escort? Have any of them returned?"

Cook's face turned a sickly green. "From what I was told, m'lady didn't take any escort. She rode out by herself."

Fury exploded within him. "This is beyond belief! With me gone, how could ye and the others permit Regan to leave here without escort?" He released her and motioned impatiently. "Go, fetch all the servants. Have them meet me in the Great Hall in ten minutes' time. I'll get to the bottom of this, I will. And, if any thought they've had an easy time of it for the past day, they'll soon rue *that* mistake.

"Aye, they'll rue it day and night until Regan's found and returns, safe and sound, to Strathyre House!"

✝

It took two days for the swelling to subside enough for Regan to see again. As soon as she looked into a mirror, though, she almost wished she could've foregone that experience for a week or two more. Her eyes were frighteningly bloodshot, and purple-red smudges encircled both sockets. There was a bruise on one cheek, and a wide, scabbed abrasion on the other. The knot on the left side of her head made her hair stand out a bit from her face, and though her hair had been washed, it was still an unsightly mess.

Her arms and legs ached whenever she moved them. There were several spots on her ribs, back, and hips that were very tender to the touch. She couldn't walk without being all but carried, thanks to her broken, splinted ankle. And her memory, even with the return of her eyesight and Mathilda Campbell's revelation that her first name was likely Regan, was as empty as ever.

The pretty silver cross the older woman had placed back around her neck hadn't jogged anything loose in her mind. Neither had its contents. That admission disturbed her far more than her probable name. The cross was obviously hers, even if it was still unclear who the little note was from and to whom it had been written.

But no more surprising, she supposed as she gazed out the bed-chamber's window from a chair they had settled her comfortably in after a breakfast of porridge and cream, than the fact she could look out on the rolling hills and verdant meadows beyond this castle and not recognize any of it. Surely she couldn't live that far from here. Yet Mathilda had assured her that her son, who was Balloch Castle's laird, knew every one of the people who lived on his lands, and didn't recognize her.

But perhaps it was her current battered state that made her face unrecognizable. Regan hoped so. This blank state of mind was most disconcerting. If only she could find her family, she'd be happy to accept any of their recollections about her until her own finally returned. Just to belong somewhere, to know who you were and where you fit into other peoples' lives, would be a comfort of sorts.

In the meanwhile, Mathilda and her servants had treated her kindly. The tall, gray-haired matriarch of Balloch Castle with the spare frame and gentle hands had seen to every detail. Regan's bed was soft and warm. The soups and fresh-baked breads had been both delicious and fortifying. Even if she had never before lived such a life, Regan knew she could easily come to like it very much.

But for all she knew, she could be some poor peasant woman, wed to a man who struggled to eke a meager living from the frequently inadequate Highland soil. She could have a brood of scrawny, ill-fed children, though she thought perhaps her flat belly at least belied *that* notion. Still, there was no way of knowing anything for certain.

There was nothing to be done for it but, as Mathilda had told her, be patient with herself, trust in the Lord, and focus first on her physical healing. When she least expected it—if she didn't try so hard—her memory would begin to return until, like some riddle, everything would finally be solved. And whatever her life had been, it would surely be as dearly grasped and loved as it was before.

There was some comfort in that, Regan thought, reaching up to clasp the silver cross in her hand. A comfort she must cling to with all her strength as she walked this dark, empty tunnel that was now her mind. Whatever the dear Lord had in store for her, surely it would lead—

Words, spoken by a voice she didn't recognize but somehow knew she should, suddenly filled her mind. *"I only pray ye choose the true path,"* the voice—a man's voice—said. *"The path that . . . will lead ye where ye've always been meant to go . . ."*

Unnerved, Regan glanced around. There was no one there but Jane, the little maidservant sent to remain with her and see to her needs. And Jane sat across the room, dozing in her chair by the door.

Her hands clenched now in her lap, Regan turned back to gaze out the window. The unexpected words had been passing thoughts, snatched from the depths of her memory. She smiled. Though the words had been cryptic, they were the first ones from her past. How long ago they had been spoken was a mystery, but it didn't matter. She was beginning to regain her memory!

Knuckles rapped unexpectedly on the door. Regan jumped almost as high as Jane, who was startled awake. She, however, didn't fall off her chair as did the rattled serving girl. From her spot now on the floor, Jane looked to her.

"Sh-should I see who it is, ma'am?"

"Aye, that'd be best, Jane," Regan replied. "I'm a guest here, after all, and since I'm fully clothed and wide awake, I've no justification to refuse any who might wish to enter."

Jane nodded, climbed to her feet, and opened the door. A man's deep voice rumbled some request, then the servant bobbed a nervous curtsy and all but danced back to swing wide the door.

"It's m'l-lord, ma'am," Jane stammered in her apparent excitement. "He wishes to pay ye a wee visit, he does."

He was tall, blond, and very broad of shoulder. That much Regan could tell from across the room. In the shadowed doorway, however, she couldn't quite make out his features, though he appeared relatively young. He was also, she well knew thanks to Jane's introduction of him, the laird of Balloch Castle.

"Pray, bid him enter, Jane." Regan straightened in her chair and plastered a smile on her face. A fleeting consideration that her appearance was far from passable filled her before she flung it aside.

Balloch's laird was but paying her a courtesy visit, and no more. His mother had already regaled her with tales of how busy he was, how devoted he was to his lands and people, and that it was the reason he hadn't, until now, been able to find the time to visit. Regan's mouth quirked at the memory of how proud Mathilda had seemed as she spoke of her son. But then, wouldn't any mother speak so?

At her request, Iain Campbell strode toward her. He wore a white linen shirt open at the throat, knee-high hose and shoes, and the belted plaid common on most Highland men. The bulk of the fabric, forming both kilt and mantle, did little to hide his long, lithe, superbly fit form—or the coiled strength and power emanating from him.

Still, if his imposing size and athletic stride weren't intimidating enough, as he passed from the shadows and into the sunlight streaming in from the window, his face only completed the effect. He looked to be in his late twenties and was one of the handsomest men she had ever seen.

His wavy hair was dark blond and brushed loosely away from his face to curl thickly down the back of his neck, almost to his shoulders. His eyes were a rich, deep blue and reminded Regan of the waters of some bottomless, inland loch. The expression in them, though, was fiercely assessing and intelligent. His brows were thick and tawny, his nose straight and strong, his jaw square with just a hint of stubbornness.

His lips were well molded, and as he finally drew up before her and smiled, she noted his teeth were white and even. It was the dazzling brilliance of his smile—warm, open, and welcoming—and how it spread all the way to his beautiful eyes that were Regan's true undoing.

She swallowed hard and forced herself to offer him her hand. "I'm honored finally to meet ye, m'lord," she said, her voice sounding tight and odd. "I've wanted to thank ye for yer hospitality. I don't know what would've become of me if ye hadn't taken me in."

He grasped her hand in a large, callused palm, gave it a gentle squeeze, then released it. "Ye're most kindly welcome, lass. But we would've never turned away anyone in need."

Regan managed a wan smile. "I know it's the Highland way, but nonetheless, I may never be able to repay ye. Even if I do have any money . . ."

"Well, with or without yer money, none of that matters. Indeed, we'd be insulted, my mither and I would, if ye ever attempted to repay us. What we offer is given freely. We serve strangers as if they were the Lord Jesus Himself. It can be no other way."

So, he was a God-fearing man, was he? The realization comforted her, as did the compassionate look of understanding in his eyes. The last bit of apprehension over being in a strange place without even the solace of her memories faded. She was safe.

"Have ye time to sit and talk with me a while?" Her gaze moved past him to where Jane stood by the open door. "Fetch m'lord a stool or something, will ye, lass? It isn't proper that he should be left standing in his own home."

Jane immediately hurried over with her own stool. "Will this suit, m'lord?"

Iain smiled. "Aye, it would, but only if ye've no further need of it. I'll not take yer own seat from ye."

"Och, dinna fash yerself, m'lord. It's past time I was folding the clean laundry, it was. So I've no further need of my stool."

The servant handed over the little seat, and Regan noted how she blushed and lowered her gaze. Regan couldn't help but smile herself. If Iain Campbell was always this considerate of his servants, she suspected half the women in the castle were secretly in love with him.

✝✝

As Jane bustled off to the far side of the bedchamber near the clothes chest and laundry basket, Balloch's laird placed the stool several feet in front of Regan and took his seat. He then lifted his striking gaze to hers.

"So, what would ye like to speak of, lass?" he asked.

Simple curiosity gleamed in his eyes, which only disarmed Regan the more. Her pulse quickened, and her mouth went dry. Then reason returned with a daunting rush.

Her response was worse than ridiculous. It was daft. No matter how attractive or gentle natured he seemed, this man was a total stranger. She was alone and, for all practical purposes, at his mercy. Or leastwise, she grimly added, until her memory returned.

"That was verra kind of ye to think of Jane's comfort," Regan said, casting about for some way to segue into the issue uppermost in her mind.

"Why? Because she's but a servant?" He shook his head. "Well, mayhap we do things a wee bit differently than some folk, but I find respect rendered is respect returned a hundredfold. And even if it weren't, I try to remember that we're all beloved by God and do my best to act accordingly. Not that," he was quick to add, likely seeing the disbelief in her eyes, "I do all that well most times. But I keep trying, knowing the Lord sees my well-meant intentions and forgives my weaknesses."

This man was too good to be true. And she *was* used to a far different way of doing things. Yet, just as soon as the realization struck Regan, she stopped short. How was it possible she was so sure, when she had no memories to support it?

An uneasy feeling filled her, and she firmly quashed it. The answers would come in time. In the meanwhile, she must get to the topic of the help she needed from him.

"Aye, mayhap I am one of those folk who are used to a different way of doing things," she said. "Yer way of doing things, though, has a great deal of merit. But I'm digressing from what I truly wished to speak with ye about." Regan paused to take in a deep breath. "I greatly desire to regain my memory as quickly as I can. And, since yer mither has informed me that ye don't recognize me, and ye know all the folk on yer lands, I can only surmise that I came here from somewhere else."

"It would seem so, lass." He leaned forward and rested his forearms on his thighs. "The mystery is why would ye have come so far, on such a miserable night, alone? Were ye fleeing from or toward something or someone?"

She tried to pierce the blackness of her mind to discover even the tiniest scrap of information that might answer his question—and found nothing. She sighed. "I don't know. And I want so desperately *to* know. Even if the truth is horrible, I want to know it. Only then can I begin to change my life. Only then can I live it in mayhap a better way."

Tears filled her eyes. She averted her gaze and angrily blinked them away. Had she always been so emotional, she wondered, or was this but a consequence of her injury? Whatever the cause, Regan hated it. She needed to think clearly, objectively, and she was far from being able to do so.

"It doesn't matter, lass," his deep voice came. "All the answers will return in God's good time. In the meanwhile, what can I do to help ye?"

Och, but there was such kindness, such concern, in his voice! It made her want to climb into his arms and weep out her fears and frustrations. But she couldn't. She didn't dare. Or did she?

Regan turned back to face the blond-haired man. "When I'm better, mayhap if someone could take me to the edges of yer lands and beyond, mayhap I might finally see things that would be familiar to me. I know it's an imposition, but I don't know what else—"

"Aye, that sounds like a fine idea," he said, cutting her off. "First, though, I thought to compose a letter to be sent to the clans nearest me, asking if anyone had come to them about a lost daughter or wife. I'd give them yer description and what ye were wearing that night. It might be enough to discover who ye belong to."

Gratitude filled her. "Aye, it might. It just might."

Balloch's laird rose then. "It may take some time to receive replies, so best I do so posthaste." He grinned of a sudden, and once more Regan was caught up in the heart-stopping beauty of him. "Who knows, lass? Ye might be back safe and snug in yer own home sooner than ye think."

✛

"So, ye finally managed to find the courage to pay our wee invalid a visit, did ye?" Mathilda Campbell said that evening as they dined. She paused to smile briefly at some comment from one of their guests at table, then took a sip of her wine, set the crystal goblet down, and turned back to eye her son. "Pray, how did it go?"

Iain chuckled. "Well enough. But then, ye already knew that. If Regan didn't tell ye, I'm sure Jane did."

"Aye, it was Jane," she admitted with a touch of impatience. "But she was across the room, and so wasn't privy to the particulars. And I want the particulars, as well ye know."

He cut a piece of the roast chicken that was the main course of the evening's meal, put it in his mouth, then proceeded to chew it slowly. Beside him, Iain could feel his mother fume, the tension building within her like water about to boil. At long last, he swallowed his now well-masticated meat and reached for his own goblet of wine. No sooner had he placed the glass back on the table, however, than his mother grabbed his wrist.

"Cut another piece of that meat, and yer life's forfeit," she muttered in her best maternal warning voice.

Eyes wide, Iain turned to her. "And what was it we were discussing then? I seem to have had a momentary lapse of memory."

"Don't play games with me, Iain Campbell." Mathilda glared at him. "Tell me about yer visit with the wee lass and be done with it."

"Och, aye. My visit with Regan." He exhaled deeply. "Well, she

59

seemed quite sweet, and of course verra concerned over her lost memory. I offered to help her search out her people."

"And how do ye propose to do that?"

"Well, this verra day I wrote letters to the chiefs of clans Murray, Menzies, Moncreiffe, Stewart, and Robertson, asking them to inform me if any of their clansmen come to them asking about a missing woman. Those clans seem the most likely lands from which she may be, after all."

His mother frowned. "It might take a time to see what comes of yer letters. What with waiting on the clan chiefs to get back to us, and all."

"Aye, but once Regan's in better health, I also agreed to send her out with an escort to see if aught looks familiar to her. And if that takes riding until they come to other clan borders and past, so be it."

"Good." Mathilda returned her attention to her plate and began to cut her meat. "That's how it should be. I was beginning to worry that ye were avoiding the lass. But now I know my fears were groundless."

One of her cousins, visiting from the south, chose that moment to ask a question. Iain's mother turned away from him. The two women were soon deep in conversation, which suited Iain well.

His mother had hit closer to the mark than she may have imagined. Though he had finally brought himself to pay their guest the requisite laird's visit, his feelings about Regan hadn't changed. On the contrary, and against all reason, now that he'd had the opportunity to talk with her, Iain only felt the more unsettled.

There was an aura of sadness and vulnerability about her that plucked at his heart. Indeed, he hadn't long been in the room with her before a strong urge to take her in his arms and comfort her filled him. To whisper words of hope and encouragement. To vow always to protect and defend her.

Even as he admitted to the ludicrous feelings, Iain wondered at his strange response. He had never felt this way about a woman before, not even about Anne. But then, he added with a wry grin, Anne was hardly sad or vulnerable. And she certainly wasn't helpless.

Not that Regan actually seemed helpless. But a few days since her nearly fatal accident, she was already struggling mightily to regain her memory and had even formulated a plan on how to go about it. Nay, it wasn't aught specific that gave rise to his strange feelings. If the truth be told, the feelings almost appeared to come from outside himself.

Och, Lord, Iain thought. *Surely this isn't the woman Ye mean for me to take as wife? I know naught about her, and might not ever know, if her memory's permanently gone. She could be a member of some clan who's the sworn enemy of the Campbells. She could even be another man's wife and a mother to his children. Or mayhap she's a murderess who was fleeing capture that night she was injured. In the Highlands, far stranger things have happened.*

Almost as soon as he finished the last thought, Iain nearly laughed out loud. He knew the Lord likely wished for him to wed and father children. It was the way of most men, and he certainly had never felt called to holy orders at any rate. But to interpret his uneasiness about being around some poor, if mysterious, woman as a sign from God that she was his soul mate was worst than ridiculous. It was daft!

The real explanation for his uncharacteristic response was far simpler. Her horrific condition, when they had first brought her to Balloch, had unsettled him more than he cared to admit. No person—and certainly no woman—should have to endure what Regan had endured. His naturally protective nature when it came to women and children had somehow reacted far out of proportion to anything he had ever felt before. And, as she healed and regained her memory, he'd regain his own emotional balance as well.

In the meanwhile, he had been wise in his initial decision to avoid her as much as possible. It was only proper, after all. To show exaggerated interest in a female guest would be unseemly, especially considering her vulnerable state. There was no need to seek her out again, at any rate. With minimal prompting on his part, Iain felt certain his mother would keep him well informed of Regan's progress.

Aye, he decided, returning to his meal with renewed appetite, it was all so simple really. He hadn't anything to worry about.

5

"M'lord will see ye now," the manservant said, even as he looked down his long, thin nose at Walter's less than sumptuous apparel, then opened the door to William Drummond's private meeting room and motioned him in.

Gritting his teeth against the impulse to backhand the man for stepping beyond himself in sneering at one of the nobility, however impoverished, Walter strode past him with head held high. The man and his opinions weren't worth his time or concern. He had bigger fish to fry.

Across the room, William Drummond was ensconced in a high-backed chair, his feet propped on a padded stool where they warmed before the hearth fire. The eldest of Regan's uncles, he was an impressively large man, a bit on the corpulent side if the truth be told, and close to fifty, if the generous gray at his temples and frosting in his thick beard were any indication. He was also, and more importantly, the titular chief now of Clan Drummond.

"Come, come, MacLaren," the older man said jovially. "Pour yerself a cup of claret over there on the sideboard and come sit with me. It's yet another miserable day to be out and about, what with this tiresomely incessant rain of late, and ye look as if ye could use something to warm yer innards."

Though Walter had no intention of allowing liquor to cloud his mind or spoil the intended purpose of his visit, he supposed one cup of claret wouldn't do any harm. He quickly poured himself a generous serving and then ambled over to the chair opposite the Drummond and sat. For a time William didn't press him, but allowed, as was proper hospitality, Walter to drink and warm himself.

Finally, though, Walter set his cup on the little side table and met the other man's eyes. "Regan's been gone for over a week now, and no one seems to know where she is. Has she mayhap come home to her clan then?"

William's eyes narrowed, and he leaned forward. "Nay, I've had no word from her since her letter about Roddy's death. Has aught happened to the lass?"

There was a gleam of almost eager anticipation in the other man's eyes, a feral light that gave Walter pause. He had known for a long while now that William, ever since he had all but assumed total power, had no desire for Regan to return to Drummond lands. Though clan holding most times passed directly to the son and heir, thanks to the ancient law of succession of King Malcolm MacKenneth, if there were no sons, primogeniture *did* allow for the oldest daughter to become heiress to her father's estates. And, even if William's close kinship also gave him some legitimacy to that same claim, it did little to negate the inescapable fact that he was—and had always been—immensely unpopular within his clan.

Indeed, in this particular case, there were likely pockets of clansmen who'd rush to Regan's side if and when she chose to assert her own right to this very house and its lands, not to mention the chieftainship. Yet until this moment, Walter hadn't fully recognized the hatred—and fear—William had for Regan.

His claim isn't as strong as he makes it out to be. Nor is his position in the clan as secure as he'd like either.

He filed the information away for possible future use. First things first. Without Regan, after all, there would never be opportunity to take over Clan Drummond.

"I'd like to think she's safe and sound, wherever she may be," Walter replied. He sighed. "Poor lass. If she isn't here, and ye've had no word that she's been seen anywhere else on Drummond lands, then I must presume the terrible events surrounding my brother's death have driven her away. But where else she'd go, I don't know."

"Well, as I've already said, Regan's not turned up anywhere in this vicinity as far as I can tell." William paused to take a deep swallow of his claret, then met Walter's gaze with a hard one of his own. "I don't wish the lass ill, but let's put aside all the niceties and speak of her future. A future I hope will never involve her return to Drummond lands."

Walter smiled thinly. *Here it comes now.* "She *is* the heiress of this house and lands, and first in line for the chieftainship."

His host gave a disparaging snort. "As if a lass, *any* lass, could rule this fractious clan! Ye know as well as I that I've no less than three brothers and five other cousins who've laid claim to the clan chieftainship. At best, if Regan returned, she'd soon become an unwitting pawn in one of their hands, until she was needed no more. And then she'd likely have an unfortunate accident."

"Not that I'd ever do such a thing to the wee lass," he hurried to explain when he apparently saw Walter's gaze darken in anger. "But what power I hold in the clan, I hold only from sheer force of will and might of sword. I can't be everywhere at once, however. And I tell ye true, MacLaren. I won't brook any opposition from her if she got it into her head to join with one of our other relatives."

"One would almost think ye're threatening Regan's life," he offered mildly.

"Take it how ye wish. Just know that, as long as she remains with ye and yers, the lass is safe. And be happy that I'm a generous, kindhearted man. The Drummonds could easily ride to Strathyre House and burn it to the ground, with ye, Regan, and the rest of yer family within."

Walter stared blandly back at him. "And is a clan feud with the MacLarens in yer best interests right now, what with all the opposition ye claim ye're dealing with within yer own clan?"

His host gave a harsh laugh, drained the contents of his cup, then set it aside and locked gazes with him. "Of course not, and I'd be the last man to wish a feud with my neighbors. I just want Regan, if the lass is still even alive, to remain with ye. Is that such a difficult thing for ye to do?"

"She's my sister-in-law. It's not proper she continue to live at Strathyre indefinitely. I'm not married, after all."

"Then find yerself a wife, man. It's past time ye were wed, especially now that ye're Strathyre's new laird."

Excitement thrummed through Walter's veins. "Aye, and well I know it. But I'll confess this to ye, and no other, that I've long loved Regan. I'll take her, and no other, to wife."

"Hmmm, that does present a wee problem." William templed his fingers beneath his chin, and his brow furrowed in thought. "It's not proper ye wed yer brother's wife."

"Aye, it'll require a papal dispensation at the verra least."

"Still, I've always thought that a ridiculous law. Ye're not really related to Regan by blood, only by marriage."

"I agree."

The other man finally glanced his way. "I might be of assistance in gaining that dispensation for ye. As one of Regan's blood family and all."

Walter smiled. "I hoped that ye would. It'd help the both of us, wouldn't it?"

His host nodded. "Aye. And mayhap, this time, the clan could provide a yearly stipend, since we've already supplied her with a dowry when she wed Roddy. A liberal amount to help keep my sweet cousin in circumstances more suitable to her true station in life."

It was a generous offer, help with obtaining a dispensation as well as a stipend. Not that William Drummond couldn't afford that and more. Clan Drummond was a wealthy clan. It would suffice for the time being, however.

"I'd be beholden to ye for aught ye might be able to do," Walter said. "I truly do love the lass and want her to remain at Strathyre."

"Then we're in agreement." William reached across the distance separating them and offered his hand.

Though Walter felt as if he were shaking hands with the devil, he did so nonetheless. Problem was, none of what had been discussed here this day could come to fruition if he didn't find Regan. And now, certain she hadn't come home to Drummond lands, he had no idea where to begin looking for her.

She watched them carry in the man on the strip of plaid, then ran toward them, halting at his side. He was deathly pale, his eyes closed, his body unmoving. She inched forward, watching his chest for any sign of movement, but she saw none. Then she touched him. He was cold. Stone cold.

A wail rose in her throat, bubbling up from the tumult roiling within her, escaping in a choked scream. And then, as if from some place far, far away, she saw herself gather the dead man to her and shriek out her agony. And saw, from that far, faraway place, the blood on his back, clotted and darkening with age, staining her fingers.

Regan awoke with a gasp. Her breath came in short, shallow breaths. Her heart hammered in her chest, and she realized she was bathed in sweat.

For a passing instant, she stared out into the blackened room, disoriented and terrified. Then her gaze snagged on the open window. In the distance, the sky was already losing its sharp edge of black and softening toward dawn.

Relief flooded her. She was at Balloch Castle, snug in her bed, as she had been every night now for the past two weeks. Jane was but a shout away, sleeping on her pallet in an alcove to the right of the door. The castle was well fortified, guarded as it was by the formidable Iain Campbell and his men. She was safe. No harm would come to her here.

But harm *had* come to the man in her dream, and she had played some part in it. How Regan knew this was a mystery, but she knew it, and knew it well. That this man had been very important to her was also clear. But who was he? A brother? A husband? Or just a dear friend?

Whoever he was, Regan sensed he was someone from her past. Whether the event in her dream had actually happened or not, she couldn't be sure. Perhaps it was but symbolic of some deep-seated fear or other trauma in her life. Still, whatever the dream represented, it held an important clue to her past. She just didn't know what it meant or how to interpret it.

Regan shoved up in bed, clasped her arms about her legs, and rested her chin on her knees. Perhaps if she calmed herself and didn't fight so, clawing frantically at the wall separating her from her former life, the memories might more easily return. She inhaled a deep breath and willed herself to relax and wait.

Minutes passed in lumbering slowness. The silence pressed down, squeezing in on her. She willed her ever-tightening muscles to loosen. *Relax,* she ordered herself. *Take in deep breaths. Keep yer mind a blank.*

Yet, as hard as she tried to block out the dream, it returned again and again. Panic filled her. Death . . . blood . . . guilt . . . Over and over the images assailed her, stretching her emotions until they were bowstrung taut.

She climbed from bed and, balancing on her good leg, lit the candle at her bedside. Then, hopping around and holding on to things, Regan proceeded to dress. Jane finally stirred awake and rolled out of bed. She padded over in night rail and bare feet.

"What's wrong, ma'am?" the servant asked, blinking groggily.

"Naught," Regan muttered, throwing a plaid over the simple dress and shoving her stockinged feet into a pair of soft leather shoes. "I just can't sleep. I need to go for a walk."

"In the dark?" It was evident from the disbelief in Jane's voice that she thought that idea a tad daft. "Shall I dress too, then, and accompany ye? Even with that tall, stout stick to lean on, ye're still a bit unsteady on yer feet."

The maidservant's question gave Regan pause. Though she had managed to become reasonably adept hopping about with the special stick old Charlie had made to help her keep her balance, it was an entirely different thing to do so in the dark. And where exactly did she plan to go at this hour, anyway, that would give her sanctuary from her terrifying thoughts?

"Aye, Jane," she replied. "I need ye to come with me and carry the candle to light the way."

"And where do ye intend to go at such an hour, ma'am?"

"Where else?" Regan asked softly. "To the chapel. I've a need to spend some time with God."

✝

As was his wont, Iain paid an early morning visit to the chapel before beginning his pre-breakfast walk around Balloch's grounds. It was the fitting start to his day, consecrating all his actions to the Lord, praying for wisdom and strength to be an able steward of his people and holdings, and just plain getting his mind centered on what was really important.

He knelt there for a time, his gaze fixed on the altar, his thoughts lifted heavenward, before turning to pick up the book of prayers he had set on the bench. As he did, out of the corner of his eye, Iain caught an unexpected movement. Instinctively, his hand dropped to the side of his lower leg, where his woolen hose held the ever-present *sgian dubh*.

In one swift, smooth motion, Iain turned and pointed the black-hilted stocking knife before him. Even then, Regan was just pushing herself upright in the pew behind him.

Her cinnamon-colored eyes widened. "Och, I'm sorry to have startled ye, m'lord," she hurried to say, clutching her hands protectively before her. "But I fell asleep and didn't hear ye come in, and then I didn't realize ye were even here until ye bumped the pew when ye leaned back. And that startled me awake, and I jumped up and—"

"Wheesht, lass," he said, shoving his *sgian dubh* back into his stocking. "Ye don't have to say aught more. It was but a misunderstanding on both our parts." He settled back sideways in the pew so he could face her, and cocked his head. "But why were ye here, sleeping in chapel rather than in yer own bed?"

A most becoming blush spread up her neck and into her face. On closer inspection, Iain noted her features were no longer swollen, the abrasion now but faint red marks, and the bruises had faded to yellow. She was quite lovely, from her high cheekbones and sparkling, long-lashed eyes, to the small chin and lush, pink mouth. Though her long mass of chestnut hair was a bit mussed from sleeping in the pew, it framed her face and complemented her eyes perfectly before falling in luxuriant waves down her back.

He had been wise to avoid her as much as possible these past two weeks, only catching glimpses of her at the evening meal, where she always sat on the other side of his mother. Even then, he had barely allowed his glance to linger on her before turning it away. In the end, though, what had he imagined he was accomplishing in the doing? Only strengthening his response to her, when next he met her like this morn?

A fierce yearning swelled within Iain. She was so very beautiful, and he wanted her. Wanted her with an intensity as strong as he had once wanted Anne Campbell.

And ye're a fool if ye lose yer heart to this woman, he savagely chastised himself. *Ye know naught about her. And, with yer unusual good fortune when it comes to women ye give yer heart to, she's either already wed or she'll not want ye in return. Have a care. Have a care . . .*

"It's . . . it's difficult to explain," Regan finally began, averting her gaze. "I woke from a nightmare and, try as I might, I couldn't shake it. So I thought to come to the chapel and spend the wee hours with the Lord, hoping He'd dispel the terrors."

"And did He?" Iain forced himself to ask, clamping down on his renewed yearning to take her into his arms and comfort her. "Help ye, I mean?"

"Aye. He gave me no insight into the meaning of the dream, but as I prayed, I felt better. So much so," she added with a soft laugh, "that I finally became drowsy and, as ye can see, fell asleep."

"Would ye tell me what yer dream was about? And was it aught that might shed some light on yer identity?"

Regan paled. "I don't know how it would help." She shuddered. "It was so horrible . . . and sad."

Compunction immediately filled him. "Then I retract my request. Truly, I've no wish to make yer experience any worse. I but thought mayhap two heads might be better than one in discerning yer dream's meaning. But ye should never feel as if ye *must* tell me aught. Yer thoughts—and dreams—are yer own."

She shot him a considering look. "I thank ye for that. And mayhap ye're right. In such a situation, two heads may well be better than one." Once more, she glanced away.

When Regan paused, Iain said nothing and continued to wait patiently. Taking a deep breath, she at last turned the full force of her open, trusting gaze on him.

"I dreamt of a man brought to me who was already dead, shot in the back somehow. And, though I didn't know who he was, I knew I must mourn him and that . . . that I'd played some part in his death." She clasped her arms tightly about her and shook her head. "But that was all, and now the unanswered questions surrounding this dream are worse than the dream itself."

Her glance turned pleading. "What am I to do? What am I to think? Och, what if I killed him?"

As loath as he was to admit it, the same thought had crossed Iain's mind. It couldn't help but do so, after his own questions earlier about her. What if she were indeed some murderess fleeing justice?

Yet, as he continued to stare deep into her tormented eyes, a strange certitude filled him. Regan was no killer. She might bear guilt over something she regretted, and mayhap her overwrought mind had translated that into a dream far more horrible than what had actually occurred, but he knew she was no more a murderer than he was.

Impulsively, palm up, he extended his hand to her. Her eyes wide and wary, she hesitated, then reached over to place her hand in his. He closed his fingers around hers.

"Don't do aught, sweet lass," he said, his voice gone husky. "At a time like this, as yer poor mind struggles so hard to sort through all the riddles and questions, all the disjointed pieces of yer returning memory, there'll likely be moments when things become unfathomable and even exaggerated. Aye, there mayhap might be clues in that dream, but I wouldn't take it at face value."

"But it seemed so clear, so real, like I'd seen it, experienced it before!"

"And do ye imagine ye're an evil person, lass? Are ye capable of murder?"

Misery clouded her beautiful eyes. "Nay, but what do I truly know about myself? What if my life until I came here was a hard, painful experience? What if I was wed to a brutal man who beat me? Or what if someone tried to harm someone dear to me? What would anyone do in such a situation?"

"The best they could, lass," Iain replied, his heart twisting at her quite evident distress. "But that wouldn't be murder then, would it? That'd be self-defense."

Regan withdrew her hand from his. "Aye, it would. And I suppose it's best if I do as ye say, and not dwell on it so. Time will tell, after all, what parts are real and which aren't."

"Ye can't do aught until ye can distinguish one from the other."

She exhaled deeply. "Aye. Ye're right. Thank ye for listening, and for yer wise counsel."

In her gentle way, she was signaling she wished to end this particular topic of conversation. Iain took her lead.

"Would ye like to remain here a time more," he asked, "or have me assist ye back to yer bedchamber?"

71

"Thank ye kindly, m'lord." Regan managed a wan smile. "But I've prayed all the prayers I have within me, leastwise for the time being. And I've also kept ye from yers far too long."

Pushing awkwardly to her feet, she balanced on one leg, then reached for her stout walking stick. Iain was far swifter, however, and came around to her pew to grasp her stick and hand it to her.

Once again, their hands touched, and neither pulled away. Her smile deepened, became warmer. "Thank ye, m'lord," she said. "For everything. Ye give me hope that, in time, all will be as it should be."

Knowing the only proper thing left him was to release the stick, break contact, and move away, Iain forced himself to do so. "It will be, lass. I know it."

She moved then, turning and leaning on her stick to hop from the pew and out into the aisle. Halfway to the door, Regan finally turned and looked back.

"There *is* one more favor I'd ask of ye, if ye don't mind, m'lord."

Iain's heart gave a great leap. "And what's that, lass?"

She grinned. "Could ye open the door so I might leave without having to hop to and fro doing so myself? It would aid me greatly."

He nearly knocked over the pews in his eagerness to do so, then watched as she made her way down the corridor until she turned the corner and disappeared from sight.

✠

Walter reined in his horse at the little parish kirk two miles down the road from Strathyre House. He hadn't been to Mass since Roddy was buried, and then only because Regan had insisted on the ceremony prior to his brother's burial. He didn't intend to attend today either, but he did plan to speak with the priest just as soon as the services were over.

At long last the chapel doors opened, Father Henry, dressed in all his finery, stepped out, and the few pious followers began to depart, greeting him as they did. Walter waited patiently in the shadow of a stand of birches growing by a nearby burn, until the old priest finally bid the last person farewell, then turned and reentered the chapel. Walter gave Father Henry and his straggling churchgoers an additional five minutes, then dismounted, tethered his horse to a tree, and headed toward the little kirk.

He found the priest kneeling at the railing up near the altar. At the sound of his footsteps echoing up the stone-paved aisle, Father Henry cast a glance over his shoulder. His eyes widened in surprise; he crossed himself and rose, then hurried down the aisle to greet him.

"And what brings ye to our bonny kirk, Walter MacLaren?" he asked with a welcoming smile.

"Naught that has to do with God, ye can be sure," Walter snarled. "I was told ye're the last one to speak with Regan the day she rode out to parts unknown. And, since it's been two weeks now since any last saw her, I was hoping ye could shed some light on where she may have gone."

"Och, I didn't know that she hadn't told anyone where she was headed." The old man sighed. "I'm so sorry, Walter. If I'd known, I'd have come to ye posthaste."

"Aye? So ye *do* know where she went?" With only the greatest difficulty, Walter managed to keep his rising anger in check. "By mountain and sea, man, tell me! She could've been taken by outlaws, or be lying in some ditch, hurt and helpless."

"We talked about ye going out to ambush Iain Campbell." Father Henry met his gaze with a calm, steady one of his own. "That there was no true justice in taking it into yer own hands. And then I left her."

"So she *didn't* tell ye where she was headed then?" Frustration filled Walter.

"Nay, not in so many words. But I heard she left soon afterward, so I can only surmise she headed out after ye, to stop ye from committing murder."

"What?" He almost choked in disbelief. "Ye sent Regan out after me, without an escort, riding straight into Campbell lands and a fierce storm, no less?"

"I didn't send her anywhere, lad," the old priest replied. "If anyone sent her, it was the Lord, working through her conscience."

Walter reached out and grasped the priest's cassock, roughly pulling the priest to him. "Ye old fool," he ground out, his fury boiling over now. "She could've lost her way in the dark. She could've gone in some entirely different direction. She could be anywhere!"

"I've kept her in my prayers ever since I heard of the lass's disappearance. As ye must as well."

Enraged, Walter found it was all he could do not to throttle the old man right here and now. But even that would steal precious time from setting out to search for Regan. He released Father Henry with a jerk, sending him sprawling backward to slam into a pew.

"Prayers never helped me, and they'll not help Regan," he cried. "Only action will help her now. But know one thing, priest."

"Aye?"

"If she's dead, she won't be needing yer prayers anymore, will she? And, in that case, neither will ye, for I swear I'll see ye dead just as soon as she's properly prayed over and buried!"

Walter turned on his heel and stalked down the aisle. "Think on that, priest," he flung after him, "when next ye say yer prayers!

"Think on *that*, if ye dare!"

6

As the summer days eased into late July, Regan's strength returned and her ankle finally healed enough to begin walking on it. Bits of old memories continued to arrive from time to time but in confusing, disjointed jumbles. She still lacked the key pieces, she realized, to join them all in some cohesive whole that would give her back her past life.

In no particular order, replies arrived from the clan chiefs Iain had first sent letters to, and none of them reported missing women matching Regan's description. She began to feel as if her family had fallen from the face of the earth. It was time, she decided, to approach Iain Campbell about the second part of their plan.

Though he seemed very busy of late, she finally managed to track him down late one morning, having seen him ride in with a group of his men. Following their voices, Regan made her way to the stables. The odor of manure and horse drew her up as she approached the large, open door, and then she realized that not only were the smells familiar, but she actually liked them. They were good, honest smells, after all, and came with horses and riding across open meadows and having the wind in your hair and the sun on your face.

A sudden image of herself astride a pretty bay mare, a dark-haired man galloping beside her, shot through her mind. She stopped short, grasping at the memory as it raced away and faded. He was the same man of that awful dream, now almost two weeks past. Until today, she hadn't recalled him again. But who *was* the man, and what was he to her?

Frustration filled her, but with a sigh, Regan relinquished the battle. Naught was served trying to force herself to remember. What came, came when it did, and she had finally learned to accept that. Most times, now, she actually did a pretty good job of it.

She knew she had the Campbells, Iain, Mathilda, and their kinsmen, largely to thank for that. They had all accepted her so readily into their midst and made her feel welcomed and loved.

Indeed, over the past weeks, Mathilda and she had grown so close that Regan felt as if the older woman had become almost a mother to her. And, though she saw Iain little enough, what she did see and hear about him from his mother and the servants only reinforced her growing esteem. Of late, he even seemed to go out of his way to stop and speak a few words with her whenever their paths crossed. And her feelings, which had at first been those of awe and respect, had gradually evolved to a great sense of ease and pleasure in his presence. Not exactly that of a brother or even a friend, because he always took great care not to be overly familiar with her, but, nonetheless, there was something special about their relationship.

Or perhaps it was just she was no different than half the women in Balloch and was simply falling in love with the handsome, generous, exceedingly kind man. Aye, that was it, Regan decided with a roll of her eyes. She was falling in love with a totally unattainable man, just like all the rest of them.

Striding into the stables before her foolish imagination next had her wed and bearing his children, Regan walked down the straw-littered aisle until she found the stall housing Iain's big horse. As expected, Iain was there, bent over, picking out his mount's hooves.

She watched him in silence until he had finished all four hooves and straightened, keeping a tight rein all the while on her thoughts about his fine, strong form. Then she cleared her throat.

Iain whirled around. "Och, it's ye, lass." Straight, white teeth gleamed in his sun-bronzed face. "I didn't hear ye come up."

"I didn't wish to disturb ye while ye were so busy with yer horse." Regan smiled. "Besides, I like being in a stable and around horses. It feels verra natural to me, it does."

He arched a dark blond brow. "Indeed? Does that mean ye're hinting ye'd like to go riding sometime soon?"

She laughed. In many ways, Iain Campbell already knew her very well. "Aye, I'd like that verra much. Which brings me to the reason I sought ye out. We've had no luck so far in discovering where I came from. I thought mayhap it was time to begin visiting the lands surrounding yers, if ye're still of a mind to assist me in that undertaking."

Iain paused to remove his horse's bridle and offer the animal a handful of hay. Then he walked from the stall and latched closed the door.

"Aye, I'm still of a mind to assist ye," he said as he ambled over to her and halted. "In fact, I've a plan to begin so three days hence, if ye're interested."

Gazing up at him, his sun-streaked blond hair and blue eyes a most pleasing contrast to his tanned face, Regan felt her stomach plummet to her toes. Och, but he was so tall and powerful and so very appealing! If only she was some noblewoman and worthy of his consideration . . .

"Of course I'm interested," she replied instead, squeezing the words past a suddenly tight throat. "I've imposed on yer hospitality overlong as it is."

"Then what say ye to imposing on someone else's hospitality for a time? A new setting and new people might do wonders for yer memory."

Though he likely hadn't meant to sound that way, Regan couldn't help the twinge of pain at what seemed Iain's sudden eagerness to send her away. To balk at his proposal now, though, would appear as if she were unappreciative of all he had already done for her.

"I'd gladly accept whatever ye had in mind, m'lord."

"Then it's done, and ye'll accompany my mither and me to visit my cousin, the Campbell clan chief, and his wife."

She stared up at his smiling countenance, struck dumb by what he had just said. He was taking her to stay now with the Campbell clan chief?

"I . . . I don't understand," Regan finally managed to stammer. "Yer cousin lives at Kilchurn Castle on Loch Awe, does he not?"

"Aye, that he does."

"But that's so far afield from any lands I may have come from. So far, indeed, as to be impossible. Why, it's at least a good two days' ride from here, it is."

"More like three, if one's in a party and traveling at a more sedate pace. Which we'll be doing. My plan's not just to pay my cousin a long-overdue visit but also to traverse a path ye may well have taken in coming here. Since it seems that ye're not from the clans north and east of us, mayhap ye're instead a Mac Nab or even a Breadalbane Campbell."

He arched a brow in inquiry. "It *is* what we'd talked about, riding out to view other areas in the hope it'd jog yer memory, is it not?"

The relief that flooded her almost made her dizzy. So, he wasn't intent on ridding himself of her. He was just trying to help her as he had promised.

"Aye, it most certainly is." Regan smiled. The time hadn't yet come when they must be parted, and she realized, with a start, that particular fear had gained great import over the past month. "It sounds a wonderful plan, m'lord."

Some emotion flickered in his deep blue eyes. He offered her his arm. "Come. We've lingered overlong in this less than aromatic place. Would ye favor me with a short walk in the gardens?"

Regan laughed then. "Och, I wouldn't say the stables lack in aroma, m'lord. Just mayhap not the most pleasant of aromas." She took his arm. "But a wee walk in the gardens would be wonderful. The roses are in full bloom now, ye know."

"I noticed that just the other day," Iain said as he began to escort her from the stable. "I go for days at a time so busy that I observe almost naught of the gentler aspects of Balloch. And then I reach a point when my heart and mind scream out for a bit of respite, and I make myself take a day or two away from the more burdensome tasks of being a laird."

"Such as today?"

"Aye, such as today." He shot her a quick glance, then looked back to the path leading to the rock-wall-enclosed garden. "And I'd like verra much to share a part of it with ye, if ye've no pressing duties."

"Yer mither and I were planning on spending the afternoon embroidering that tapestry she's making."

Iain chuckled. "Somehow, I think I can prevail upon her to allow me an hour or two with ye. It'll soon be time for the midday meal, and I thought that afterwards ye might enjoy a wee ride. It's past time ye begin reusing yer riding muscles, or ye'll find our impending journey rather unpleasant for the first day or so."

Regan giggled. "Aye, I imagine I would at that."

They reached the garden gate and paused while Iain slid the bolt and pushed open the little door. Then, after another pause while he closed and bolted the gate behind them, they set out down the flagstone footpath.

The garden was large, consisting of herb and vegetable beds near the back door leading to the kitchen. A waist-high boxwood hedge delineated the herb and vegetable portion from the flower gardens, in which they now walked. Purple clematis climbed high wooden trellises behind fragrant lavender bushes. Deep, purple-pink bell heather grew among bright yellow broom bushes and silver green artemisia. Cobalt blue bachelor buttons nestled among white lilies and daisies. It was the myriad rosebushes, filling the two opposite sides of the garden, however, that always caught and held Regan's attention.

As soon as she reached the first roses, she slipped her hand from Iain's arm and knelt to cup one of the light crimson blooms. She inhaled deeply of its sweet fragrance.

"Do ye know aught of roses, lass?"

She glanced up at Iain standing there smiling down at her. "Verra little, I'm sorry to say. Wherever I came from, we must not have raised them."

"Well, that particular rose is what is considered a Gallica rose," he said. "Romans and Greeks used to grow them, so of course they're verra ancient. And that particular one is known as the Apothecary rose. It can be turned into jellies, powders, and oils, and was believed to cure a multitude of illnesses."

"Indeed?" With renewed interest, Regan glanced back at the beautiful flower. "I didn't know roses were so verra useful, aside from making perfumes and as cut flowers."

"Then now ye know differently. Would ye care to learn about some of the other varieties we're fortunate to grow here at Balloch?"

"Och, aye!" Accepting Iain's proffered hand, she climbed back to her feet. "In addition to all yer other considerable talents, I didn't realize ye were also a gardener."

He chuckled softly. "I hardly have the time to tend this formidable garden, but when I was a lad, my mither taught me about the roses. She's the gardener in the family, though even she now has help in the services of a full-time gardener." He tugged on her hand. "But come, let's move on to the next variety.

"Mither liked to plant the same types of roses near each other," Iain said as he drew up next before a bush of particularly striking, crimson and pink-and-white-striped roses with bright golden stamens. "This is also a Gallica rose, called Rosa Mundi. It's said to be named after Fair Rosamund, the mistress of King Henry II of England."

He removed his *sgian dubh*, bent, cut a flower free, then handed it to her. "A fair rose for a fair lady."

She could feel the heat steal into her cheeks but said nothing and accepted the lovely blossom. Lifting it to her nose, Regan breathed in its perfume. Then, because Iain continued to stare at her with a most intense expression, she smiled and, using the rose, pointed past him.

"Are there more? More varieties of roses, I mean?"

For an instant longer, he stared at her. Then, as if rousing himself, he nodded. "Aye. Come along and I'll show ye."

They spent another good half hour touring the garden, examining and discussing roses. Regan found it the most delightful experience. She learned of the Damask rose, thought to originate in the Middle East, likely near Damascus, that was brought back to England by the Crusaders and was used for the production of attar of roses in perfumes. And she couldn't help but be equally taken with the pink and red varieties of those highly fragrant roses, especially with the one Iain called the Autumn Damask, which had a wonderful, exceptionally fragrant wine scent.

"How did ye come to own so many roses?" Regan asked after they had completed a walk around the flower garden and she had learned of yet another variety of roses, the Albas. By now, her hands were full of samples Iain had cut for her. She held a shell-pink Maiden's Blush that had an exceptionally sweet fragrance, a creamy white Alba Semiplena, as well as the Rosa Mundi and an Autumn Damask.

"Well, it began with my grandmither, actually, and my mither learned the art from her when she wed my father and came to live at Balloch. I think, aside from me, they were one of her few comforts living here."

Regan frowned. "But Balloch's a wonderful castle. Why would yer mither not find many pleasures—" She cut herself off. "Och, I beg pardon, m'lord. I didn't mean to pry into something not of my concern."

His lips went tight for an instant, then he sighed and shook his head. "It's all right, lass. It's no secret what kind of man my father was, or that he died trying to steal the clan chieftainship from my cousin, Niall."

"Och, I'm sorry to hear that. It must have been a great source of pain to both ye and yer mither."

"To be sure," he muttered, his expression going dark. Then, as if shaking off the unpleasant memories, he turned back to her and smiled. "But then, we all have our difficulties in life to overcome, don't we? And what matters is that we don't let them embitter us or turn us from the Lord and His loving ways."

At that moment, gazing up at his beautifully hewn face and into eyes that burned with such fierce resolve, Regan thought him the most wonderful man she had ever known. How she knew this, unable as she was to recall all the men of her past life, she couldn't say, but she knew with an unshakable certainty. And knew at that moment, as well, that she truly was falling in love with him.

Not that she cherished any illusion she was a fitting mate, or that Iain viewed her as aught more than a poor waif whom he, in his tenderhearted kindness, had taken in and intended to help. But she didn't care. She'd love him from afar and urequited, for she couldn't help it. What woman could, if ever she had opportunity to know him as she had?

"Aye," Regan softly replied, gazing down once again at the lovely flowers she held. "We all have difficulties to overcome. The Lord grant us all, though, the courage to find our way past them to His truths and love."

Just then, the bell rang out for the midday meal. She looked up and gave him her brightest smile. "We'd best be going, m'lord. Cook doesn't like her food to get cold, waiting on stragglers."

He laughed then. "Aye, best we should. But one thing first, lass."

She angled her head. "Aye, m'lord?"

"My name's Iain. Would ye call me that from here on out?"

Regan's gut clenched. "Aye, if ye wish, but it seems an impertinence, ye being the laird and all."

"It's no impertinence if I give ye leave, is it?" he asked, moving to her side and taking her by the elbow.

"Nay," she slowly replied, "I suppose not."

"Good. Then it's settled." And with that Iain set out, guiding her through the summer-sweet garden toward the kitchen door.

✝

Breathless with excitement, Walter paid the man and sent him on his way. After all this time, nearly five weeks since Regan had seemingly disappeared off the face of the earth, he finally had information that she was alive. He had sent out several of his clansmen north into various parts of Campbell and other neighboring clan lands, with orders to inquire after a missing lass. And all but one man had finally returned with no word of Regan.

All but Fergus MacLaren, who had stumbled onto a Murray laird with news worth every penny of the bribe money Walter had given each of his men. Though his heart had nearly stopped in his chest when he had learned the name of the Campbell who had sent out letters inquiring about a lass who fit Regan's description, one of which had come into the Murray laird's possession, it was, in the total scheme of things, of little import. What mattered was Regan was alive!

Still, it was most strange that she now resided at Balloch Castle with Iain Campbell and his mother. And, Fergus had next informed him after taking the initiative to then ride to Balloch and spy out the situation a bit further, from all appearances, Regan seemed quite happy there. She wasn't being held prisoner and could come and go quite freely. She even went out on rides with Iain Campbell himself, no less.

After some thought, and about four cups of wine later, Walter finally hit on the answer. Rumor had it that Iain Campbell had once been in love with Niall Campbell's wife, who, for a time at least, had been suspected of witchcraft. Indeed, she had barely escaped burning at the stake after being tried and convicted as a

83

witch. Perhaps Iain was in league with her, had become a warlock to her witch, and had cast a spell over Regan.

It seemed the only plausible explanation. Regan was as loyal as they came. She'd never willingly remain in the lair of her worst enemy, the man whom she imagined had killed her beloved husband.

The trick, though, would be in extricating her from Balloch Castle. Walter couldn't, after all, just ride up and demand her release or lay siege to the place. Not only did he lack sufficient men and arms, but any attack would soon bring Niall Campbell and the rest of his clan down on them.

Nay, Walter realized, he needed to find some other way to rescue Regan. But how?

✠

The day they set out for Kilchurn was clear, bright, and warm. Iain and Charlie took the lead, with Regan and Mathilda riding directly behind them. Jane had been chosen to accompany the two women as a serving maid to be shared between them. Two pack animals carried the necessary clothing, including extra cloaks in case of rain. Bringing up the rear were eight more armed clansmen as escort and protection.

Iain was heavily armed as well, with his huge claymore slung across his back, a shorter sword hanging from his belt on one hip, and a powder horn and bag of shot on the other. In addition, he had a pair of "daggs" or heavy, single-shot, wheel-lock pistols in large, leather holsters attached to the front of his saddle on each side.

He had shown the daggs to her earlier, after she had asked about the key on a long cord that he wore around his neck. The pistols' wheel-lock mechanism would fire by spinning against a piece of flint, he explained, creating a spark that would then ignite the powder. The steel wheel was spring loaded, however, and required the key or "spanner" to wind the spring each time it was to be fired. "Lose the spanner," he then added with a grin, "and ye're out of luck, laddie."

She could barely repress a shiver as she looked at the long, silver barrels with their fine wooden handles. Imported from Holland, they were, Iain said before shoving them back into their holsters, and worth a pretty penny to boot. Still, at close range, they had proven their value several times already, and likely would again.

Regan knew he spoke true. Even a journey that would take them primarily through Campbell lands was one fraught with danger. The powerful Campbells weren't without enemies, and then there was the always very real threat from thieves and bands of broken, clanless men who roamed the Highlands. Somehow, though, she felt perfectly safe in Iain's company. From all she had heard at Balloch, he was as fearsome a warrior as he was a prosperous laird. He hadn't been chosen the Campbell chief's tanist and chosen successor without good reason.

"Ye're looking deep in thought this day, ye are," Mathilda's voice intruded just then. "Are ye already trying to discern if aught around us appears familiar?"

"Och, it all appears familiar just now." Regan grinned and glanced over at the older woman. "We've only just left sight of Balloch, and Iain and I've ridden this direction several times already. But it didn't appear familiar the first time I rode out with him, if ye're wondering that. Not here, or for mayhap a good half day's ride in this direction, which is as far as we've gone until today."

"Well, that'd make sense. Considering ye were found nearly that far away when ye had yer accident." Mathilda sighed. "Likely there's no chance then of ye living closer than a half day's journey from here in any direction."

Regan opened her mouth to ask a question that had been plaguing her of late, then closed it, then decided to ask it anyway. "What if . . . what if I never fully regain my memory or discover who I truly am? Or is that even possible?"

Iain's mother shrugged. "I don't know the answer to that, child. I suppose it's possible." She smiled. "But dinna fash yerself. It's only been a bit over five weeks since ye came to us. There's still time."

"It's not as if I don't want to remember," Regan said by way of explanation. "But I can't continue to live off yer generosity much longer. It's not right or honorable."

"And has anyone at Balloch led ye to believe ye've worn out yer welcome? Because if they have, I want to know and I'll soon silence such inhospitable chatter."

"Och, nay!" Regan flushed in embarrassment. "No one has said an unkind word. But *I* feel badly about this, I do."

"And exactly what would ye be suggesting then?"

She suddenly didn't know. "Well, mayhap if there's some servant's position at Balloch that I might fill. That young kitchen helper—Bessie's her name, isn't it?—is soon to be wed. Will she be staying on after that?"

Mathilda laughed. "So, ye've got designs on poor Bessie's job, do ye? Well, though ye're willing to do aught that's asked of ye, I'm not thinking ye're suited for kitchen drudgery. Not to mention, I doubt Iain would hear of treating ye in such a dishonorable way."

"But I've my honor too!" Regan cried in frustration. "And I'm not some fine lady unsuited to hard work. Indeed, I'm not verra fine at all."

Her companion arched a graying brow. "Aren't ye? I saw yer hands when ye came to us. Soft and refined beneath that mud and grime ye were dragged through. And ye can read, lass, not to mention yer clothes, though not of the most costly fabric, weren't those of a simple crofter's either."

"Then why hasn't anyone come looking for me? Even a simple crofter's wife or daughter deserves better than that!"

Mathilda shook her head. "I don't know, child. It's most puzzling." She sighed. "Well, mayhap the answers lie just over the next horizon. Or mayhap someone will recognize ye at Kilchurn. Far more folk pass through there, seeking audience with the Campbell for all sorts of favors and resolution of grievances. If naught else, ye'll be exposed to many more faces there than ye ever would if ye'd remained hidden away at Balloch."

"Aye, I suppose so," Regan muttered even as she thought that, as long as Iain was there, she wouldn't mind staying hidden away the rest of her life.

"Och, don't go on so, child." Mathilda laughed. "Ye can't imagine the fun ye'll have at Kilchurn. Anne's close to yer age, if mayhap a few years older, and Caitlin, Niall's sister, is likely but a few years younger, so ye'll have two young women with similar upbringing and interests to spend time with. Much as ye seem to enjoy my company, surely by now ye're yearning for a few friends yer own age."

"I've been verra happy at Balloch, m'lady." Regan shot her a quick smile. "And I feel verra comfortable in yer company."

"I'd like to think we've become friends."

There was a note of pensive yearning in Iain's mother's voice. It surprised Regan. It almost sounded as if the older woman sincerely desired her friendship.

"Och, aye," she said. "I cherish yer company, m'lady. That I do. I just didn't want to presume . . ."

"Well, it's settled then," Mathilda stated firmly. "We're friends, and friends don't speak of imposing on each other. Agreed?"

She had been tricked and maneuvered into ending the issue of her overstaying her welcome at Balloch, Regan realized with no small amount of chagrin. Not that it didn't please her to be considered Mathilda Campbell's friend. It just wasn't right to become a useless burden anywhere.

There was naught more she could do about the problem just now, though, so best she leave it be. But only for a time more.

Regan turned to Mathilda and nodded her acquiescence. "Agreed."

7

It indeed took them three days to reach Kilchurn. Three days spent out in the warm sunshine and fresh air, enjoying the wildflowers blooming in the meadows, the heath washing the hills in lavender and pink, the sparkling burns flowing through the glens, and the eagles soaring overhead. Three days that she spent in Iain's company, if not actually riding at his side, and cherishing every minute of it.

Not once, however, did Regan recognize any village or town they passed; nor did any terrain appear familiar. Perhaps it should've upset her more than it did, but she was becoming used to, if not comfortable with, the memory gaps of her past. It was almost as if she had resigned herself to building a new life in the here and now, a life that day by day was fashioning a past of its own.

Since inns in the Highlands were almost nonexistent, nights on the road were spent within the safe, snug confines of the homes of local if lesser Campbell lairds or tacksmen—she, Mathilda, and Jane in one bedchamber, the men all in another. She imagined she and the other women got the best of that bargain, knowing most of the men ended up sleeping on the floor wrapped in their plaids. Not that such arrangements were unusual for Highlanders. That was how most of them slept when away from home and out of doors.

At twilight of the third day, to the eerie plaint of the peesweep and harsh call of ravens, they finally approached Kilchurn Castle.

That great stone fortress of Clan Campbell, perched on a spit of land jutting into freshwater Loch Awe, was dominated by the towering twin peaks of Ben Cruachan, which, Regan knew, was the inspiration for the Campbell battle cry of "Cruachan!" Her gaze lifted from the mountain's wooded, lower slopes, until the trees thinned and disappeared, revealing a bare, lumpy peak split into two cones. Mighty Ben Cruachan, a fitting symbol of the majesty and might of what was now one of the most powerful of Highland clans.

One side of Kilchurn's earthen-hued edifice was surrounded by grassy meadow and trees. The other sat close to the gently lapping waters of the loch. Regan thought she could easily spend hours visiting Loch Awe in the days to come, shaded by some of the trees that grew close to its edges a ways down from Kilchurn. She had always found great peace, she realized, sitting by a loch, gazing out onto deep waters.

The loch that came to mind, however, wasn't Loch Awe or even Loch Tay, which Balloch Castle overlooked, but some other loch entirely. A much smaller loch, to be sure, but studded around its edges with scattered forests and presided over by its own towering mountain peak.

For a moment, as they rode toward Kilchurn's huge wooden gates, Regan closed her eyes and gave herself over to the image in her mind, trying to put a name to the place. And, as always, even as she struggled to bring it into sharper focus, the image began to crumble at its edges and fade. Finally, with a sigh, she let it go.

As they rode through the gate and its high curtain wall defended by round towers at each of its corners, their party was greeted with a courtyard ablaze with light. Myriad torches encircled a large area that led to the steps of the keep. On those steps stood a tall, dark-haired man and an auburn-haired woman, their arms entwined about each other's waists. Beside the woman stood a girl with long, ebony hair.

"That's Niall and Anne," Mathilda whispered, leaning toward Regan. "And the girl is Niall's sister, Caitlin."

Her stomach aflutter with sudden nervousness, Regan could manage only a nod in response. As they drew to a halt, servants ran over to hold their horses. Iain and Charlie quickly dismounted. Charlie came around and graciously helped Mathilda down. Iain walked up to Regan.

"May I be of assistance, lass?" he asked, looking up at her.

She flushed. "Thank ye, m'lor—Iain," she said, not wishing to appear ungrateful for his gallant offer. She surrendered her reins to the boy who had come up to hold her horse. Then, leaning over, she extended her arms to Iain.

He took her to him without any apparent effort, swinging her gently down until her feet touched ground. His gaze was tender, and he didn't release her right off but continued to grasp her arms as if he didn't want to let her go. For a few precious seconds, with everyone bustling around them, Regan felt as if she were in a sweet, secret world that included only her and Iain.

Then he released her and stepped back.

"Come, lass," he said, offering her his arm. "It's past time ye were meeting my cousin and his family."

Hungry for some continued contact with him, Regan eagerly took his arm. "I'd like that verra much."

With Charlie escorting Mathilda alongside them, they proceeded to march up the steps, halting only when they were but two steps below their hosts. Niall Campbell grinned, then fisted his hands on his hips.

"Ye were wise to pay us a visit when ye did, cousin," he growled. "I was about to send my men to drag ye here to fulfill yer proper duties."

"Were ye, indeed?" Iain laughed. "Well, then as always, my timing's perfect."

Niall's mouth quirked in amusement. "Aye, in the past ye always were verra good at showing up at the most inopportune times. Or, leastwise, at the times *I* didn't want ye around. But nowadays, when

I *do* want ye around, ye ride off to sequester yerself at Balloch for months at a time."

"No one about anymore to take yer ill temper out on, is there?"

"Exactly!" And then Niall threw back his head and gave a shout of laughter.

"That'll be enough of the manly blustering, husband." Anne Campbell stepped forward. "Ye and Iain can arm wrestle or flay each other over a game of chess later. For now, our guests languish out here on the steps, and it's time we were asking them to come inside."

"Och, aye." The Campbell shot Regan a look of curiosity. "First, though, it's only proper Iain introduce us to the bonny lass he has on his arm. Eh, cousin?"

"This lady's name is Regan. She's been our honored guest for the past month and a half." Iain graced her with a quick, reassuring glance. "Now, may we enter and mayhap have something to rinse the dust from our throats?"

"Och, ye'll get more than that," Niall said. "We've prepared a fine feast to welcome ye, we have."

"But first," Anne injected, "we'll see ye settled in yer proper bedchambers, where ye can wash, change yer clothes, *and* have a wee drink before the supper meal's served in an hour's time."

With that she turned her husband around. Together, they led the way into the keep.

Iain grinned down at Regan. "Not much for formality, are they?"

She chuckled. "It's good to see that ye're so close, ye and Niall."

"Aye," he muttered wryly as he began to lead her up the last few steps and through the keep's open doorway, "and if we were verra much closer, we'd be celebrating our reunion rolling around on the ground, beating in each other's heads."

✝

The next morn as she lay in bed, savoring the comfort of the feather mattress after the last two nights on straw-stuffed mattresses at the various inns, Regan glanced languidly around her bedchamber. Everything in Kilchurn was so beautiful and fascinating, from the magnificence of the building itself to her bedchamber with its big tester bed, stunning wall tapestry of a forest and lake, carved clothes chest, and cupboard for toilet articles, with its prettily painted pottery basin and ewer and pewter chamber pot. In anticipation of their arrival, the stone floors had been swept then strewn with fresh rushes mixed with lavender and rosemary clippings. Everything was clean and sweet smelling. Once again, as at Balloch, she couldn't help but revel in what seemed like the height of luxury.

Kilchurn's five-story keep was large, spacious, and even more sumptuously appointed than Balloch's quite ample environs. Essentially a large tower house enclosed by a good-sized courtyard, with a private garden on the house's backside situated between the keep and the outer walls, it was similarly structured with a belowground cellar, dungeon, and servants' quarters.

The ground floor housed the kitchen and additional workrooms; the second floor, which the outside stairs led up to, was comprised of a large entry that opened on one side to the Great Hall and on the other to a library and two small reception rooms. A wide staircase at the back of the entry led to the next floor and two corridors of bedchambers, as well as the chapel. From that floor, in the rear of the building, a turnpike stair climbed to a combined garret with several large windows and the attic.

The contrast between the wealth in which she now lived and that which had apparently been lacking in her past life, however, was of little concern anymore. If the truth be told, Regan was beginning to care less and less if she ever regained her memory. Some instinct warned she might well be disappointed when she did. And, even more than losing the accommodations and the company of the refined people she now enjoyed, she dreaded the very real possibility of having to leave Iain in the bargain.

She soon tossed that daunting consideration aside and, throwing back the covers, sat up on the side of the bed. Her movement must have alerted Jane, who was busy stoking the hearth fire against the morning chill.

"Och, ye're finally awake, ma'am," the little maidservant said. She climbed to her feet, wiped her hands on her apron, and ambled over. "So, what's it to be? A nice hot bath to wash off all the road grime, or breakfast?"

"A bath, of course." Regan grinned. "If ye can rouse the kitchen staff to heat water at this early an hour."

Jane chuckled. "It's not as early as ye imagine, ma'am. It's just the mists lie heavy this morn and make it seem grayer. Sunrise was well over four hours ago."

"Truly?"

Regan felt her face go hot. She never slept so late. What would her hosts think of her? Yet she had stayed up until nearly midnight, listening in avid interest to Iain, Mathilda, Anne, and Niall's animated conversation. And that after a day's ride that had begun at first light, so as to reach Kilchurn before dark.

"Aye, truly, ma'am."

"Then breakfast is long since past. I'll have to wait until the midday meal now."

"Nay, the lady Anne sent up some food a few hours ago." Jane pointed to the covered tray sitting atop the clothes chest. "She said not to wake ye, though. That she knew ye must be verra weary after such a long journey and all."

Gratitude for the other woman's kindness filled Regan. "Then more the reason to get on with my bath. I need to seek out the Lady Anne and thank her."

"I'll be off to the kitchen to fetch yer bathwater then." With that, Jane bustled across the room and out the door.

An hour later, her hair still damp from her bath, Regan headed downstairs. She halted the first servant she encountered. "Is yer mistress about?"

The old woman nodded. "Aye, ma'am. She's in the kitchen, talking with Maudie, the head cook."

"And which way would be the kitchen?"

"Down the stairs. Ye'll find it easily enough by the smells." The servant indicated a hallway just beneath the wide wooden staircase. "Ye'll find the stairs at the end of the hall, ma'am."

"Thank ye . . ." Regan paused. "I'm sorry, but I don't yet know yer name."

"It's Agnes, ma'am." She smiled. "I'm Lady Anne's serving woman."

"Well, it's verra nice to make yer acquaintance, Agnes." Regan returned the old woman's smile. "Now, if ye don't mind, I'd like to find yer mistress before she leaves the kitchen."

"Aye, ma'am." Agnes curtsied, then turned and continued on her way.

The back stairs were easy enough to find, as was the kitchen. And, true to Agnes's prediction, Kilchurn's hostess was indeed there. Regan waited just inside the doorway until Anne and Maudie were finished discussing the menu for the evening meal. Then, as Anne turned to go, Regan joined her.

"Well, ye look quite refreshed and rested," Anne Campbell said, quickly surveying her. "I take it the bed was to yer liking?"

"It was heavenly, m'lady." Regan smiled. "As was the wonderful bath I had this morn. And the breakfast."

"I'm glad. And if there's aught more ye need, don't hesitate to ask. Ye're our honored guest, and we want yer stay to be pleasant in every way."

Are all of Iain's relations so gracious and warm? Regan wondered. If so, he was indeed blessed. She paused to study the other woman. In the brighter light of day, Regan realized Anne Campbell was even more beautiful than she had imagined last night.

Her long hair was a rich auburn and plaited into one thick, fat braid to hang down her back. Her skin was ivory and flawless, her nose straight, short, and charming, her lips full and pink, and her figure slender but womanly.

It was Anne's arresting silver-gray eyes, however, that drew Regan time and again. Framed by thick, dark brown lashes, they gazed back at her with an open honesty. There was no guile or subterfuge in Anne Campbell, Regan realized. She felt she could trust her and, given time and familiarity, easily become friends.

She paused to glance around the big kitchen. A huge, arched hearth with an iron spit and two chimney cranes to swing pots into position over the fire stood at both ends of the long room, as well as an attached brick oven for baking. A large wooden table filled the center of the kitchen, at which four assistants now stood, two chopping vegetables and two kneading bread. A huge washbasin was inset on the outside wall, its drain emptying into the garden.

Myriad pots hung from an iron rack over the worktable, and in a tall, open cupboard, Regan could see chafing dishes, frying pans, graters, mortars and pestles, in addition to piles of plates and platters. Several wooden boxes stacked atop each other on one shelf likely held the eating utensils. A block of wood in the middle of the table contained all the cutting knives.

"I can't think of aught I'd need that hasn't been provided," Regan said, turning her glance back to that of Anne's. "I'd like verra much, though, to be of any assistance I could in yer household. What with the extra guests, I'd imagine yer staff's a bit overtaxed. And I'm no fine lady, though Iain and Mathilda have treated me as one since I first came to them."

"And so will we, for ye're their friend and our guest. But yer generous offer's most appreciated." Anne laid a hand on her arm. "I could use some help in the garden, though, if ye're of a mind for a short walk outside. I thought to cut flowers for the high table for this eve's meal."

"Och, aye, m'lady." Regan could barely contain her eagerness to be of help. "And I'd dearly love to see yer garden, as well. Iain has taught me much of the flowers that grow in Balloch's garden. I'd be verra interested in seeing what kinds ye grow in Kilchurn."

"Then come, let's be gone." Anne turned and, leading the way, hurried across the kitchen to the back door. It opened directly onto the garden.

Regan followed her outside, then halted, taking in the abundance of flower beds and hedges, all radiating from a large round fountain at the center. "Och, it's so verra beautiful, m'lady."

"Anne. Pray, call me Anne."

"What?" Regan wheeled around. "Och, but I couldn't. It'd be too forward of me."

"Yet ye call Iain by his given name. How's it any different?"

The question gave Regan pause. "Well, I suppose there's not much difference, save that ye're the Campbell's wife and all. And I'm . . . I'm not sure who or what *I* am."

Compassion flared in Anne's striking eyes. "Iain told me a bit this morn of yer predicament. It must be verra hard, not remembering who ye really are or where ye came from. And yer poor family. They must be beside themselves with worry."

At mention of her family, Regan felt a twinge of guilt. She'd not willingly cause anyone pain, and especially not those who loved her. But over time and what with the few bits of memory that had returned, she had begun to doubt she had been that much loved, or even missed. It was a terrible observation to broach to anyone, though, and so she hadn't—and wouldn't. She felt the certitude, nonetheless, to the marrow of her bones.

"Aye, it's been verra hard," she said, looking down. "But living with Mathilda and Iain and being the recipient of their kindness has made it bearable. Indeed, there are times, not being altogether sure of where and from whom I came, that I almost wish I might never know." Regan lifted her gaze. "It must sound strange, me saying that, but I cannot help but think I've never been so happy as I've been at Balloch. Or, leastwise, not for a verra long time."

In spite of herself, her eyes filled with tears. "I don't mean to sound as if I'm taking advantage of Mathilda and Iain. Truly I don't. But the longer I'm with them, the harder it becomes to imagine leaving them. I . . . I just care for them so."

Anne's grasp on her arm tightened. "Come. Let's sit for a time and talk. There's no rush in getting the flowers."

"A-aye," Regan whispered, savagely swiping away her tears. "I wouldn't want anyone else to see me weeping. Especially not Iain."

They walked down the footpath until they came to a rose arbor just large enough for two people to sit within. Deep enough to hide their presence, it provided the perfect shelter from curious eyes.

"Now, tell me why you'd think anyone would imagine ye're taking advantage of Mathilda and Iain?" Anne asked as soon as they were both seated. "And why ye wouldn't want Iain to see ye weep? He's one of the most tenderhearted men I know, and wouldn't take offense. Indeed, knowing him, he'd be the first to take ye in his arms and comfort ye."

Regan sucked in a strangled breath, then proceeded to choke on it. Her face, which she knew had immediately colored at mention of Iain taking her in his arms, only turned the redder with her prolonged bout of coughing. Finally, though, she was able to catch her breath.

"Aye, Iain's most certainly a tenderhearted man," she said as she brushed her freshened tears away. "But I've been enough of a burden to him in the past weeks and don't wish to cause him additional distress." She paused then, reluctant to reveal more of her private thoughts about Iain. Thoughts like how she never wanted to leave him, yet knew she must.

Anne leaned back, a considering look in her eyes. "The way he talked about ye this morn, not to mention how protectively he acted about ye last eve, I'd wager a guess he doesn't view ye as a burden. Not any burden at all."

Regan swallowed hard. "He's but an exceedingly kind man. He'd treat any person in need exactly the same way."

"Well, to some extent, that *would* be true." Her hostess smiled. "But I know Iain, and it's different with ye. Would ye think me too forward to ask ye how ye feel about him?"

Panic seized Regan, and all she could do was stammer. "I . . . I don't . . . He's a dear friend . . . And who wouldn't find him the most wonderful . . . ?" Frustration filled her. "Och, it doesn't matter how I feel about him! I'm so far beneath him that even to dream of aught more is presumptuous, not to mention a fool's quest."

"Yet ye cannot help what yer heart tells ye, can ye?"

The softly couched question drew Regan up short. *Dear, sweet Lord,* she thought. *Anne knows. Och, she knows!*

Suddenly, she couldn't look at her companion. Regan's head dropped, and she stared down, unseeing, at her lap. "I don't know why I told ye what I did. I hardly know ye, after all." She looked up and met Anne's understanding gaze. "I'd beg ye, though, not to say a word of this to Iain. I'd die of the shame, I would, and it'd ruin what friendship we do have."

"And why would it ruin it?"

"Because it'd change everything! And . . . and I couldn't bear his pity." She reached out and took her hostess's hands in hers. "Och, please, Anne! I know ye're first and foremost Iain's friend, as well ye should be. But it'll do him no harm not to know this. Indeed, it'd only distress him, not knowing how to act around me anymore. And I couldn't bear it. If his friendship's all I'll ever have, it's enough."

"Ah, but there ye're wrong, my friend. It won't be enough. It'll only tear out yer heart in the end, and ye may even come to hate Iain for not returning yer affection."

"Nay!" Regan shook her head with fierce resolve. "I'll never hate him. I'll leave him before I ever let that happen!"

For a long moment, Anne studied her with thoughtful deliberation, then sighed. "Well, this doesn't concern me at any rate, does it? What will happen between ye and Iain will happen if it's meant to. But I will say a prayer for ye. That ye find what ye're truly seeking."

Once again, similar words rose in her memory, and this time she saw the face of a man of God speaking them. Father . . . Och, his name was on the tip of her tongue! But whatever his name, his words seemed just as cryptic as Anne's did just now.

"What ye're truly seeking . . ."

Indeed, what *was* that? Only one thing was becoming increasingly clear. It wasn't just her memory that had been lost. There was a big, gaping hole in the middle of her chest, the result of something very dear being ripped away.

Regan only wondered if that hole would be filled anew and her life be complete once more when her memory finally did return.

✠

"Ye and I must have a wee talk, and we must do it here and now," Mathilda Campbell informed her son a week later.

Iain paused to glance up from the document he was poring over in Kilchurn's large library and eyed his mother with no small amount of exasperation. "And this is something that can't wait a time, until I discover the information Niall's asked me to find for him? I'm here to assist him, as any tanist must, ye know, and my days at Kilchurn should be spent in his service, not my own."

"And since when is Niall some unfeeling despot, driving ye mercilessly from dawn to dusk?" His mother walked around the table, pulled up a chair beside him, took her seat, then met his gaze. "Not to mention, I *am* yer mither, and ye owe me the proper respect."

"Fine." With a resigned sigh, Iain rolled up the parchment scroll, retied it with a piece of ribbon, and laid it aside. Then, folding his hands on the tabletop, he looked to her. "Now, what's so important that ye insist we must speak of it here and now?"

"What else but Regan?"

He eyed her in puzzlement. "And what's the matter with Regan?

Last I saw her, which was just this morn, she looked hale and hearty."

Mathilda rolled her eyes. "Och, and why is it the man's always the last to know?"

The first stirrings of unease rippled through Iain. "Know what, Mither? Has her memory returned? Or does something else altogether trouble her?"

She gave a snort of disgust. "Och, aye, something indeed troubles her. *Ye* trouble her."

"What?" Iain's gut clenched. "What've *I* done? Tell me, and I'll straightaway seek her out and make amends."

"And can ye mend a heart that's fair to breaking over love for ye? If so, ye're a far better man than any I've known in my life."

His gut did more than clench this time. It twisted, flip-flopped, then did backspins. *Regan loves me? It isn't possible.*

"I think yer imagination's a wee bit overwrought here, Mither," he finally found voice to say. "We're but friends."

"And is that *yer* feeling for her, or yer perception of how *she* feels for ye?"

Iain opened his mouth to reply, then caught himself before he flung himself unheeding into her trap. A trap he couldn't escape without either lying or admitting to the true depth of his affection for Regan. And, though he wasn't ashamed of his growing love for her, the matter was best settled first between them before sharing the news with others.

"This is a private issue between Regan and me, Mither," he finally ground out.

"Och," she cried, throwing up her hands. "I knew it. I knew it!"

He sucked in an irritated breath. "Stay out of this, Mither. It's none of yer affair."

Mathilda wheeled about in her chair to face him. "Isn't it? Don't I love ye both? Indeed, Regan's like the daughter I never had. And ye tread on dangerous ground here, lad. Ye truly know naught about her. What if she's already wed? What will ye do then, when her memory finally returns?"

"Do ye think I haven't thought about that, agonized over such a possibility?"

"Ye must guard yer heart, lad." She laid a hand on his arm. "I know it's a difficult thing to do. Regan's a dear, sweet lass, without a shred of meanness or guile in her. But ye must keep yer distance—for her sake as much as for yers."

"I *am* trying, Mither," he cried. "Even knowing, from the first time I saw her, there was something verra special about her. And ye yerself chided me in the beginning for what ye imagined was my rudeness in avoiding her. Yet even then I knew. I knew . . ."

"Knew what, lad?"

"That she was the woman the Lord had chosen for me."

Mathilda paled. "Nay. That's but yer heart shaping things to justify what ye want. Ye can't be certain the Lord has chosen her for ye. Not two years past, ye were madly in love with Anne. Did ye then imagine the Lord had chosen her for ye as well?"

He shot her an exasperated look. "Two years ago, I wasn't as concerned about what God did or didn't want for me in my life. Ye know that, Mither."

"Aye, I do." She sighed. "Have a care, though, lad. Just because ye now seek to do the Lord's will doesn't mean it's that much easier to know it. And the desires of our hearts can trick us into doing *their* bidding, rather than that of the Lord's."

"I'm doing the best I can," Iain muttered, nearly at the end of his patience. "How long must I wait then for Regan's memory to return before I can reveal my true feelings to her? Another six months? A year? Five years? And what if her memory never returns? What then?"

"She asked me the same thing, about her memory not returning, as we journeyed here. She wondered what would happen then. She even," Mathilda added with a chuckle, "offered her services as one of our servants, so distressed was she at continuing to profit from our hospitality, now that she was again physically able."

"I hope ye told her to banish such thoughts from her head. I'll not have her repaying us by working as a servant."

"Aye, I told her. But she's an honorable lass, and I fear she won't let the matter lie for long. Indeed, Anne told me that Regan offered to help in Kilchurn's kitchen the morn after we arrived."

He cursed softly.

"She's trying to make a new way for herself," his mother said. "Though I think she loves us both like family, she also knows we're *not* her true family. The true family who has apparently made no effort to try and find her. And that hurts her verra much."

"Well, that settles it. Just as soon as we return from our visit here and the harvest's in, I'm taking Regan and we're going to ride until we find that blasted family of hers, even if it means covering the entire Highlands!"

"An overly ambitious plan, to be sure." Mathilda released his arm and leaned back in her chair. "But it won't hurt to have tried everything ye can to find Regan's family, even if that takes some extended journeys. And if ye start soon after harvest and travel out mayhap in a hundred-mile radius from Balloch, well, that's a good four to five days' travel in every direction. It's verra unlikely she could've come from any farther away than that."

The plan heartened him. If luck was with them, they'd be back at Balloch before the heavy snows came. And mayhap, just mayhap, if Regan *did* bear some affection for him, they could even be wed by Christmas.

"Aye, it's verra unlikely Regan's family would live even that far away, but at least it gives us a fair range," he replied, well aware his hopes and dreams were getting away from him. "And surely, if her memory hasn't returned by then, it isn't coming back. By then, if she's willing, she'll be mine for the taking."

"It'd seem a fair and reasonable plan." Mathilda pushed back her chair and stood. "So we're agreed then, are we? That you'll neither do nor say aught to encourage the lass until all efforts to discover her past have been exhausted?"

Iain looked up at his mother. She was a clever one, and no mistake. Once again, she had maneuvered him into another trap. If he agreed, it would likely be another four months, at the very least, before he could approach Regan about his true feelings. Four more long, frustrating months.

"I'll do my best, Mither," he said, meeting her searching gaze with an equally resolute one of his own. "For Regan's sake, if not for my own."

✝

Five days later, Anne asked Mathilda, Regan, Iain, and Caitlin to meet her and Niall in the library just before the evening meal.

"Do ye have any idea what this is all about?" Mathilda asked her son as they descended the stairs from their bedchambers.

He smiled and shook his head. "Nay. But all will be revealed in good time, won't it?"

"Aye, I suppose so." She immediately turned to Regan, who was walking on her other side along with Caitlin.

"And what of ye, child? Have ye any inkling of what this meeting's about? It's all so private that I worry there might be bad news."

Though Regan did indeed have an inkling, she wasn't about to ruin Anne and Niall's surprise. In the past days, once she had learned of Anne's special skills as a healer, she had begged her to teach her some of the healing arts. In the process of the lessons, which generally began early in the morn when most herbs were best harvested, she had soon discovered that Anne had been suffering for several weeks now with a queasy stomach.

"I'd imagine, as much that goes on here, Niall being clan chief and all, that it could be one of several things," she replied. "But I haven't seen any long faces of late, so I'd wager the news will be good."

The older woman harrumphed, then admitted Regan was likely

right. Mathilda next turned to query Caitlin, but just then they drew up outside the library.

Iain opened the door, motioned them in, then followed, closing the door behind him. Anne and Niall awaited them before the curtained windows. Mathilda wasted no time in hurrying over to them.

"Well, what is it?" she immediately demanded. "I've been dying of worry ever since ye sent word to meet ye here, and that ye'd something of utmost importance to tell us."

Anne looked to Niall, and their gazes locked momentarily in joyous anticipation. Then, as Iain, Regan, and Caitlin drew up at last at Mathilda's side, Anne turned to them.

"I'm with child," she said, breaking into a breathtaking smile. "We're going to be parents sometime in early February."

As Mathilda staggered backward and would've lost her balance if not for Regan and Caitlin's quick response in catching her, Iain leaped forward to take Anne into his arms. "Och, lass, lass," he whispered, holding her close. "I'm so happy for ye. So verra, verra happy!"

"And why is it ye're always grabbing my wife and so conveniently forgetting all about me?" Niall groused from behind them. "I vow if I didn't like ye so well, cousin, I'd be taking great offense right about now."

With a laugh and quick kiss to Anne's cheek, Iain released her and quickly strode over to Niall. They grasped each other, hand to forearm, and grinned.

"Ye always were a jealous lout," Iain said. "Not that I ever had a chance with Annie at any rate. But my heartiest congratulations nonetheless. Ye're going to be a father then, are ye?"

Niall returned his grin, though it was one of sheepish bemusement. "Aye, so it seems."

By then Mathilda had regained her composure and had replaced Iain at Anne's side, hugging her in happy excitement. Caitlin rushed up and threw her arms about her brother.

"Och, lass," Iain's mother all but wept. "I'm so verra happy for ye. Whatever ye need, ye just have to ask. And if ye wish me to attend ye at yer lying-in, just say the word and I'll be at yer side. Och, lass, lass!"

Watching them, Regan couldn't help but smile. They were such a close, loving family, and would do aught for each other. It would be so verra good to belong amongst them.

But she must not let herself long so desperately for what wasn't hers to have. She must be content even having the opportunity to get to know them and share in this happy moment. Knowing now of Niall's loss of his first wife and son in childbirth, she could guess that the news Anne was carrying his child was bittersweet for Niall. Yet life, love, and renewed hope had given him the strength to go on, until he had once more been granted another chance at fathering a family. Love and hope in his beloved Anne—and in the Lord.

Someday, *she* might have that same chance to begin anew. Not with Iain, of course, but perhaps with some other man. Some man she might even already know and had yet to rediscover. But to do that, she also needed to place her hope and trust in the Lord. In the end, that was all she *could* do.

Amidst the excited chatter and congratulations, it took a moment for Regan to realize someone was knocking on the library door. One glance back at her friends and she knew they were unaware of the unexpected visitor, so she headed across the room and opened the door.

Charlie stood there, a worried look in his eyes.

"Is there aught I can do for ye?" Regan asked.

His glance strayed past her to the jubilant gathering across the room. Then he looked back to her. "Er, Brady the stableman just brought me this sealed document. Seems some rider delivered it but a few minutes ago, with orders for it to be delivered to m'lord."

Regan hated to have Anne and Niall's happy moment inter-rupted just then. "Can't it wait for a time? Until at least after the evening meal?"

The old man shook his head. "Nay, ma'am, it can't. The messenger said this letter had to be delivered immediately. And, since he was sent from the queen, I daren't disobey."

"The queen? Queen Mary?"

"Aye, the verra same."

She stepped aside, wordlessly waved him in, then watched as he hurried across the library. As he approached Niall and the others, they seemed finally to notice him. All fell silent. Regan closed the door and followed in Charlie's wake.

"A letter, m'lord," Charlie said as he drew up before the Campbell. "A letter from the queen."

His expression gone serious, Niall accepted the missive, opened its sealed leather case, and extracted the rolled parchment. He lost no time unfurling it and reading the contents. The seconds ticked by in the now stone-silent room, and Regan could hear her heart pounding in her ears.

Finally, after what seemed an eternity, Niall lifted his gaze and met that of his wife. A slight smile twitched at the corner of his mouth. "We'll be having a royal houseguest in two weeks' time. Seems the queen is paying us a visit."

8

Every letter from Fergus of late, Walter thought, crumpling the latest missive and throwing it into the fire, seemed to convey increasingly worse news. It was bad enough that Regan appeared to be developing a close relationship with Iain Campbell and had made no attempt to escape. But now Fergus had recently watched them depart for what appeared to be an extended visit to Kilchurn Castle, the seat of Campbell power. Regan was not only getting farther and farther away from him, but he feared she was also coming so deeply under Iain Campbell's spell that he might never be able to bring her back.

It was time he cease hiding behind his spies, Walter resolved, and try and make contact with Regan himself. Kilchurn, after all, saw all sorts of strangers pass through its gates, most in the hopes of gaining some special favor from the Campbell. He might just as easily pass through them unnoticed and finally speak with Regan.

What he hoped to accomplish if she truly *were* bespelled, Walter didn't know. But there was a local healer who might have some charm to protect him, as well as some magical potion to remove Regan's ensorcelment. Still, even the consideration of drawing near to such devilish taint made Walter's skin crawl. There was naught to be done for it though.

For the sake of his bonny Regan, he was willing to risk even that.

✠

Though he found the act distasteful, if not downright cruel, Iain managed successfully to limit the amount of time spent in Regan's company for the next week to an hour or two during and after the evening meal. And that time was spent in the presence of others, forcing his conversation with her to be general rather than personal. The rest of each day, he either buried himself in the library researching documents or holed up in private conference with Niall, interspersed at times with riding with him to survey Campbell landholdings or to meet with Niall's various lairds and tacksmen.

Regan, however, must have found the brief interactions with him as frustrating as he did. On the morn of the seventh day, almost as if she were lying in wait for him to appear, she hurried down the keep's front steps just as he led his horse from the stables.

"And where are ye going this fine morn?" she asked, finally drawing up before him. "Another ride out to survey Niall's domain for him? Or mayhap he's sent ye on yet another mission altogether?"

A wry smile tugging at the corner of his mouth, Iain gazed down at her. Her cheeks were most becomingly flushed, and her chest heaved from what was likely her race to catch up with him before he departed. But there was a fire in her eyes as well, and he wondered if it wasn't fueled by anger. But whether it was anger at him for his failure to spend much time with her of late—which he secretly hoped was the case—or from some other cause, Iain didn't know.

"Actually, I'd planned a wee ride around Loch Awe to one of my favorite spots," he replied. "Niall's busy with Anne at the moment, fine-tuning the plans for Queen Mary's visit. And, as complex as that will be, what with all her royal needs, I'm free for the morn."

Her face fell. "Och, so ye'll be wanting some peace and quiet for yerself then, won't ye?"

He knew he should agree with her assessment, even as he sensed she wanted to spend some time with him, but suddenly Iain didn't care what he had promised his mother, or what was likely the best and honorable course to take with Regan. What harm could possibly come, after all, from a wee gallop together around Loch Awe?

"Would ye like to ride with me, lass?" He angled his head and smiled. "Because if ye would, I'd be most pleased to have ye along."

Regan's expression brightened. "Aye, I'd like that verra much." She hesitated. "But can ye wait fifteen minutes more, while I go and prepare myself?"

"Sounds like just enough time to tack up yer mare." Iain made a shooing motion. "So get along with ye, then. The morn draws on even as we stand here and blather."

With a laugh, Regan gathered her skirts and raced back toward the keep.

True to her word, fifteen minutes later she returned, dressed in a simple, blue wool gown and Campbell plaid wrapped around her shoulders and fastened in place with the smaller silver version of the Campbell clan crest he had gifted her with just before they had departed Balloch. With her long, reddish-brown hair plaited into a single braid and then twisted into a tight bun at the nape of her neck, she looked so lovely, and so much a Campbell lass, that she took Iain's breath away.

He had an instant's misgiving about agreeing to take her on the ride, then shoved it aside. He was a grown man, after all, and could well control his more carnal impulses. Besides, he'd never intentionally do anything to cause her harm or pain.

Iain helped Regan mount, and they were soon galloping through Kilchurn's massive gates and out and around the loch. It was a glorious early August day, the heavens scrubbed to a fresh, clear blue from last night's rain and the windswept clouds shredded bits of white strewn across the sky. They rode for a time, content in each other's company and in the beautiful day. Finally, though, not quite across the loch from Kilchurn, at a spot where they were just able to catch a glimpse of one of its towers, Iain halted.

Swinging off his horse, he dropped the reins to let the animal graze on the verdant grass and walked over to her. "Come down, lass," he said, lifting his arms to her. "I want to show ye one of my favorite places at Kilchurn."

She tossed down her own horse's reins and gladly came to him. Unlike that eve they had first arrived at Kilchurn, as soon as her feet were firmly on the ground, Iain lost not a moment putting her away from him. He tried to ease what might be taken as avoidance by grabbing her hand and tugging her forward, down to one side of a small burn that eventually emptied into the loch.

Huge, ancient oaks spread their gnarled arms across the chuckling little stream, the sunlight piercing their foliage in spots to send bursts of dazzling brilliance glancing off the water. Summer wildflowers, including lavender-hued wild orchids and purple thistle, grew in the rich, green grass. In the distance behind Kilchurn stood mighty Ben Cruachan, its bare, wind-scoured peaks jutting toward the sky.

She turned to him. "It's lovely. I can see why ye like to come here. Thank ye for showing this spot to me."

"I brought Anne here, just after she'd first arrived at Kilchurn. In those days, she'd just agreed to handfast with Niall in order to bring an end to the feud between her clan and ours."

"Aye, Anne told me of yer kindness in those early days, and the quick bond ye formed." Regan grinned. "Indeed, if I didn't know she was madly in love with her husband, I think I'd almost be jealous of yer special friendship."

Iain chuckled. "Would ye now?"

"I might, if I didn't know yer first love was Clan Campbell and aiding Niall in every way ye can. No woman, even the likes of Anne, can ever hold a candle to that."

He frowned at the slight edge to her voice now. "And why would ye say that, lass?"

She shrugged, disengaged her hand from his clasp, and turned to gaze out over Loch Awe. "Why else? Save for Niall, no one has hardly seen ye this week except for the evening meal. Or is it just me? That ye no longer have time to spend with me?"

And how was he supposed to answer that? Iain wondered. To tell her he was purposely avoiding her because he feared the consequences of revealing his true feelings for her would only complicate things for the both of them. Yet to admit he didn't wish to be around her was a lie.

"It's verra complicated, lass," Iain replied, choosing to take an entirely different tack in the hope she'd fashion an alternate reason for his continued absences of late. "It's been over two years now since my father, Niall's first tanist, died. In the aftermath of that death, several of Niall's lairds and other kinsmen cautioned him about his plan to name me his next tanist. I was, after all, the son of the traitor who had plotted and planned for years to seize the chieftainship, not only from Niall but from Niall's father, my father's own brother. Who was to say that I, too, didn't secretly covet Niall's position?"

"And it'd be dangerous for Niall to keep ye too close," Regan offered, turning back to him, "and hold ye in the private confidences he'd need to if ye were his tanist."

"Not to mention, as long as Niall had no heir, and I was his chosen successor, if aught happened to him, I'd automatically be next in line for the clan chieftainship."

"Yet he chose ye nonetheless."

"Aye, he did, and for a time, several lairds looked none too favorably on me."

"So what did ye do? Just wait them out?"

Iain nodded. "In a sense, aye. I returned to Balloch and lay low, aiding Niall as best as I could from afar. Indeed, in the two years since he first named me tanist, this is only the second time I've returned to Kilchurn. Hence," he added with a grin, "why there's so much work when I do pay Niall a visit."

She smiled. "And it explains, as well, some of his rather barbed comments toward ye when we first arrived. I wondered why Niall chided ye so about sequestering yerself so long at Balloch, and threatened to send his men to drag ye here."

"Aye." Iain sighed. "Mayhap I did wrong in not advising him of my plan to stay away for a time, but I didn't want to add to his burdens. He didn't need the sight of me hanging about, stirring up his other lairds, who feared another Duncan Campbell, albeit a younger version, might be in their midst."

"It must be hard, two years since yer father's death, still to be paying the price for his deeds."

"Och, in some ways, I fear I'll be paying the price for him the rest of my days!" he said with a sharp laugh. "As will my mither, in the pain he caused her. It's why she finally left him, when I was almost a man. She did her best all those years of my boyhood and youth to protect me from my father's cruel, callous acts, even as she silently suffered as his wife. Indeed, whatever sort of man I am today, it's because of my mither and her loving ways. But never, ever, thanks to aught my father did, for he never had any time or interest in me. Or, leastwise, not until I was a man and could be used to further his own ambitions."

Suddenly, all the old frustrations and seething anger swelled anew. Iain couldn't bear for her to see him like this, so he walked the few feet more to stand at the edge of the loch. A sudden breeze whipped the water's surface, sending agitated ripples across its darkling expanse. Just like the state of his soul just now, he realized. A soul that, for the most part, was at peace with his failed relationship with his father, but so easily stirred once again to discontent and restlessness with but the slightest touch of memory.

"I thought—hoped—I had forgiven him when I gave my life over to the Lord," he said, hearing Regan come up to stand behind him. "But over and over, with but a passing reminder or provocation, the anger rises anew, and I know I've never fully forgiven. It's a thorn in my flesh, it is, that I've a limit to the amount of times

I can be hurt or betrayed before I forever pluck a person from my heart. It seems I lack the courage—or love—sufficient to forgive seventy times seven."

Anguish flooded him. "Och, what must the Lord think of me, Regan? That I'm a coward, a liar, a false friend? And why can't I finally and forever let my father go?"

Of a sudden, her arms came around his middle to hold him, and he felt her small body press against his. She laid her cheek against his back.

"I read something once, or mayhap it was something someone told me," she said. "About forgiveness sometimes being a journey. A journey as much directed inward as it was outward toward the person we were to forgive. And that, as we circled ever deeper and deeper toward self-knowledge and toward God, we came to forgive more completely. In a more Christlike, totally self-forgetting way."

He placed his hands over hers and clasped them to him, savoring her nearness, her touch. "Then I've a verra long way to go on my journey to God. I think that realization, more than aught else, is what distresses me so in times such as these. Not that I'm far from the holiness the Lord wishes of us all, but that I've failed Him."

"He understands, Iain," she whispered, her voice now clogged with tears. "After what ye've been through at yer father's h-hands . . ."

Dismay filled him. He pulled her hands free to turn and face her. Regan tried to hide her countenance from him, but he grasped her chin and gently forced her to look up. As he had suspected, she was indeed weeping.

"Lass, lass," he cried, his gut twisting at her pain. "It's not as bad as that. Och, I shouldn't have told ye all this! I never meant to make ye weep!"

She gazed up at him with tear-bright eyes. "It's fine. *I'm* fine. But just for a moment, the image of ye as a wee lad crossed my mind. Of ye running to yer father to show him something ye'd found—a pretty pebble or a cleverly fashioned bit of wood—and having him turn and walk away. A-and ye were such a bonny wee lad, with yer pale yellow hair and rosy cheeks and bright blue eyes, and I imagined the look on yer face, and it f-fair to broke my h-heart."

"Ah, sweet lass," Iain crooned, pulling her to him. "Whatever I experienced, it's over now. And all of us have our special hurts as we grow, but we don't have to allow them to twist us into the poor, unhappy folk that inflicted them. I told ye all this once before, and I meant it." He paused, cursing the self-pity that had led him to this moment, even as it touched his heart that she seemed to care so much for him. "In most ways I'm content with my life. I'm blessed with such abundance in my home and lands, my family and friends, and in the knowledge that, in spite of all my missteps and failings, the Lord Jesus will never cease to love me."

"Och, Iain," Regan whispered, "and I'm so blessed in knowing ye." She leaned back in his arms. "Ye're the most wonderful, honorable, loving man I've ever known!"

Her beautiful brown eyes were filled with such ineffable tenderness that, for a passing instant, Iain was undone. Almost as if drawn to her by invisible cords, his head lowered toward her soft, slightly parted lips. And then, as if Regan finally realized that he meant to kiss her, she closed her eyes and tilted her head back in willing acquiescence.

Then one of their horses, grazing nearby, must have trod on its reins. The animal snorted, jerked back, and shook its head. Leather squeaked; a bit jingled.

The spell was broken. Realizing what he had almost done, Iain released Regan and took a quick step back. Her eyes snapped open.

"We need to return to Kilchurn," he barely managed to grit out through clenched teeth. He forced himself to glance toward the sun, nearly at its zenith. "As it is, we'll just make it back for the midday meal."

With that, Iain turned on his heel and strode over to gather up both horses. It was a long while later, however, before he could banish from his mind that look of wounded disappointment on Regan's face and the heady memory of her eager mouth lifted to his.

✝

Four days later, Walter watched the party depart Kilchurn. Two men and women rode out, followed by another man driving a cart. If the empty cart following in their wake were any indication, they were likely bound for the village of Dalmally, just two miles down the road, and its Saturday morning market. One of the women he recognized as Regan. Like some leech who couldn't long survive without his source of sustenance, Iain Campbell rode at her side. The other woman, who rode behind them with an older man, he guessed to be the Campbell's wife, if her famous flaming hair were any indication.

"Och, lass," he whispered from his hiding place in a thick stand of birch trees, "between the witch and her warlock, ye haven't a chance. It's past time I speak with ye. Past time I try and break their devilish spells."

He allowed them to pass and, after a short wait, set out after them. Wherever they were headed, it was evident their outing was but for the day. And he could easily follow their tracks, wherever they led.

Aye, one way or another, Walter resolved, today was the day he'd rescue his beloved Regan from the clutches of her unholy captors.

✝

"Och, look, Regan," Anne exclaimed in excitement as they stood in the midst of Dalmally's bustling market. "What do ye think of these candles? The proprietor claims they're made of the purest beeswax. Do ye think the queen would find them pleasing in her bedchamber?"

Regan stepped over to examine the candles. Tall and thick, they gleamed with a creamy luster that bespoke the highest quality. These candles would fill the room with a delightful fragrance, not drip or smoke, and burn for a good hour or more with a warm glow. They were also, Regan knew, very costly.

"I doubt Mary would find any better candles in the land," she said, looking back to Anne.

"Aye, that's what I was thinking as well. And Niall said to spare no expense, so I think I'll buy them."

The man wrapped six candles of various sizes in soft cloths, then placed them in the wicker basket Anne carried. She paid him and turned to Iain, who had just rejoined them.

"These are verra heavy." She smiled up at Balloch's laird. "Would ye be a dear and carry them to the cart so Regan and I can continue our shopping?"

Iain accepted the now candle-laden basket. "Gladly. It *is* why Niall asked me to come along, after all. As escort and errand boy."

"And ye do both as admirably well as ye do everything else," Anne said with a laugh.

He grinned and, wheeling about, began to thread his way through the ever-thickening crowd.

Regan watched him until he finally disappeared from sight. Strange, she mused, how she never tired of seeing him, being near him. Indeed, every time she was with him, it seemed she discovered yet another endearing aspect of his personality. Given the rest of her life with him, she thought she always would.

Still, since that day he had taken her to that favorite spot of his, Iain had once again been avoiding her. And avoid her he had. She knew that now. A soft smile touched her lips. No matter how hard he had tried to cover up his intent, her woman's instincts told her he *had* meant to kiss her. And, she knew as well, it was only a matter of time until he actually did.

"Enough of pining after Iain," Anne's amused voice cut into her reverie just then. "He won't long be gone, and ye've still the entire ride back to be with him."

Embarrassed to be caught in a daydream, Regan whirled around. She couldn't help the hot blood in her cheeks, however, no matter how hard she pretended surprise over Anne's comment. "I'd dearly appreciate it," she muttered, glancing down, "if ye'd quit teasing me about that."

"Why? Afraid Iain might hear me sometime?"

Regan jerked up her head. "Ye promised ye'd not say a thing to him!"

"Well, actually, I didn't promise. Ye just asked me not to do so, and I haven't. Though I don't see what a terrible thing it'd be, Iain knowing and all."

"Anne, please!" she wailed in dismay. "Please don't!"

Her friend chuckled and laid a hand on Regan's arm. "Och, I won't. But I think *ye* should tell him. If ye did, I wager ye might be verra pleasantly surprised."

For a fleeting instant, Regan was tempted to ask Anne why she thought so, then quashed the impulse. It didn't matter. Until she regained her memory and knew who and what she truly was, she had naught to offer a man such as Iain Campbell. To do aught else would be cruel and self-serving.

"Mayhap I will, when the time's right," she replied instead. "But it must be when *I* feel it's right."

Anne shrugged and smiled. "Suit yerself. Now,"—she paused to glance around her—"there's still a passel of foodstuffs to buy in order to feed the queen and the entourage she's sure to bring with her." She tore her parchment in half. "Here, ye take this"—Anne handed one piece of the list to Regan—"and start shopping for those items, and I'll proceed to find what's on mine. That way we can purchase everything in half the time."

Regan glanced down at her list. She needed to buy ten pounds of sugar, five different kinds of spices, forty pounds of flour, and about ten each of halibut, salmon, and cod. "Just as soon as the men return, will ye be sure and send one to aid me?" she asked, meeting her friend's gaze.

"Hmmm, and which one of the two would ye like to serve as yer errand boy?" Anne furrowed her brow in exaggerated thought. "Hmmm, Charlie or Iain?"

"Och, and well ye know who I'd choose!" Regan replied with a laugh. "Send me Iain, of course."

With that, the two women parted. Regan spent the next fifteen minutes haggling with the itinerant spice merchant over the cost of cloves, cinnamon, ginger, nutmeg, and pepper. When she was finally satisfied that she had extracted the best possible prices, she had the man fill individual leather pouches full of the spices and tie them closed. Once back at Kilchurn, the valuable spices would be locked in a wooden spice box for safekeeping.

As she finished paying the merchant and tucking the spice bags into her basket, a hand settled on her shoulder. Someone leaned close to whisper in her ear.

"Don't make a scene, lass," a masculine voice said. "Just turn around as if ye're going about yer shopping, and come with me."

The voice was familiar, yet Regan knew she hadn't heard it in months. A memory flashed through her. She was standing in a courtyard, gazing up at a man. He wore a blue bonnet decorated with one eagle feather, identifying him as a gentleman of the nobility.

"I'd crawl back on my hands and knees, I would," he'd said, *"to return to a bonny lass such as ye."*

Walter!

Her heart thudding beneath her breast, Regan forced herself to do as he asked. Already he was striding away, headed toward an alley between two of the wattle-and-daub-constructed buildings. Wracked suddenly with uncontrollable shivering, she glanced about for Anne or Iain. It was now the height of market day, however, and she failed to see them among the jostling bodies crowding around nearly every stall and table.

Well, mayhap that was for the best, she told herself. Time enough later to find them, once she met and talked with Walter. Walter

. . . her brother-in-law. Walter, a MacLaren, which made her, as well, a MacLaren.

As soon as Regan neared, he grabbed her arm and drew her into the shadowed alley. For a long moment, he said nothing, only searched her eyes.

"Ye don't look bespelled," he muttered at last.

She stared up at him, bewildered. "Of course I'm not bespelled. Whatever would make ye think such a thing?"

"And what other reason would there be, then, for ye keeping company with Iain Campbell all these past weeks? The verra man who murdered yer husband."

Her husband?

For an instant Regan's mind was so filled with memories, coming now one after another in rapid succession, that she feared her skull might explode. The face of the dead man in her dreams appeared before her, and this time she knew him. *Roddy! Och, Roddy, Roddy!*

Nausea seized her. The world spun suddenly around her. Her knees buckled, the basket dropped from nerveless fingers, and, if not for Walter's firm grip, Regan would've gone down.

"Now, none of that, lass." He gathered her into his arms and carried her to a rickety old bench. Placing her there, he shoved Regan's head between her knees.

"Take some slow, deep breaths," he ordered, his voice now sounding curiously far away. "And keep yer head down until it clears."

Three separate times, Regan did as she was told. Then, just when she thought she was finally feeling better, like a sharp punch to the gut, all her long-lost memories would return. Once more dizziness and nausea would overwhelm her, and she'd have to put her head back down. Finally, though, the chaotic onslaught of her newfound recollections sorted themselves out a bit, and she began to calm.

"Let me up," she croaked at last. "I'm . . . I'm feeling better."

He released her, and she slowly straightened. For a second or two more, everything twirled about her, then settled. She looked to Walter, managed a wan smile.

"It's so good to see ye again." Tears welled. "So verra, verra good!"

"What happened to ye, lass?" He leaned close, touched her cheek, his dark eyes filled with worry and compassion. "Why didn't ye come back home to Strathyre House?"

She felt the moisture trickle down her cheeks but didn't care. "I-I couldn't. That night I went out to find ye, I fell from my horse and hit my head. And, when I awoke in Balloch Castle, I found I'd lost all memory of my past life."

"Sounds to me more like witchcraft, it does," he growled.

"Och, nay. I was sore injured, with a huge knot on my head and a broken ankle, not to mention all my other scrapes and bruises." Regan took his hand. "Blessedly, though, I was found by one of Iain's clansmen and brought to Balloch, where Iain and his mither most kindly took me in. It's where I've been all this time, healing, while I struggled to regain my memory."

She paused as additional memories assailed her of that night she had ridden into that storm, trying to catch up with Walter and his men. "What happened? I tried to reach ye, to stop ye from lying in ambush for Iain, but I never found ye. And it's evident ye failed in yer attempt to kill him."

He gave a snort of disgust. "They never left Balloch. Seems the foul weather put them off. And then the men began to grumble, so I decided it best to try again some other day."

"Och, if only ye, instead of that Campbell crofter, had found me! I wouldn't have spent these past two months not knowing who I was . . ." And not ever knowing and coming to love Iain, either, Regan realized. The man who may have killed her husband.

"Well, what's past is past," Walter replied, interrupting her anguished thoughts. "All that matters is ye now know who ye are, and we can head back to Strathyre this verra day."

Head back to Strathyre? Leave Iain and Anne and Mathilda? Regan swallowed hard. The thought sent a shard of agony piercing clear through to her heart. Yet wasn't this what she had been working toward and praying for all these weeks? Finally to know who and what she was?

"Aye, mayhap that'd be best," she said, her voice strangely tight. "But first, I must find Anne and Iain and tell them what's happened, that my memory's returned." She stood, walked to where she had dropped the basket, and retrieved it. "Aye, that's what I must do. I owe them that much at the verra least."

Walter leaped to his feet and hurried to her side. "Nay, lass. Ye daren't tell them! They're in league, they are, bound by the evil craft they both pursue. If ye tell them—indeed, if ye even dare return now to them—they won't *let* ye leave. It'd break the spell they've cast about ye, it would!"

She eyed him with puzzlement. Whyever did Walter continue to go on so about witchcraft and spells? It made no sense.

"Anne and Iain aren't witches, I tell ye." Regan dug beneath the neck of her gown and withdrew her mother's cross. "And, even if they were, this would protect me. But ye needn't worry. Both Anne and Iain are good, God-fearing folk. They'll be happy that my memory's returned. It's what they've all wanted for me since I first came to them."

"Regan! Where are ye, lass?"

From the market stalls fronting the alley, Iain's deep voice came. It was filled with concern, and Regan's heart twisted. She'd never wish to cause him worry or pain.

Instinctively, she turned to go to him, only to have Walter grasp her arm and pull her back.

"Ye'd return to him then? Yer husband's killer?" he rasped in her ear.

His words drew her up short. Once more, roiling confusion muddied her thoughts. Iain . . . Iain had killed Roddy? Then she remembered. *The pistol shot to Roddy's back as he and his men tried to escape the Campbells . . . Campbells led by their laird. Balloch's laird. Iain Campbell.*

"Regan! Answer me, lass!"

Once more Iain cried out for her, his beloved voice washing over her heightened awareness like honey flowing over the tongue. She yearned to go to him, to see once again that boyishly endearing smile, to beg him to take her and hold her close. Och, to hide away in the haven of his arms, to drink deeply of his strength and reassurance that all would yet be well . . .

Perhaps that dream was gone forever, crushed beneath the terrible weight of her hard, heavy memories. It was too soon to be certain of that, though. And too soon to turn her back on what yet lay before her.

"I cannot go with ye today," she said, looking at Walter. "I need time to think, to sort it all out."

"And that can only be done within the Campbells' foul lair?"

"For a time more, aye." Resolve hardened within her. "Can ye meet me this time two days' hence?"

A joyous, eager light flared in his eyes. "Where?"

His question gave her pause. Where could they meet that would be safe from prying eyes? Inspiration struck her.

"Not far from Kilchurn, on the shores of Loch Awe, there's a small burn whose banks are lined with huge oaks. Ye can just see the trees from Kilchurn's gates. Meet me there."

"Gladly."

Regan had turned to go when Walter's grip tightened. "Aye?" She cast a glance over her shoulder at him.

"One thing more. Whatever ye do, don't tell the Campbells, and especially not Iain, who ye are or that yer memory's returned. Best ye wait a bit on that, until ye've sorted everything out."

She considered his advice for a moment, then nodded. "Aye. Ye're right. Best I wait."

He released her then, and Regan made her way back down the alley toward the market stalls.

9

For the next two days, Regan felt as if she were in a waking nightmare. Nonetheless, when she wasn't hiding in her bedchamber, staring out the window and crying, she went about her usual daily routine if for no other reason than to avoid unnecessary questions or concern. Everything she did, though, felt forced, drained of all joy or energy.

Not that anyone appeared to notice, what with all the busy anticipation of Mary's arrival on the morrow. Which was just as well, Regan thought, once more in her bedchamber shortly after the midday meal on the day she was to meet once again with Walter. If Anne or Mathilda had even touched on her less than happy countenance, she feared she'd have broken down right there and confessed everything. And if Iain had had the opportunity to speak with her in any context, she might have begun shrieking at him and never stopped.

Regan felt strung so tightly she thought she might snap at any moment, pulled first one way and then the other. All memory of her past life had now returned, its recovery set into motion by her encounter with Walter. She *had* been wed before, but no longer. She *had* loved Roddy, but never, ever like she had come to love Iain.

Yet Walter claimed Iain had killed Roddy with a single, well-placed pistol shot to the back. And Iain owned not one, but two, fine silver daggs. He had also led, according to Walter and several of their clansmen, the Campbell party that had pursued them. All evidence pointed to Iain as Roddy's killer. Few others, save the wealthier nobility after all, could afford such expensive weapons.

It still strained belief that Iain would've committed such a cold-blooded, brutal act, that he was a murderer. He had spared the MacLarens when his superior force had overwhelmed them, then sent them on their way. Why would he then choose to shoot Roddy in the back?

Yet he was apparently the only one with pistols.

For hours on end Regan struggled with that dilemma. Perhaps Iain thought he had reason for what he did. Perhaps he imagined, at the last minute, that Roddy and the others were turning back to attack them. Perhaps it was best just to confront him and demand the truth.

But could she believe it—*would* she believe it—if he denied his involvement in Roddy's murder? Or would the doubts hang between them for the rest of their lives?

One thing was certain. Roddy deserved justice. Deserved that his killer be punished. But not as Walter had intended that day he had ridden off after Iain and set this whole, convoluted, painful mess into motion. Nay. Only a court of law could sort through it all and arrive at a just verdict.

But who'd dare convict a member of one of the most powerful clans in the Highlands? A man who was an influential laird in his own right, not to mention the Campbell chief's cousin as well as tanist? Only a king—or a queen—might dare look past the Campbell clan's trappings of power and wealth to the eventual truth.

Regan's heart commenced a trip hammer beat. The queen would arrive on the morrow. The timing was so perfect as to be almost a divine intervention. They had come to Kilchurn at the most opportune time; she had met Walter and regained her memory just two days ago, and now the queen would soon be here.

It was a bold plan, but likely Regan's only chance to win justice for Roddy. And, though the accusation would humiliate Iain, the resulting investigation might well exonerate him as it uncovered the true killer. Or it might convict him.

The consideration chilled her to the bone. Was she willing to risk seeing Iain sent to trial, found guilty, and sentenced to hanging or worse? Dear, kind Iain, the man she loved?

Or rather, had once loved. Perhaps she had never really known him. Perhaps he was but a superb dissembler, a handsome, charming man who had long ago learned how to manipulate and deceive others. If the truth be told, he'd had a superb teacher in his father, the faithless, callously ambitious Duncan Campbell. Perhaps Iain had learned from him all too well.

Hot tears stung her eyes. What was she to do, to think? What was truth, and what were lies? It was beyond her ken, she well knew. But it wasn't beyond the Lord's.

Regan swiped away her tears, rose from her window seat, and headed across her bedchamber. Kilchurn's chapel was on the same floor and but a quick five minutes' walk away. Surely, in one of His holy sanctuaries, God would listen and answer her prayers.

Thankfully, no one was about in the chapel. Regan hurried down the aisle until she reached the first pew and slipped into it. Kneeling, she clasped her hands before her and gazed at the altar in fervent supplication.

Och, Lord, she prayed, *help me, I beg of Ye. I'm torn between Roddy and Iain and don't know what to believe, what to do. Is Iain a killer? My heart tells me nay, but the evidence against him is so damning. A part—a verra selfish part—wants to let it be, pretend I know naught about Iain's possible guilt. To allow things to take their natural course, which, now that I remember who I am and that I'm free to take another husband, could well lead to a marriage between Iain and me.*

He loves me, Lord. I know he has yet to speak the words, but I saw it so surely in his eyes that day by Loch Awe. But if he's guilty, of what value is his love? And what of my first commitment to Roddy, to seek a just retribution for his death? What manner of woman am I if I shirk my responsibilities, my honor?

She pressed her forehead against her now fisted hands and clenched shut her eyes. *Help me, Lord. Och, help me!*

The minutes in the stone-silent chapel passed with lumbering slowness. The sweet, clean scent of the beeswax tapers on the altar filled the air. An errant fly buzzed in some dark corner. And Regan's heartbeat pulsed in her ears.

But no whisper, no still, silent voice came to fill her with hope or reassurance. To fill her with the answers she craved. Not then, or later, as she knelt there until she was stiff from kneeling and numb from the cold.

At long last, Regan rose and left the chapel. If God wouldn't tell her what she must do, then she'd have to decide on her own. And it was past time she rode out to meet Walter.

✝

It was harder than Regan had anticipated, leaving Kilchurn in the middle of the afternoon. But then, at the time she had made the arrangements with Walter, she was inundated with all the market chaos and noise, Iain was nearby, calling her name, and she had just barely reestablished some semblance of equilibrium after having her memory, rife with all sorts of momentous implications, return. Fortunately for her, everyone was still preoccupied with all the last-minute preparations, and no one questioned her as she tacked up her horse and rode from the castle. Equally as fortunate, she hadn't seen either Iain or Niall at the midday meal, which likely meant they were holed up somewhere in some sort of deep discussion.

Only when she was a goodly distance from Kilchurn did Regan finally begin to relax. She wasn't some prisoner, after all, and had every right to go for a ride. If questioned later, she'd just claim she hadn't wanted to impose on anyone, what with them being so busy and all.

Still, Regan couldn't escape the stab of guilt at her deliberate deception. She *was* sneaking off to plot and plan with Walter. The act made her feel dishonorable, but she could see no other option. She couldn't do what needed to be done alone, yet she daren't risk seeking an ally in Kilchurn.

Mathilda was Iain's mother and loved him dearly. Anne was his fiercely devoted friend. And Niall was not only Iain's cousin, but he was also a loyal chief to his tanist. There'd be no support or understanding from any of them.

But Walter understood and would support her. He wanted Roddy's killer brought to justice just as dearly as did she. And if, after the accusation was taken to the queen, something should "accidentally" happen to silence her, Regan at least had the comfort of knowing Walter would still be out there to raise a hue and cry.

Not that she truly expected the Campbells to stoop to such a dastardly ploy as having her killed to protect Iain, Regan thought as she rode along. Anything was possible, but she believed Niall and Anne to be honorable people. And she was, after all, a guest in their home, protected by the Highland code of hospitality. Notwithstanding the fact that such a powerful clan as the Campbells would be unlikely to risk such a horrible stain on their honor, to do so in the very presence of the queen would be unthinkable.

Nay, Queen Mary's presence guaranteed her safety. What Regan dreaded was the inevitable moment of confronting Iain, of looking into his eyes as the accusation was made. Of facing Mathilda, and Anne and her formidable husband. Of the recriminations for her lack of gratitude for what they had done for her, especially Mathilda and Iain for taking her in and caring for her.

She had so cherished their kindness and friendship. Friendship that would be forever swept away in the impending floodtide of shock, disbelief, and pain. It would never, ever be the same again.

For a fleeting instant as Regan caught sight of the burn flowing down to Loch Awe and glimpsed Walter and his horse in the shadows of the oaks, she wavered once more in her resolve. She had known such joy and contentment in the company of the Campbells these past two months. A joy and contentment she well knew, with the return of her memory, that she had never experienced since her parents' deaths. Even with the satisfaction of gaining justice for Roddy—*if* that ever happened—she'd never find that again, leastwise not at Strathyre House.

But, in the end, she wasn't doing this to obtain joy or contentment. She was doing this because her honor would tolerate no less. She was doing this for the sake of justice. And she was doing it in order to assuage her guilt over her part in Roddy's death. She had been his wife. This was the last thing she could ever do for him.

Walter hurried over as Regan drew up and dismounted. Meeting his excited gaze, she knew he fully expected her to return to Strathyre House with him this very day.

"I've decided what I must do," she said, lifting a hand to forestall the question she sensed was forthcoming. "Queen Mary arrives at Kilchurn on the morrow."

A look of impatience flashed in his eyes. "Aye, it's all the talk in Dalmally. But what's that to us?"

"I intend to bring my demand for justice for Roddy's death to her. And ye can be sure I'll include the evidence against Iain in my accusations."

He went pale. "I don't like it, lass. It's too dangerous for ye. There's got to be some other way."

"Such as going back to yer old plan of lying in wait to ambush Iain?" Regan shook her head. "Nay, I've already paid a terrible price for that escapade of yers. And I won't stoop to the same despicable actions of the man who killed Roddy. His murderer *must* be brought to trial."

"But once ye accuse Iain Campbell of such a vile deed, yer life's well forfeit. If naught else, the Campbells stand by each other. Not to mention, with their powers of witchcraft, yer death can be made to look an accident." Walter took her by the arms. "Och, I won't hear of it, lass. I'll not lose ye as well as Roddy."

"Dinna fash yerself. I'll be in no danger. The queen will protect me. And besides, just as soon as I set this all into motion, I intend to depart Kilchurn. The Campbells, for their part, will be more than happy to send me on my way."

"So ye want me to await ye here in Dalmally? Is that it?"

Actually, Regan realized with a stab of disappointment, she had wanted Walter to offer to accompany her back to Kilchurn. She had then intended to set her plan into motion by first revealing her memory had returned and that Walter was her brother-in-law. Next, on the morrow, she hoped to have him stand beside her as she begged for Mary's aid in finding Roddy's killer and told her of Iain's possible involvement in that death.

But then, Regan quickly reminded herself, if, in spite of her certainty that nothing would happen to her, something did, she needed Walter on the outside. And surely he had already thought of that and assumed she had too.

"Aye," she replied, her mind made. "That seems the best plan, unless ye can think of aught better."

"The only better plan *I* can think of is ye discarding this daft idea and returning to Strathyre with me posthaste. Molly's been beside herself these past months, missing ye, crying her wee heart out. She needs ye, Regan. Needs ye verra badly."

An image of a cherubic, pink-cheeked face flashed across Regan's mind. *Ah, Molly, Molly,* she thought with a sharp pang. *How could I have forgotten about ye?*

"I'll soon be back home with Molly," she said. "This only postpones our return by another few days at the most. I didn't say I wasn't riding back with ye. Just not today."

"But think on it, Regan." His grip on her arms tightened, and once again the excitement flared in his eyes. "If the Campbells don't even know yer memory's returned, they don't know who ye really are. And, since MacLarens rarely if ever have opportunity to see them under normal circumstances, they might never know what became of ye. Ye can plead yer cause to Queen Mary just as well through letters, and the Campbells won't ever know it's ye."

His quite evident concern for her touched Regan's heart, banishing the last, lingering doubts over what seemed his unwillingness to stand at her side when she went to the queen. He was her true family, he and little Molly. And they both loved her and wanted her back home.

Walter's idea was very tempting. She'd not have to confront the Campbells, see the pain in their eyes, hear their angry protestations and counterattacks. Indeed, his proposal was more tempting than she cared to admit. But it was also cowardly, dishonorable.

"Nay, if I haven't the courage to look them straight in the eye and face them down, then I don't deserve to accuse them. And an accusation through letters will also give our cause less weight with Mary, I'd wager." Regan met his dark gaze. "This is the best of all plans, Walter. I'm certain of it."

He released her then with a sigh and stepped back. "Have it yer way then, lass. I just have a bad feeling about this. A verra bad feeling."

"Naught about this sad, sorry mess is going to be easy or pleasant. Ye must have faith that justice will prevail." She managed a smile. "Now, I daren't stay overlong outside Kilchurn or someone's bound to notice my absence. I must be going."

"I'll await ye in Dalmally then, at the lodging of the town butcher," Walter called to her as she turned and headed back to her horse. "And don't tarry in yer task, lass. Remember, Molly needs ye. And so do I."

Regan reached her horse, mounted, then met Walter's suddenly piercing glance. "I won't forget. I promise." With that, she turned her horse and set off back toward Kilchurn.

✠

Queen Mary's arrival the next afternoon, though she brought only the most minimal retinue, threw all of Kilchurn into an uproar. Regan pled a sick headache and didn't even go down for the formal greetings. The queen, after all, had come to visit Campbells, and she wasn't a Campbell.

It also didn't sit well with her to stand beside them, pretending an allegiance she no longer felt. Not that she held Anne, Niall, and Mathilda guilty of any blame. Far from it. She just knew, in such a close-knit family, to turn against one Campbell was to turn against them all. And it was past time she begin distancing herself from them, physically as well as emotionally.

There was no way she could avoid attending the grand feast welcoming Mary to Kilchurn that eve, however. She only hoped she could fade into the background, what with all the attention and talk turned to the queen. That and retire early, just as soon as was proper.

Mathilda had apparently been waiting for her outside the Great Hall. She hurried over just as soon as she caught sight of Regan descending the stairs from the bedchambers.

"Och, there ye are, child," Iain's mother said. "I was sorry to hear ye didn't feel well enough to attend Mary's arrival, but it's just as well. There was so much confusion and folk milling about that ye likely wouldn't have been able to greet her anyway." She paused to search her face. "Are ye feeling better? Ye look a mite pale, ye do."

Regan forced a smile. "Aye, or leastwise well enough to attend the feast. I may not be up to a late night of it, however."

Mathilda patted her on the cheek. "Dinna fash yerself, child. Mary will understand."

Regan glanced down to hide the sudden moisture that sprang to her eyes. *Och, don't be so kind to me,* she thought. *I don't deserve it.*

The fiddlers, who were to play during the meal, began a lively jig, signaling the meal would soon begin. Mathilda grabbed Regan's hand.

"Come, child." She began to pull her along. "We need to take our seats, as the queen will enter last. And ye're to sit beside me, four seats down from Mary on her left."

Dismay filled Regan. She had assumed, what with all the dignitaries present, she'd be at the end of the main table or even seated at one of the lesser ones. Four seats down from the queen was not at all conducive to fading into the background.

"Och, I couldn't take a seat from someone far more worthy to sit at the main table," she protested. "I'm not even a Campbell, after all."

"It was Iain's wish, child," the older woman said briskly, "and he'd brook no protest. So ye sit next to me."

Regan swallowed hard. Iain. Why, oh why, did he persist in his kindness to her? It only made the coming confrontation so much harder to bear. But then, once the truth was out, she expected she might finally see what he was really made of. And that would almost be a relief.

The Great Hall was ablaze with light, from the sputtering pitch torches on the walls to the thick candles on tall, iron spikes standing at each end of the main table to the pretty centerpiece of a single, pure beeswax candle surrounded by pine boughs, summer flowers, and the strongly aromatic bog myrtle, clan plant of the Campbells, placed on the table where Mary would sit. A long, white linen cloth covered the length of the main table, which was placed upon a dais above the other tables and set with pewter plates and cups, linen napkins, spoons, and finger bowls.

Regan followed Mathilda and took the seat she indicated. Gazing out at the assemblage of diners already at the four long tables below, she drew in a deep breath. The room was filled to capacity with invited guests, and Regan was nearly overcome by an impulse to get up and run from the room. She didn't belong here. Didn't deserve the honor being paid her.

In that irrational, panicked instant, she almost hated Iain for putting her into this position, knowing it would make her ultimate betrayal of him—for treachery it would be in the minds of Clan Campbell—all the more reprehensible. Yet it was so unfair. All she was trying to do was obtain justice for her murdered husband.

Closing her eyes, Regan took several long, deep breaths, then opened her eyes again. *But a few days more,* she told herself, *and it'll all be over. But a few days more for Roddy . . .*

Then, with a dramatic flourish, the fiddlers abruptly ended their song. All eyes turned to the doorway at the end of the Hall. Mary, queen of all Scotland, stood there, her hand in her escort's, the ever-loyal Lord Seton. She was tall and beautiful. Everyone inhaled in admiration.

Once more, the fiddlers began to play, a solemn, regal piece that filled the room with music. Mary looked to Lord Seton and then, as one, they entered the Great Hall.

✠

The next afternoon, after another private conference in the library with the queen and Lord Seton, Niall and Iain headed out together for a short ride along the shores of Loch Awe. The ride was as much for the freedom to speak their minds in private as it was for the opportunity to remove themselves for a short time from all the ongoing chaos of the queen's presence and the resultant constant agitation of Anne and Mathilda, who were striving to care for Mary's needs in every way they could. For a while, both rode in silence, mulling over the queen's current plight and her plea for their support.

"She can't get in a much worse position," Iain finally said, glancing over at his cousin. "The lords at Court dare to murder her personal secretary in her verra presence, with her husband's full support no less, and now Mary's all but estranged from him because of it."

Niall made a disgusted sound. "Darnley was always a dissolute, irresponsible man. Likely he began to fear he was losing favor with the queen and blamed poor David Rizzio for it. I'll wager it didn't take Lord Ruthven and the rest much to convince Darnley after that. Still, ever since, Mary has aligned herself with Bothwell, and I'm not so certain that won't ultimately be a mistake as well. In his own way, he's a verra ambitious, self-serving man."

"But ye'll support Mary nonetheless?"

His cousin sighed. "Aye. She's now mother of our future king, as well as ruling queen in her own right. I fear, though, what this next year might bring. Mark my words. Between Darnley and Bothwell, her position's not as stable as it once was."

"She needs to divorce Darnley," Iain muttered.

"That'd be the wisest course, to be sure."

Once more, they fell silent, enjoying the late summer's day. Already, Iain could see a change in the leaves as the days began to grow shorter. Autumn wouldn't be long in coming.

"Anne says ye're verra taken with yer ward," Niall of a sudden said. "That ye're in love with her."

Iain shot his cousin a startled glance. Niall had never been known for playing the matchmaker, so his unexpected observation likely had some other motive behind it. "And what of it?" he asked at last, well aware there was no point in pretending ignorance. He did make a mental note, though, to have a wee talk with Anne at the verra next opportunity. "Regan's a bonny lass and suits me in every way."

"Well, I suppose ye cannot play on the young ward ploy too much longer, even if she is, what—ten or so years younger than ye? Considering she came to ye under such mysterious circumstances and all." He looked at Iain, squarely meeting his gaze. "But aren't ye treading a thin line, cousin, in giving yer heart to a woman ye know absolutely naught about? What if she planned this loss of memory, with the intent to win ye over all along? Or what if her memory returned a while back, and when she saw yer interest and the fine life she'd have as yer wife, decided to continue to play the helpless maiden to yer gallant rescuer?"

Iain could feel his anger begin to rise, but he clamped down hard on it. Niall meant well, he told himself. Though it was none of his concern, he meant well.

"I know all I need to know about Regan," he muttered. "With or without a memory, her true essence, her soul, shines through

as brightly as sunlight off a polished sword blade. And I trust her
to tell me when her memory does return. Indeed, I think she has
feelings for me too, and but waits as I do to regain her past."

"Mayhap." Niall shrugged. "Just have a care for yer tender heart.
Anne's worried about ye, ye know. And, for some reason," he added
with a grin, "she has a great need to see ye settled and happy."

Iain chuckled. "Aye, she does. If all goes as planned, come Christmastide, I may be well on my way to that verra state of wedded
bliss."

"Indeed?" Niall asked with an arch of a dark brow.

"Indeed," Iain replied, then settled back to enjoy the ride and
lose himself in happy contemplation.

✝

Standing at Queen Mary's side in the private study just off what
was currently the royal bedchamber, Regan waited in rising dread
for Niall and Iain to put up their horses and answer their sovereign's
summons. It had taken her until just before the midday meal,
directly after Niall and Iain had finished their first meeting of the
day with the queen, to get a note requesting a private audience with
Mary. Three hours later, to Regan's astonishment, the queen's lady-
in-waiting had come for her, saying Mary would see her now.

Gazing into Mary's sympathetic eyes, Regan found it a surprisingly easy thing to tell the queen all that had happened to her in
the past three and a half months, from her marriage to Roddy,
to his death, to how she had come to Balloch Castle and finally
regained her memory. Mary was, after all, only seven years older,
and had had her fair share of trials—indeed, more than any young
woman deserved.

Mary's expression, however, as Regan proceeded to tell her of
Iain's possible involvement in her husband's murder, gradually
changed from that of open regard to a more shuttered one. And,
when Regan's tale finally ended, Mary had rather flatly stated that
it was only fair that Iain be brought before them to share his side

of the story. She had next sent off her lady's maid to fetch him and the Campbell chief. Fortunately—and not—the two men had just returned from a ride and sent word they'd meet with Mary posthaste.

As the seconds ticked by, Regan's heart pounded ever more rapidly beneath her breast. Her palms grew clammy and her throat tight. The moment she had so dreaded was nearly upon her. She began to fear she might soon faint or empty the contents of her stomach, shaming herself before them all.

Help me, Lord, she prayed with all her might, hoping at least this time He'd hear her and respond. *Grant me the courage I need to see this through. It's the right thing to do, after all. Seeking justice in a legal way. And it's how Ye'd want me to do it, isn't it?*

The prayer gave her fleeting comfort, just long enough to keep her there, standing at Mary's side, until a knock finally came at the door and the lady-in-waiting rose to answer it. And then Niall and Iain were walking in. Almost immediately, Iain's gaze slammed into hers, and his eyes widened.

Niall next caught sight of her. He frowned slightly and glanced at his cousin. Iain shrugged and shook his head.

It didn't take them long to cover the short distance to stand before the queen. Both men bowed, then straightened. Niall looked directly at the queen.

"We came as ye requested, Majesty. What is it ye desire?"

Mary turned to Regan. "This young woman has just told me a most disturbing tale. A tale of memory lost and finally found. Of a man wed and murdered, shot in the back one night when he was out reiving cattle. Worst of all, though, she now accuses a Campbell of doing the dastardly deed."

Queen Mary paused then, her gaze shifting to Iain's. "She accuses you, my friend. So I ask you now. What have you to say in yer defense?"

10

It was almost as if Iain hadn't heard the queen speak to him. He continued to stare at Regan in stunned disbelief. Finally, though, he found his voice.

"Yer memory's returned then, has it? When?"

She glanced nervously to the queen, who, with a slight nod, gave her permission to answer. "But f-four days ago," she stammered.

"And why didn't ye tell me, lass? Why?"

His dark, sorrowful gaze seemed to pull her in, dragging her down into the anguished depths of his heart. Regan opened her mouth and found she had no words.

"I'll tell ye why she didn't tell ye," Niall snarled, his voice filling the tension-fraught silence. "It's as I warned ye, Iain. She's known all along who she really is. She but awaited the right moment to drive her claws into ye. And, even if she'd planned it from the start, Mary's visit here couldn't have given her a more perfect opportunity."

Regan jerked her glance from Iain to meet Niall's furious countenance. "Nay," she said, struggling to throw off the almost mind-numbing pain she had seen in Iain's eyes. "I spoke true. Until four days ago, I didn't know who I was. But then—"

She caught herself before she revealed meeting Walter at Dalmally's market. Best she leave him out of it for as long as she could. "But then," Regan forced herself to continue, turning back to Iain, "like water rushing over a fall, it all came back, one memory after another. I remembered I was Regan MacLaren, that I'd been wed to Roddy MacLaren. And that he and his men had ridden out on our wedding night and ended up in far more mischief than was wise. And that . . . and that he came back to me, dead from a single pistol shot, and ye were there when he died. And ye own two pistols."

"Aye, I own two pistols," he replied hoarsely. "I've never hidden the fact from ye. And I was there that night. Roddy MacLaren was trying to lift Campbell cattle. Of course I'd be there. But I didn't shoot yer husband. After all this time, I thought ye knew me better than that. I thought ye—" He caught himself, clenched his jaw, then shook his head. "Apparently I was mistaken about a lot of things."

Pain, reproach, and the first flickerings of anger shone now in his eyes. Though Regan had known it would come to this, that Iain would forever close his heart to her, until this moment as she saw him emotionally withdraw, she could only imagine how it would feel. But now she knew. It was as if a dark shroud had fallen between them. As if all the light and life had flickered out, died.

If she had been anywhere else, Regan thought she might've fallen to her knees and shrieked out her sorrow. But she was standing before the queen, facing two men who had likely just become her worst enemies. Only her instinctual need for self-preservation held her together now.

"As was I, m'lord," she said softly, catching and sending back the meaning-laden barb he had cast at her. "Mistaken about a lot of things."

Mary, apparently desirous that the unfortunate meeting move back to its original purpose, chose at that moment to clear her throat. Three gazes swiveled in her direction.

"Allow me to review what I think has been said here," she began. "Regan has accused Iain of murdering her husband. And you," she said, looking to Iain, "claim you didn't. Have I perceived everything correctly so far?"

Both Regan and Iain nodded.

"Well, we all know how costly daggs are these days," Mary then continued. "So it's safe to assume few, if any, other men that night carried them. And Regan has already informed me of the single shot in the middle of her husband's back that apparently killed him, for he bore few other wounds, none of which would've been fatal. All, however, including your admission you were present the night Roderick MacLaren died, is but circumstantial evidence." Slowly, Mary moved her gaze from one person to the next, finally alighting on Regan. "It'll take more evidence than that to convict Iain, I'm afraid."

Regan's heart sank. Her worst fears had come to fruition. No one, not even the queen, would take a stand against a Campbell. Righteous anger rose within her.

"I'm not asking for Iain to be convicted, or not convicted, from the evidence I've presented," she said, clamping down on her fury and frustration. "All I'm asking is that my husband's death be investigated more thoroughly. *Someone* killed him. That someone should be brought to justice. If he's guilty, even if he's a Campbell, he deserves punishment."

"Even if he's a Campbell!" Beside Iain, Niall Campbell's face purpled in rage. "And exactly what is that supposed to mean? We've never put ourselves above the law, and certainly don't mean to do so now, even for the sake of some young fool who brought his own death upon himself. Iain was within his rights to kill or imprison them all when he and his men caught up with those thieves. But instead, he just retrieved his cattle and let those reivers go."

"Mayhap he did," Regan replied, glaring back now just as fiercely at Niall as he was at her. "All I'm asking is that *whoever* murdered my husband be brought to justice. Unless ye'd just like to sweep away the whole sordid affair and risk a clan feud."

Niall gave a harsh laugh. "Now, that's a thought. Clan MacLaren threatening Clan Campbell."

Something went cold within Regan. *The arrogant dog! How dare he be so belittling?* "In case the entire import of all this has yet escaped ye, *m'lord,* I'm also heiress to all the lands and the chieftainship of Clan Drummond. And Clans Murray, Mac Nab, and Menzies are our sworn allies. So though ye may look down yer nose at the MacLarens, I say think twice about doing so at the united strength standing behind Clan Drummond!"

"Och, and don't you look like two banty roosters about to do battle?" Mary chose that moment to interject with a chuckle. "You Highlanders are all far too quick to threaten feuds and retribution, you are. And I never said I wouldn't investigate further into your claims, lass. I just find it very difficult to believe Iain would back-shoot anyone. He doesn't need to. His battle prowess is unrivaled. Not to mention, I've never met a more honorable man."

Relief surged through Regan. "Then ye'll oversee this investigation and bring in impartial reviewers? That's all I've ever wanted, Majesty. That no Campbell influence taint the inquiry."

"There ye go again," Niall growled, "insulting Campbell integrity."

"Let it go, cousin," Iain tersely cut in just then. "Regan says naught that other clans not friends of Clan Campbell wouldn't say. Let the truth see the light of day. I know my innocence. I'm not afraid."

"Aye, but well ye should be. An impartial investigation's in the eye of the beholder. Especially at Court."

"It's in the Lord's hands, cousin. Let it be."

Regan watched the two men lock gazes, saw the battle of wills that raged between them, and saw, as well, the deep love they had for each other. Her throat clogged with tears, knowing she had set a course of events into motion that might have long-reaching, even horrific, consequences. Nay, she quickly corrected herself, the *murderer* had set the events into motion. *She* had but moved those events along, after they had nearly foundered in fear and apathy.

"Then we're all agreed," the queen said, looking once again at each of them. "An official investigation will commence immediately, led by Lord Seton. His loyalty is first and foremost to me, so I trust his impartiality implicitly. In the next two weeks, I'm certain he can thoroughly question all Campbells involved in that lamentable night, both the ones who accompanied Iain here and the ones yet at Balloch. Then, under Campbell escort, he can next ride to your home." She paused and glanced to Regan. "Where did you say you and your late husband lived, lass?"

"Strathyre House, on Loch Voil, Majesty."

"Yes, Strathyre House." Mary nodded. "Another week or so there, and Lord Seton should be able to return with his verdict. I'll await him here in the meanwhile, if it's no hardship on you, m'lord?" she asked, turning next to Niall.

Niall straightened. "No hardship at all, Majesty. We'd be honored to have ye for as long as ye wish."

"Good. I must confess I've more than one motive in that request. Not only do I think it best to have this matter settled before I leave, but I'm also in no hurry to return to Court and have to deal again with my husband." Her mouth quirked. "Still, my prime concern is to lay to rest threats of a major clan feud."

"Aye, Majesty." Niall shot a narrow glance at Regan. "That's a prime concern for us all."

"I ask leave to return home to Strathyre House, then, Majesty," Regan said, deciding this was the proper time to broach that subject. "So as to make arrangements to have all those concerned on the MacLaren side identified and gathered for Lord Seton's arrival. It'd expedite his investigation, it would."

"Rather, Majesty," Niall immediately spoke up, "in the cause of justice and impartiality, I think it better if the lady remained *here* throughout the investigation. Not being certain of her true motives, I'd prefer she not have opportunity to return home and 'poison the well,' so to speak."

Regan sucked in an indignant breath. "How dare ye—" She halted as the queen held up a hand.

"And how, pray tell, do you see her doing that?" Mary leaned forward. "You tread in dangerous waters here, m'lord."

"Aye, true enough, Majesty," Niall replied with not, Regan noted, a shred of compunction in his eyes or voice. "But my cousin's life may well be in jeopardy here, and we all know how evidence can be twisted in the wrong hands." He gestured toward Regan. "Long have I already puzzled over the strange circumstances surrounding this woman's arrival at Balloch Castle, and of her growing relationship with my cousin, which now has taken such a villainous turn. It is all *most* puzzling, and *most* suspect."

Her brow furrowing in thought, Mary settled back in her chair. In the ensuing silence, which seemed to drag on and on, resentment at the unfairness of it all filled Regan. Of any of them, she was the most innocent, the victim, yet Niall had cleverly managed now to make her appear almost as suspect as Iain. And all because she had ridden out that day to try and prevent Walter from ambushing and killing Iain!

But to reveal the true reasons behind how she came to Balloch would be to implicate Walter. And she wouldn't do that. As wrong as he had been in his plan to seek retribution in such a manner, at the time he hadn't been thinking clearly. His judgment had been clouded by his grief for Roddy. She'd not risk bringing down Clan Campbell's wrath on him as well.

Finally, the queen exhaled a long, considering breath. "Your words have merit, m'lord. I think it best, for the sake of impartiality," she said, meeting Regan's gaze, "that you remain here until the investigation's finished."

Regan felt the blood drain from her face. "To remain here now is to dwell among my enemies," she whispered.

"And do you feel, in doing so, your life's in danger?"

The queen had given her the perfect opening to hie herself fast and far from Kilchurn. Regan knew it, and so did Mary. But there was something deeper being asked here than just what appeared on the surface. Was she truly convinced Iain was capable of murder? And did she believe, in her heart of hearts, that Niall was a dishonorable man?

In that moment of hesitation, Regan's gaze skittered to Iain. He stared back at her, calm, guarded, appraising; and overlaying it all was that deep, dark pain. *Och, if I'm wrong, Iain, I beg pardon,* she silently cried, her heart's remorse in her eyes. *I beg yer deepest pardon!*

Yet even as she opened her mouth to answer the queen, Regan knew she couldn't lie. Not even to please Walter, not even to escape the long days and nights to come with only her own doubts to keep her company. Not even if her very life depended on it.

"Nay, Majesty." Regan wrenched her gaze from Iain's and turned back to the queen. "My life's in no danger, leastwise not from Campbells, if I remain here."

✠

"Haven't ye aught that needs attending to at Balloch?" Niall asked, sidling up to Iain two days later as he stood on the roof walk, gazing out over Loch Awe. "Lord Seton's well done with questioning ye and Charlie, and is set to leave for Balloch on the morrow. Mayhap ye could be of service to him there, easing his way in the investigation and all?"

Iain turned to meet his cousin's innocent gaze. So innocent as to be suspect, it was. "Tired of my company already, are ye? If so, why not just come out and say it? I've never known ye to mince words before."

Niall rolled his eyes. "Ye need to stay away from that MacLaren woman. And, to my mind, the farther ye are from her right now, the better!"

"She won't even see me, much less speak to me, Niall. I'm in no danger."

"Aye, mayhap for a time she won't, but I think she but plays upon yer kind heart. She'll come around to ye soon enough, she will."

"And whatever for?" Iain expelled a frustrated breath. "To force a confession from me, mayhap? Because there's not much more Regan can do, is there? I've already dictated and signed my statement of the events of that night, and it's now in Seton's possession."

"I only wish ye hadn't mentioned that ye'd fired both yer pistols that night," Niall muttered. "It lends further credence to the possibility that one of them was used against MacLaren."

"Even if they were both fired earlier, when we first engaged them?" Iain gave a sharp laugh. "Well, I refuse to lie. Besides, everyone knows the likelihood of me having time to reload is next to impossible. And if Seton's smart, he'll now know to inquire at Strathyre for any men who may have received gunshot wounds that night."

"And what if ye missed both times ye fired? It was verra dark. Ye said that yerself."

"Then mayhap we both should lift a wee prayer that the Lord guided my aim that night." He sighed and shook his head. "I said what I did, and I'm at peace with it. Let it be, Niall."

"Fine. I suppose it *is* pointless, repeatedly revisiting that night." His cousin leaned on the waist-high wall enclosing the roof. "Will ye at least consider returning to Balloch with Seton then?"

Iain couldn't help a smile. "Nay. Just as ye didn't think it fair to permit Regan to return to Strathyre, just in case she'd try to manipulate the evidence, it's no more fair for me to be at Balloch during Seton's investigation."

Niall fell silent for several seconds. Finally, though, he turned to Iain. "If ye imagine she's finally playing fair, ye're mistaken. Even now, she continues to scheme behind yer back."

He shot his cousin a sharp look. "What are ye saying?"

"She's had some sort of contact outside Kilchurn, with someone it appears she has been communicating with, if not secretly meeting." Niall smiled, but the smile never quite reached his eyes. "I've had her watched since the day she accused ye. Yesterday, she apparently paid one of the stable boys to deliver a message to someone in Dalmally. Unfortunately, my man lost the lad in the market crowds. By the time we found the boy back at the stables, learned where he had been in Dalmally, and returned there, the man was gone."

"Could the lad at least give ye the man's name?"

Niall shook his head. "Nay. Regan was too clever for that. She only told the boy to deliver the message to the man lodging at the town butcher's home. And, not surprisingly, the butcher didn't know his guest's name either. Whoever he was, he was a clever one, and no mistake."

With heavy heart, Iain turned back to gaze out over Loch Awe. It was a gloomy day, with ominous clouds building in the west. Trees swayed to and fro in the gusting winds, and choppy waves rippled in endless succession across the lake. A storm was on the way.

He felt as unsettled as the day, pulled to and fro by wild, chaotic emotions. On one hand, there was the still raw wound of Regan's sudden change of heart, of her not only rejecting him but also all but naming him a murderer. And, on the other, there was that stubborn hope that, beneath it all, somehow she still loved him. He had seen *something* in her eyes that day they had stood before Mary. Sadness, remorse, even a look of entreaty. It hurt, and hurt badly, that she hadn't trusted him enough to come to him and tell him the truth. But he knew, as well, that she was as much a victim in this sad, sorry mess as was he.

Or, leastwise, he tried to believe that. But now . . . now to learn Regan had been in communication with someone outside Kilchurn was almost more than Iain could bear. Had Niall been right all along? Had Regan planned all of this—even her loss of memory— from the start? And had she always had an accomplice?

"There can be several explanations for the presence of that man in Dalmally," Iain replied at last. "Indeed, the man, whoever he is, could've been the one to plant the seeds of doubt about me. Mayhap he even had a hand in her husband's murder."

"By mountain and sea!" Niall threw up his hands. "Do ye hear yerself? That woman all but has her ring in yer nose, and ye convinced that she can do no wrong, no matter how many times she stabs ye in the back and then twists the knife deeper!" He grabbed Iain by the arm. "Does yer mither realize how besotted ye are with this woman? Does Anne?"

Fury exploded in Iain. He jerked away. "Keep them out of this, Niall! It's bad enough ye're so involved. And I'm not so besotted that I can't think straight."

"Ye are when it comes to Regan!"

Iain shook his head, the pained bewilderment swamping him yet again. "It's almost as if, of a sudden, she's two different women. Yet still I see, hidden deep within this woman whom she has apparently always been, the woman I first came to know. I see the inherent goodness in her, buried as it now seems to be beneath years of hurt, confusion, and life's cruel vagaries."

"The way she was before she lost her memory—if she truly did—is how she really is, cousin. Ye must face that, or set yerself down the road to yer own destruction. Even more importantly, even if she finally does accept yer innocence, can ye ever fully trust her again?"

"I don't know. The Lord admonishes us to forgive our trespassers."

"Aye, that He does, but does forgiveness also entail having once more to trust that person? To my way of thinking, forgiving doesn't require us also to become fools."

"Mayhap not." Iain straightened. "Ye've given me a lot to consider. And consider it I will. Now, if ye'll excuse me, I think I need to spend some time in the chapel."

Niall smiled. "Aye, that *is* the best place to find answers, isn't it?"

He nodded. "It is." With that, Iain turned and headed for the stairs.

No one was in the chapel, which didn't surprise him considering it was well into the afternoon. With a warm sense of having come home, Iain slipped into one of the pews midway down from the altar. He clasped his hands, lowered his head, and closed his eyes.

Just then, the door opened and closed behind him. Normally, he wouldn't have turned but instead given the visitor his privacy. But some instinct, some sense of a special someone, told him to turn. His gaze locked with Regan's.

For a long, wordless moment, they stared at each other. Shock, anguish, then tears filled her eyes. He half rose, opened his mouth to beckon her to him, when she wheeled about, wrenched the door back open, and fled down the hall.

✜

From her bedchamber window, Regan watched Lord Seton and an escort of armed Campbells ride out the next morn, headed, she well knew, to Balloch Castle. From that same window, eight days later, she also saw him return. Allowing for two days hard riding to and from Balloch, she knew he had spent a total of four days there.

Whether or not that had allowed him sufficient time to thoroughly question all who might have accompanied Iain the night of Roddy's death, Regan didn't know. She hoped so. In the end, she knew she'd have to trust in Seton's word that it had. So much of this was, and had always been, out of her hands. That realization frustrated her. Frustrated her greatly.

At least Iain hadn't accompanied Lord Seton back to Balloch. She had almost suspected he would, or if not him, Niall. But both men had remained at Kilchurn. Perhaps they had done so in the cause of fairness. Or perhaps they knew the verdict even before the investigation had barely commenced. Who'd choose, after all, to believe a woman from some minor clan over the Campbell chief and his tanist?

A knock came at her door. Since no one in the past week and a half had demanded to see her, Regan supposed it was just Jane bringing in some fresh linens or another pile of wood for the fireplace.

"Enter," she called out, not even bothering to turn to greet the maidservant. There was no point at any rate. Nowadays, Jane spoke only when spoken to, and the rest of the time she was tight-lipped and averted her gaze.

The door opened, then closed. Leather-clad feet crossed the bedchamber and came to stand behind her.

Regan sighed. "Aye, what is it now, Jane?"

"It's not Jane, Regan. It's Anne."

With a gasp, Regan wheeled around. Niall's auburn-haired wife stood there, gazing solemnly back at her.

"I-I beg pardon, m'lady," Regan choked out, rising to her feet. "If I'd known it was ye, I would've answered the door. But aside from Jane, I've not been receiving visitors of late."

"Ye've never been confined to yer room, Regan," Anne gently replied. "And I *have* tried to visit ye, several times in fact, but ye never answered until today."

"I-I didn't know it was ye." She lowered her gaze. "But then, I didn't wish to speak with anyone, even through the door. Especially if it were Niall or Iain." Realizing how her words might be construed, Regan looked up. "Och, I didn't mean aught against yer husband, m'lady," she hurried to explain, "this being his home and all. There was just naught more to be said that wouldn't have been hurtful, and I've caused enough pain as it is."

"Aye, and I'd wager ye've tasted yer fair measure of that pain as well." Anne paused. "I'd like to stay a time and speak with ye, if ye'd be willing. There are yet some unanswered questions that still gnaw at me."

The last person—well, *almost* the last anyway—Regan wanted to speak with was Anne. Anything she told her would go straight back to Niall, and perhaps even Iain. Yet Regan wouldn't lie.

She indicated the chair she had been sitting in. "Ye may sit there if ye wish, and I can bring over a stool. But I tell ye true, there's not much more to be said. Leastwise, naught I'd care for others to know."

"If ye don't wish me to tell Niall what we speak of, I won't. I just can't bear to think of ye up here all alone and bereft of anyone to talk to. Indeed, if ye want, we can just speak of other things entirely, like two friends."

Regan's gaze narrowed. Did she dare believe her, or was Anne pretending concern so as to lull her into revealing something that might be of use to Iain? Still, aside from speaking about Walter's involvement, there wasn't anything else she could inadvertently reveal that wasn't already known.

"Have it yer way then." Regan headed across the bedchamber to retrieve the stool, which she then placed across from Anne's chair. "Sit, if ye will," she then said, indicating the chair.

They sat there for a time in silence, Regan not having any idea what to say next. Finally, Anne spoke up.

"I think my wee bairn moved yesterday."

Regan couldn't help a smile. "Indeed? And how did it feel?"

With a dreamy look in her eyes, Anne looked out the window and into the distance. "Like the flutter of a butterfly's wings. It was so swift and so slight, the first time I didn't think aught of it. But then it came again, deep within my belly, and I knew. Knew it was my bairn."

Such a simple, commonplace, happy event, Regan thought, a mother's first sense of new life within her. And perhaps even more so for Anne, who had struggled for the past two years to conceive the children and heirs her husband so deeply desired. Niall had already endured the loss of one bairn and wife in childbirth. Anne didn't want him to suffer, on top of that loss, with a barren second wife.

But no more. The Lord had finally blessed their union with the first conception of what they hoped would be many children. Their happiness—and life—would soon be complete.

For a long, anguished moment, Regan was overcome by such an intense yearning to have *her* old life back, to just have things the way they once were, that she thought she'd cry out from the pain. Anything was better than what she had now, which was nothing but a huge, gaping hole where once had beat her heart. Her heart

. . . Iain . . . Mathilda . . . Balloch Castle . . . and the friends she had made.

She blinked back tears. "I'm verra happy all goes well with ye and yer bairn. Truly, I am."

"I know ye are, my friend." Anne reached down and laid a hand on Regan's cheek. "I know."

At the gentle, caring touch, something disintegrated in Regan. Walls crumbled, floodgates opened, and tears, long held in check, burst through. She began to weep, and try as she might to call back the tears, she couldn't. Cradling her arms about her head, Regan buried her face in her lap and sobbed uncontrollably.

With a soft sound of compassion, Anne was on the floor beside her, gathering her into her arms to hold her close. Which only made Regan weep the harder, so starved had she been in the past week for kindness and human companionship. Weep until all that remained were body-wracking, hiccupping sobs that finally dissipated into renewed silence.

"Och, lass, lass," Anne crooned as she tenderly stroked Regan's head. "I'm so sorry. So verra, verra sorry all this has happened to ye. It tears my heart out to see ye in such a way. As it does Iain, who's equally worried about ye."

At the mention of his name, Regan tensed. She drew in a deep, steadying breath, then pushed Anne's hands away and sat up. "Is that why ye came here, then? To find some way to speak to me of Iain?"

"I care about ye both, and hate to see the two of ye in such pain over this matter."

Regan gave a harsh laugh. "The only pain *he* feels is the fear he might yet be found guilty. One way or another, though, Iain's washed his hands of me. If he feels aught for me now, it's hatred."

"And do ye care? If he hates ye now?"

She blinked in surprise. "What does it matter what I care? I knew the consequences of accusing him. But I had to, Anne. I've never admitted this to anyone, but I drove Roddy away on our wedding night, when he came to me drunk and tried to take me in a less than gentle way. I hid from him, and when he couldn't find me, he rode out to reive some cattle for a bridal gift. In the hopes of making it all up to me." Suddenly, the shame was too much to bear, and the tears began to flow again. "He'd be alive to this day, he would, if I hadn't refused, in my pride and stubbornness, to go to him when he called for me."

"So it was yer doing, was it, that made Roddy try to steal someone else's cattle?" Anne sighed. "Och, Regan. Roddy was a grown man. He made the choice that led to his death, not ye."

"Then why do I feel so . . . so g-guilty?" she sobbed. "As guilty as the man who actually killed him?"

"Because ye're a good, moral person, and ye loved Roddy and regret what ye see as yer unkindness to him that night. And ye didn't get to say good-bye, and ye feel cheated. And because ye've no way left to make amends now, save to bring his murderer to justice."

Regan took out a handkerchief and blew her nose, then managed a sad little smile. "It's all verra complicated then, isn't it? Guilt, I mean."

"Aye, it frequently is," her friend said. "Guilt, however, can also cloud one's judgment and make one do illogical things. Like mayhap refuse to see the truth about Iain and his innocence."

"As can affection also cloud one's judgment and prevent one from doing the right thing, no matter how hard it may be!"

She knew where Anne was headed with this, and she refused to revisit the painful considerations again. Indeed, she should've known better than to allow Anne to lead her back to the topic of Iain's innocence. Of course, Anne's first loyalty would always be to him.

"Och, if ye only knew how long and hard I agonized over what I felt I must do!" Regan cried, her frustration and sense of Anne's treacherous manipulations searing her heart. "Despite what anyone—especially Iain—thinks, my decision wasn't one easily made."

"I never thought it was."

Angrily, Regan brushed away the remnants of her tears. "Well, then ye're the only one who doesn't."

"Despite what ye may imagine, Iain also realizes the difficulty of yer situation. And he doesn't hate ye. He's not a fickle man. He doesn't flee love for hate as easily as some."

Regan stared, dumbfounded, at Anne. Had she heard her correctly? Nay, she must have misunderstood. No man, and certainly no Campbell, would tolerate a betrayal such as hers.

"If what ye say is true," she finally found the words to utter, "then I'm grateful for his understanding. But it doesn't change what I must do. I'm committed to discovering my husband's killer."

"As would I be," Anne said, "if the same had happened to Niall. But what will ye do if Lord Seton's findings exonerate Iain, or at worst, don't present conclusive enough evidence to bring him to trial? How will ye feel about Iain then?"

Regan lifted a puzzled gaze to the auburn-haired woman. "If Lord Seton can offer indisputable proof that Iain's innocent, then I'll be satisfied. I don't wish Iain ill. But to convince me that Iain didn't kill Roddy, Lord Seton must also bring proof that another is the murderer."

Anne sighed and shook her head. "Sometimes it's not as easy as that, my friend. Sometimes the real killer is never discovered. Must Iain then forever bear that taint in yer heart?"

Regan climbed to her feet and walked the short distance to stare once more out the window. "And if he must," she asked softly, "what does it matter? He'll be free, and I'll return to Strathyre. And that'll be the end of it."

11

Lord Seton remained at Kilchurn two days, then left once more, this time for Strathyre House. Regan didn't expect to see him again for about another week, and she settled down to her now usual routine of avoiding Kilchurn's residents as much as she could. She took to saying her prayers in the chapel before sunrise, followed by a brisk stroll around the roof walk in the first light of dawn. The rest of the day was spent in her room.

With a late afternoon nap to fortify her, she'd then venture from her bedchamber at about 10:00 at night, when most if not all the residents were abed, and after more time spent in the chapel, she'd risk a few hours in the library. It wasn't much, but it kept her from going mad, cooped up constantly in her bedchamber.

Her schedule permitting, Anne also began spending a part of each day with Regan. The two women would talk and embroider or play a game or two of chess. Though they hadn't spoken again of Regan meeting with Iain, Anne nonetheless kept her apprised of all the castle's goings-on, including what Iain was doing. Regan wasn't able, however, to gain any information on what Lord Seton had garnered from his visit to Balloch. Anne didn't know, nor did anyone else save perhaps the queen.

The question, however, was foremost in Regan's mind. She woke with it and went to bed at night with it still hovering at the edge of her thoughts. And now that Seton was likely at Strathyre, she mused early one morning as she began her walk around the roof's confines, it seemed she couldn't keep her mind off the investigation.

How was Walter holding up beneath Lord Seton's questioning? And had the queen's man yet uncovered *any* information that shed conclusive light on the murderer's identity? As she walked along, she clenched her hands in frustration. Och, but the waiting, the not knowing anything, was beginning to erode not only her patience but also her tightly held control. Indeed, it wouldn't take very much at all anymore—

A sound—footsteps—echoed suddenly in the deep silence. Regan wheeled around and realized someone was coming up the stairs. She panicked, glanced wildly around for someplace to hide, but there was none. Aside from a stone bench placed at the best vantage point overlooking the loch, and the small, enclosed stairway entrance, the entire roof was out in plain sight.

"Easy now," she whispered in an attempt to calm herself. "Likely it's but Jane or Anne, searching for ye."

And then her worst nightmare exited the stairway enclosure. Iain paused, glanced around, and found her. If the truth were told, at that moment Regan wanted nothing as desperately as to faint dead away.

Unfortunately, her usually well-appreciated, strong constitution failed her most miserably. The best she could manage was total loss of her tongue and an inability to move.

Iain, however, appeared to suffer no such infirmities. His gaze turned resolute, his shoulders squared, and he strode toward her.

"So, Jane was right," he said, drawing up before her. "Ye do take clandestine, early morning walks up here."

Though her heart was clamoring in her breast and her knees were quaking, somehow Iain's particular choice of words irked Regan enough that anger gave impetus to her speech. "My walks are hardly clandestine," she managed to choke out, not quite looking at him. "I just prefer my privacy, that's all. Now, if ye don't mind," she added, gathering her skirts and beginning to sidle around him, "I'm finished with my walk and must return to my bedchamber."

He neatly stepped in her way. "And what's the hurry? It's not as if ye're all that busy these days, going hither and yon about Kilchurn."

He had moved close, and Regan found her eyes at chest level to him. She didn't want to meet his gaze but knew there was no way now of avoiding it. Ever so reluctantly, she looked up.

Deep blue eyes stared back at her. Eyes that held neither a look of hatred nor affection, but rather were mildly amused and considering. She wasn't so sure, though, that she liked that any more than she would animosity or compassion.

"We've naught to talk about, and well ye know it, Iain Campbell!" Regan finally spat out. "So, unless ye find some sort of cruel pleasure in tormenting me, let me go." She made a quick move then to dash around him, but he was quicker still.

"On the contrary, sweet lass," he said, taking her now by the arms, "we've quite a lot to talk about. And since I tire of waiting for ye to come to me, I thought it time for me to come to ye."

She hadn't realized how much she had missed him. Missed hearing his rich, deep voice. Missed his touch. Missed his manly scent of sandalwood and leather and wool.

At this moment, as she stood so close she could feel his heat, hear him breathe, soak in, even if just one time more, that bright, wonderful energy he always seemed to exude, Regan thought it surely worth whatever was next to come. She had been so long bereft of him, and needed, oh, how she needed, the sustaining essence, the soothing balm that was Iain! Almost as if some force drew her, Regan leaned toward him, her need for bodily contact all but overwhelming her.

Then, like the chill splash of water on an icy morn, reality returned with all its sudden, disconcerting might. She reared back. "Let me go, I say!" she cried, twisting in his grip. "Ye've no right to lay hands on me, much less hold me here against my will!"

His grip on her tightened. "Are ye such a coward, then, that the strength of yer convictions isn't enough to provide sufficient courage? Indeed, it speaks verra poorly to the rightness of yer cause if ye cannot face me and hear what I've to say."

He wouldn't let it be, Regan thought. He must persist in reaping yet again and again a harvest of anger and pain and hard words, when all she wanted to do was spare him whatever she could.

"Fine," Regan said with a sigh of resignation. "I suppose, since the last time we spoke we were in the queen's presence, I robbed ye of the opportunity fully to vent yer spleen on me. So pray, get it over with. Tell me of yer anger, yer disgust and hatred. That I'm the most ungrateful and unfeeling woman ye've ever known, and a liar and backstabbing traitor in the bargain." She paused to drag in a swift breath. "Have I left aught out?"

To her surprise, he chuckled. "Nay, that pretty much sums it up or, leastwise, what *ye* imagine I think of ye."

Regan didn't know what to say. Her mind raced, trying to anticipate what Iain's game might be, and when and how he'd drive the knife of his own attack into her. For a game it must be. No man would tolerate what she had done without retaliating. Leastwise, no man *she* had ever known.

Roddy had a quick and violent temper, and his pride would brook no dissent or disloyalty. It was an anger quickly over, though, if one survived the initial attack. Walter's anger, on the other hand, was of a far quieter and more lethal kind, long simmering as he considered every possible way to take his revenge. And, when his vengeance came, it was always far more vicious and enduring. It also frequently appeared at the most unexpected time, long after the slight had been forgotten and the other party had moved on to other things.

Which way would Iain react? Well, one way or another, she'd soon know.

"Then get it over with, will ye?" she demanded, glaring up at him. "Obviously, I haven't a notion what ye're really thinking. Tell me what ye came to say and be done with it!"

"I don't hate ye, lass." His eyes burned with a fierce intensity. "I'm hurt, confused to be sure, but I don't hate ye. I just want to understand . . . understand why, after all the time we've spent together, after what I thought was growing between us, ye'd imagine I was capable of murder. That's all, Regan. That's all I want to know."

He only asked what she had asked herself over and over again in the past few weeks. Yet what answer could she give him, save the same ones—that all evidence pointed to him, that it wasn't personal, that she just needed to obtain justice for Roddy's death. But Regan realized now, perhaps just because Iain had finally asked it, that the answer was a lot more complex than just that.

She wasn't the same person she had been before, when her memory was gone and everything seemed far more simple. She was now the old Regan, wary and self-protective, mightily guarding the portal of her heart. She had closed herself off from others and backed away, choosing to keep a wide distance. And an empty ache deep within her throbbed. Och, how it throbbed!

"I'm not the woman ye first knew," Regan finally replied. "Indeed, I was never truly that woman. So ye don't know me, Iain. If ye did, ye'd understand why I'm capable of accusing ye of murder. And ye'd see that I'm not at all the sort of woman ye'd ever care for, much less love."

"Och, but of course ye are, lass!" He pulled her to him, held her tight. "Ye're both those women, to be sure. The part of ye I saw when ye'd lost yer memory is how ye'd have been if yer life had taken a different course, with different people to love and care for ye. And aye, I see how ye're now, marked as ye were by different people and experiences. But both women are parts of ye, lass. I know it'll be difficult, but nonetheless it's up to ye to choose which aspects to keep and which to discard."

She clung to him, though she knew she shouldn't, drinking in the feel of his big, strong body, hearing the reassuring beat of his heart, encircled in the safe haven of his arms. Here, at this moment in time, Regan almost imagined what he said was possible. That she wasn't forever bound to the old habits and ways of seeing things, that she could choose who and what she wanted to be.

But she also knew Iain saw the world far differently than she did, that old Regan whom she had known the longest. She was safe, comfortable in her old skin. She knew how to react, what to do and think. And that happier, more innocent girl she had temporarily been was already beginning to recede, to shred and dissipate. Indeed, even now, Regan could barely remember her.

The only part of *her* that lingered on was her love for Iain. Somehow, that had remained strong and clear, never wavering, no matter how hard she tried to kill it. But kill it she must. The real Regan MacLaren wasn't worthy of a man the likes of Iain Campbell. How could she be? Her parents had left her, her own clan didn't want her, and she had all but driven her husband to his doom. At the very least, she was death to any who dared love her.

Breaking contact with Iain, Regan pressed against the barrier of his arms. "Ye don't understand," she said, forcing herself to meet his gaze. "I *have* chosen who I want to be. And I'm not the woman for ye. Leastwise, not anymore and, in truth, not ever."

For the first time since he had found her here, pain twisted his features and uncertainty darkened his eyes. She could see the battle he waged, the doubts, the questions, the fear. At any second, Regan thought, Iain would arrive at the same conclusion, and the wall would finally rise before his heart.

A wild impulse to stop him, to call back her lie, shuddered through her, and she almost succumbed to it. But if she did, where would that leave Roddy's retribution? Where would it leave Walter and, even more importantly, little Molly, who saw her as the only mother she had ever had?

She knew how to be Regan MacLaren. She didn't know how to be that girl Regan, the clanless, family-bereft waif Iain and his mother had taken in. And she would never know how to be the sort of wife a man like Iain Campbell deserved and needed.

"And I think ye're wrong, lass. About not being the woman for me," he said softly, even as he released her. "Verra, verra wrong."

She stepped away from him. "Let it be, Iain. I've caused ye enough pain. Let it be."

"And what of yer pain? Do ye really wish to return to that, to live the rest of yer life with it?"

"And why not?" Regan's laugh was strained and strident. "It's all I know, after all."

"But it doesn't have to remain that way."

Och, but he spoke so sweetly, and the look in his eyes fair to took her breath away. But he didn't understand. How could he? He was so very, very different than she.

"Will ye force me, then, into some mold ye've formed for me?" she whispered.

"Nay! Never!" Iain gave a savage shake of his head. "Never would I do that to ye!"

"Then let me be, Iain." Tears filled her eyes, and she didn't bother to hide them. "Let me be."

With that, Regan darted around him and fled toward the stairs. This time, Iain didn't try to stop her. She started down the steps, weeping now, and almost collided with someone in the staircase. With a mumbled apology, Regan eased past the woman.

Only later, when her tortured thoughts had had a time to settle, did she realize the woman had been the queen.

✠

A week later, Lord Seton returned late in the afternoon. No sooner had he dismounted and his horse was led away than Niall escorted him into the queen's presence. Regan began to pace the confines of her bedchamber, her anxiety mounting with each passing minute. Finally, an hour later, Anne came to fetch her.

"Have ye heard aught?" Regan asked her as they headed down

159

the corridor toward the main stairs. "About what Seton found or what his final conclusions are?"

Niall's wife shook her head. "Nay. Seton immediately sequestered himself in the library with Mary. Even Niall wasn't privy to their discussion. And now he's busy fetching Iain even as I've come for ye. We'll all hear the results of Lord Seton's investigation together."

The sudden realization that Iain's fate would likely be decided this very eve filled Regan with a curious mix of apprehension and dread. She wanted very much to know who had killed Roddy, to see that person punished. She just didn't want it to be Iain.

Not that there was anything she could do now to change the outcome of Seton's findings. That die had been cast the instant she had opened her mouth to accuse Iain. There was naught left her but to see this whole, sorry mess through to its natural end, and accept the outcome.

"I'm so afraid, Anne," she whispered. "I don't know anymore what I want out of this."

"No more afraid than I, my friend," her companion whispered back. She reached over and took Regan's hand, giving it a quick squeeze. "It's in the Lord's hands now, as it's always been. We must trust in Him."

They reached the stairs just then and began to descend them. Below, and off to their right, Niall drew up with Iain at the library door. Both men paused to turn and gaze up at them.

There was some indefinable light in Iain's eyes as his glance met hers. Not fearful. Not angry. Regan puzzled over it for an instant and decided it was one of acceptance. Whatever the findings, she realized, Iain was already at peace with them.

She only wished she felt so calm. Instead, her heart pounded almost painfully in her chest, and fear clutched her insides with a cruel, twisting grip. Her head spun with conflicting emotions until she almost feared she was on the verge of losing her mind.

They halted a few feet from the two men. Niall all but impaled her with a steely glance, then turned and opened the door. Mary and Lord Seton sat across the room, the queen at the head of the long, oak table with Seton in the chair to her right. Three rolled and ribbon-bound parchments lay before him. Once they were all inside and Niall had shut the door behind them, Mary indicated the chairs lined up down the length of the table.

"Come," the queen said. "Seat yourselves and we can commence. Lord Seton has been most thorough, and I'm well pleased with his work."

As she took her place on Anne's other side, Regan could only wonder at what Mary meant by that comment. Did it imply Seton had actually discovered the identity of Roddy's killer? Or was Mary just satisfied with the outcome, whatever it was?

For some reason, Iain ended up directly across from her. Regan had no recourse but to meet his gaze, however briefly. He smiled at her, a kind, concerned smile without any trace of anger or rancor. She managed a swift, wan smile of her own, then immediately fixed her attention on Lord Seton.

The nobleman waited until all were settled and quiet. Then he cleared his throat, shot Mary a questioning look, and began speaking after she nodded to him. "The past three weeks have been long and arduous. I have tried, though, to the verra best of my ability, to be thorough and leave no stone unturned." He paused, reached over to the parchments that lay before him, and took up one. After unrolling it, he began to read.

"Report of my findings at Balloch Castle. All men queried agreed that the night in question was dark, due to heavy cloud cover that only rarely parted to shed any moonlight. Though several admitted to hearing pistol shots, there was great discrepancy as to how many shots were fired and when. Some claimed to hear two gunshots, others, three. Some thought two were fired in close succession, some thought two were fired at different times during the course of the fighting, and some thought two were fired in close succession and then one more at a later time."

As Regan listened to Seton's Balloch report drone on, she realized that no conclusive information would come from it. Finally, Lord Seton finished reading that parchment, rerolled and tied it, and set it aside. He then picked up a second parchment.

"This is my report from Strathyre," he next began, and proceeded to deliver an almost identical report. "A survey of all wounded MacLarens," he finally said as he neared the end of the document, "revealed one man—in addition to the deceased—who had suffered a pistol shot. No one saw anyone in their midst with a pistol. No one, including Walter MacLaren, the current laird, admitted to owning a pistol, and once again there was great disparity as to the amount of gunshots heard that night. All agree, however, that all shots were heard in close proximity to the other, suggesting only that the shots had come from either or both the Campbell and MacLaren camps."

He finished, rerolled and tied that parchment, and picked up the third and final one. As Regan watched him, her thoughts raced. So, two or three shots had been fired that night, yet it was unlikely Iain had had sufficient opportunity to reload his two pistols. Two men had received pistol wounds—Roddy and another MacLaren clansman. If only two shots had been fired, all evidence pointed to Iain, even though he claimed he had fired both pistols in rapid succession earlier in the fighting, long before Roddy was shot. If three shots had been fired, and Iain's claim were true, Iain may have missed once and hit one man, and the third shot had come from somewhere else. The third and last shot that likely killed Roddy.

"A summary of my findings and conclusion are as follows," Lord Seton finally spoke up again, and essentially began to repeat exactly what Regan had just surmised on her own. "In conclusion, due to the poor visibility that night, the discrepancy in accounts as to the number of gunshots heard, and that no eyewitnesses as to who fired the pistol used to kill Roderick MacLaren are available, only circumstantial evidence now links Iain Campbell to the murder. And circumstantial evidence, as ye well know, isn't sufficient to convict."

With that, he rerolled the parchment, tied it, and added it back to the pile. In the sudden hush, all gazes turned to the queen. She closed her eyes, looked down, and for a long moment was silent. Then, with a sigh Regan couldn't help but imagine was at least partially one of relief, she glanced up and opened her eyes.

"So, no one has been found guilty?" she asked, meeting Lord Seton's gaze.

"That'd be correct, Majesty."

"Then you're no longer a murder suspect, Iain." She turned to smile at him. "Congratulations."

His face expressionless, Iain answered with a slight nod. "Thank ye, Majesty."

Niall grinned. "In that case, if there's no further work to be done here, may I suggest we adjourn to the Great Hall? From all the savory scents coming our way, I'd say the supper meal's nearly ready to be served."

"One moment more, m'lord." Mary placed her arms on the table and leaned forward. "There's yet one small matter to discuss." Her glance moved from Iain across the table to Regan. "You're a widow now and, as the Drummond heiress, will soon be considered by many as a potential wife. What are your plans, lass?"

All eyes turned to Regan, and she could feel her cheeks flush fire hot. "Why, they're just as I'd mentioned before, Majesty," she managed to reply. "Return to Strathyre House. The MacLarens—Walter and his sister, Molly—are the only real family I have. I can hardly remember any Drummond relatives, after all, and few have ever visited me over the years I remained at Strathyre, much less ever requested I return home."

"Yet you cannot wed Walter MacLaren. He's your brother-in-law."

"Aye, that's true, Majesty." She shrugged. "I suppose, in time, some suitable man will take me as his wife. However, I'm in no hurry to wed again."

"Nay, I suppose you're not," Mary replied. "Still, I'd prefer you wed well, rather than poorly. And, if someday you wished to try and reclaim Drummond lands from your mess of squabbling relatives, it'd be wise to have a strong husband, from a strong clan, to aid you, wouldn't you say?"

Regan wasn't quite sure where the queen was going with this, but some instinct warned she'd had some plan in mind all along. "Aye, a strong husband from a strong clan would be ideal. I'll be sure to keep that in mind, when and if that time comes."

"Ah, but it has, lass." Mary's mouth lifted in a triumphant smile. "Now that Iain has been cleared of all charges against him and found to be innocent as he has always claimed, I cannot think of a finer man for you to wed. Indeed, it's my greatest desire for you to marry him."

The blood drained from Regan's face. She stared, open-mouthed, at the queen.

"Och, don't look so shocked, lass." Mary laughed. "There are women aplenty who'd swoon from happiness at the chance to take such a fine, handsome man as Iain Campbell to husband. I only wish I had given him more serious consideration myself when I was contemplating a second marriage. But I was headstrong and determined that wiser folk wouldn't tell me who to wed. And who, indeed, *was* to tell me otherwise? But you . . . you're fortunate. Wiser folk can, and will, tell you otherwise."

"But yer Majesty," Regan all but whispered, so tight now was her throat, "I don't want to marry Iain. Though he wasn't proven to be Roddy's killer, he also wasn't really proven not to be, either. And I could never marry him while there was still doubt."

Mary's mouth tightened. "Well, in my mind, there is no doubt, and that's all that matters. As is my will that you two should wed."

The room and faces before her began to whirl about. Regan felt hot, then cold, then hot again, and feared suddenly that she might be sick.

Wed Iain? Nay, it could never be. All she wanted was to leave behind him and that illusory life she had once, for a short time, lived at Balloch. All she wanted was to return to Strathyre, to abide once more among folk who were like her, who understood her and would always accept her.

Yet she was also well aware that the queen's will was tantamount to an order. To refuse her was potentially to bring down her wrath not only on Clan MacLaren but on Clan Drummond as well. There seemed no way, absolutely no way, to decline.

But what of Iain? How did he feel about this? If he were also unwilling, surely the two of them together might sway the queen. Regan looked up, snared his gaze, and sent him a silent entreaty.

He stared back, his glance steady but lit from within by a fierce, burning fire. A fire that was both joyous and exultant. She knew then, even before Mary next turned to him, that her fate was sealed.

"And what of you, Iain Campbell?" the queen asked, at last riveting the full force of her gaze on him. "Are you equally adverse to the idea of wedding a woman who still doubts your innocence in the murder of her husband?"

As he wrenched his attention from Regan to Mary, his mouth quirked sadly. "It pains me greatly that Regan still mistrusts me, Majesty. I can but hope that, over time and close association, she'll eventually see me for the man I am, a man who'd never commit such a dastardly deed. So, in answer to yer question, nay, if it's yer will, then I'm not at all adverse to taking her as my wife.

"I am, after all," he said, inclining his head toward Mary, "yer most loyal and devoted servant."

12

Though she could have demanded that Regan attend the supper meal, Mary apparently took some small measure of pity on her. Which was likely for the best, Regan thought as she hurried upstairs to her bedchamber. As tumultuous as were her emotions and the state of her stomach just now, if she had been forced to sit at table and even watch the food brought in, she feared she might become physically ill before them all.

It had been difficult enough to endure Seton's endless droning as he laboriously read through all the parchments, when he could've summarized his conclusion in a few, brief sentences. Indeed, he might as well have just said Iain was innocent and been done with it. In her heart of hearts, Regan had suspected that would finally be the case at any rate.

But she had never anticipated that, once the investigation was finished, she'd be all but commanded to wed the prime subject of the investigation. It was beyond belief, much less understanding! And it was so unfair.

Not that a queen had to worry about what was and wasn't fair, Regan thought sourly as she finally reached her bedchamber door and entered. *She* could do whatever she wished, and they must all obey. But Mary was a woman as well as a queen and must surely understand a woman's horror of being forced to wed against her will. Why, oh why, had Mary chosen to turn on her like this?

Regan all but slammed the door closed, only to have someone give a squeak of surprise behind her. She whirled around. For some reason, Jane was there, sitting before the fire apparently warming herself against what had turned out to be a rather chill, mid-September night. Regan, however, was in no mood for company.

"I won't be needing ye further this eve," she forced herself to say in what she hoped was a polite tone. "Ye may go, Jane."

"But won't ye be wanting something to eat later?" the maidservant asked. "Considering ye don't seem to be attending the supper meal?"

Regan choked back a laugh she feared might end up more a scream than anything else. "Nay," she ground out, walking over to stare out the window even as she fought to hide her sudden surge of tears. "I thank ye for yer consideration, but nay, I've no appetite, and likely won't for a long time to come."

Jane finally must have taken her turned back and extended silence for a dismissal. "As ye wish, ma'am," she said at long last and departed the room.

Almost as soon as the door closed, Regan's tears came. They weren't, however, tears of sadness, but ones of fury and bitter frustration. They were all in a conspiracy against her! Mary, Niall, and Iain. Perhaps they had planned all this from the start.

Anne was the only one whom Regan doubted had had a hand in this. Regan had seen the shocked look on the other woman's face, a look that quickly turned to one of compassion and concern as she had met Regan's gaze after the queen's startling pronouncement. Next, Anne had swung her glance to that of Iain, her gaze puzzled and questioning. Not that her friend had gained aught for her effort, Regan thought angrily. Iain's expression had gone carefully blank by then.

Och, but she hated him, she did! Regan pounded her fists on the stone windowsill. He was a devious, cold-blooded manipulator. And he had likely been maneuvering her to his own purposes from the start.

But why? Of what possible use was she to him? The MacLarens had naught to offer. She held no right to any of that clan's lands, or even Strathyre House. And, though Drummond lands were far larger and more profitable, was Iain really that interested in them? It seemed unlikely, leastwise for any wealth he might think to procure.

Though historically Clan Drummond had always been staunchly loyal to the Crown of Scotland, her cousin William Drummond was known to favor the faction of lords at Court who seemed to be distancing themselves from the queen. Perhaps Mary hoped to regain the allegiance of the Drummonds through Iain and his marriage to the Drummond heiress.

Iain had, after all, admitted he was the queen's loyal and devoted servant. Perhaps it was his way of agreeing to all Mary was—and wasn't—saying.

The sense of a trap closing around her filled Regan. Not that that should surprise her. She had been well aware that the exceedingly generous dowry William had sent to honor her marriage to Roddy had been a bribe. A bribe to keep her firmly bound to Clan MacLaren and far away from Drummond infighting and machinations for the chieftainship.

Nay, Regan had known but had chosen to pretend ignorance. She had, after all, wanted the marriage to Roddy. She had wanted to stay where she knew she was welcomed and loved.

But she was also tired of being used as the pawn of ambitious men, as well as now of a queen who was struggling to keep her crown. The problem was how to extricate herself from this newest and most untenable situation. If there were indeed any way to do so.

Walter would have no influence with the queen, especially not against the Campbells' overwhelming strength. And even if Regan could assure Mary that Clan Drummond would be loyal to her, with Regan as its chief, there seemed no way for her to secure that chieftainship all on her own. William wasn't the only relative who'd prefer never to see her step foot in Drummond lands again.

Like a wheel turning on its axis, it all came back around to Iain. Regan's brow furrowed in thought. If his main motive in wedding her was to gain Drummond support for Mary, perhaps there was some way to bargain with him. If she could procure Campbell aid in winning the chieftainship, with the assurance that she'd then keep Clan Drummond loyal to the queen, perhaps that would suffice to prevent this forced marriage.

It would solve so many problems. She'd avoid wedding Iain. She'd still be free to pursue an investigation of her own as to Roddy's killer. And, if ever she discovered who that person was, even if it were indeed Iain Campbell, she'd then possess a certain amount of power to seek justice in her own right.

The problem lay in convincing Iain that he didn't need to marry her to demonstrate his loyalty to Mary. All he had to do was support her in her quest to regain the Drummond chieftainship. There had never been any true affection for her in his heart, though he had been supremely adept at pretending it was so.

She smiled grimly. Iain Campbell was indeed his father's son.

Regan lifted her chin, inhaled a deep breath, and made up her mind. Somehow, some way, she must convince Iain of the many advantages of her plan. Advantages that would serve both of them well. And, one way or another, Regan knew she must do so this very night.

He was, after all, her only hope of convincing Mary to change her mind.

✠

As Iain rose to join the queen, Seton, Niall, Anne, and his mother for some after-supper talk and fellowship before the huge hearth fire at the end of the Great Hall, one of the servants ran up and slipped a note into his hand. He stared at the lad in bemusement, but the boy simply shook his head and hurried away. Only Niall saw the surreptitious act and lingered nearby while the rest of their party headed across the Hall.

"A secret admirer?"

Iain shrugged and proceeded to open and read the note. As the words registered, excitement rippled through him. "Hardly," he replied with a grin, meeting Niall's intent gaze. "It's from Regan. She asks to speak with me in the library."

Niall gave a snort of disgust. "Have a care, cousin. She's had time to reconsider and regroup. In fact," he added, a hard look darkening his eyes, "I'd better come with ye. Ye're so besotted with her and the idea ye might finally take her to wife that ye're in desperate need of a clearer perspective. A perspective from someone who won't be distracted by a fetching face and form."

Iain had had all the unkind remarks about Regan he could take from his cousin. "And I thank ye kindly for yer offer. Her request, though, was to speak with me in private, and I intend to do so. Now, if ye'll give my regrets to the ladies . . ."

"Wait." Niall grabbed him by the arm, halting him.

Pointedly, Iain looked down at the hand on his arm, then up to Niall. "Leave it be, cousin," he growled. "I know what I'm doing."

"Ye forget the queen has already made her will in this clear."

"On the contrary, I've forgotten naught. And, despite what ye may think of me of late, I'm no fool."

With a sigh, Niall released him. "Most times, nay, ye're certainly no fool. But when it comes to this particular woman . . ."

"She's to be my wife, whether she wishes it or not," Iain said softly. "I don't need to grant her aught, and I'll still have what I've desired for a long time now."

"Aye, true enough, but I know ye too well. Ye want more than her body. Ye want her love. And ye've a long way to go to acquire that, my friend. The question is, how much will ye sacrifice in the hopes of attaining it?"

"I'll sacrifice everything." At Niall's startled expression, Iain grinned. "Everything but my clan, my queen, and my soul, that is."

The look of relief on his cousin's face almost made Iain laugh out loud.

"Och, in that case," Niall said, "I suppose it's safe to send ye on yer way."

"Aye, it most certainly is." With that, Iain turned on his heel and headed for the entry hall and the library.

He found Regan already there, standing before the hearth fire, her slender form silhouetted by the leaping flames. His throat went dry with longing, and his palms were suddenly damp, but Iain forced the unsettling thoughts from his mind, focusing instead on the confrontation to come. For a confrontation it would most certainly be, considering the stakes to be won or lost this night.

She must have heard him close the door. Regan turned. From across the room, their gazes locked. He felt something hot and powerful arc between them, but what it was he wasn't sure. For all he knew, it could well be hatred, leastwise emanating from Regan.

There was naught to be done for it, however, but meet the battle head on. Iain strode toward the hearth and came to stand before her. She didn't flinch or back away, only stared up at him with those incredibly rich brown eyes of hers, eyes, he noted, that were still a bit red and swollen, most likely from weeping.

"I came as soon as I received yer message," he said softly, filled with remorse that he had been the cause—at least partially—of her pain. "What do ye wish of me, lass?"

She looked down to stare into the fire. "I need yer help."

He almost imagined that the entreaty had been all but physically wrenched from her. "If it's within my power, ask and I'll do it. But I cannot—I won't—go against the queen's desire for us to wed."

"Why not?" Regan jerked up her head to impale him with a piercing stare. "In the end, what matters is that Mary have what she wants, and not the manner of how that's achieved."

He angled his head to eye her. "Exactly what do ye imagine she really wants, lass?"

"What else?" She gave a shaky laugh. "She wishes to ensure the stability of her position. She wishes to gather as many allies about her as she can. But that can be done without forcing us to wed, Iain."

So, he thought, *now we get to the heart of the matter.* "How would our marriage help Mary in that regard?"

"Ye know as well as I that she stands to lose Drummond support if my cousin William has his way. But if I was chosen clan chief—an undertaking only possible with Campbell support—she stands to regain Drummond allegiance."

"Aye," he agreed slowly, "that might well be part of her plan. A wise ruler hopes to gain more than one advantage from a political marriage. Somehow, though, I think Mary also possesses a tender, romantic side. I think she hopes our marriage will be a more successful and far happier one than she's ever been blessed with."

"Then she doesn't know us verra well, does she?" Regan muttered through taut lips.

"On the contrary, she has come to know *me* reasonably well. I've been at Court several times now over the past five years of her reign here in Scotland. My mither, after all, spent four years at Court with her, as well as with her mither before her."

"And yer point is?"

Iain chose to ignore the anger blazing in her voice and gaze. "My point is, Mary's a friend, and friends help each other the best they can. True, she needs my loyalty and cooperation. But she also cares what becomes of me, cares for my happiness."

"Well, she's mistaken if she imagines ye'll ever find happiness wed to me!"

"Indeed?" Iain couldn't help it. Regan's vehemence filled him with amusement. "Yer hope for our wedded bliss is dismal, to be sure, and we've yet to speak our vows."

"And why shouldn't it be dismal?" she cried, rounding on him. "Not only am I still unconvinced of yer innocence in Roddy's murder, but now ye conspire to marry me for political reasons. Whyever would ye imagine I'd be happy to take ye as husband?"

"Och, I don't know." He shrugged. "Mayhap because I love ye and would wed ye even without the queen's command? Because I loved ye even before I knew ye were the Drummond heiress, not that I care one way or another about that even now."

She glared up at him for a long moment, speechless, then turned away. "Well, I don't believe ye. Ye're naught more than a far more charming replica of yer father. And ye well warned me about him many times already, so I'm forearmed."

Pain stabbed through him, and into its gaping hole came fury. "I didn't tell ye about him so as to have ye turn my words against me, or to feed yer doubts and suspicions," he rasped. "Instead, I trusted ye with some of my deepest fears and failings."

For several seconds, Iain found he couldn't go on, his sense of hurt and betrayal was that strong. Then reason returned. Regan had just been commanded to marry; she'd had no say in the matter whatsoever, and this coming on the heels of being widowed, losing her memory for a time, and then learning that the man who had taken her in might well be her late husband's murderer. Her turning his words against him just now hardly mattered in comparison.

He dragged in an unsteady breath. "Forgive me for my anger," he said. "I'd imagine, at a time like this, my professions of love *would* mean little to ye. But, laying all that aside, the queen's command is still an insurmountable obstacle. As I said before. I cannot—will not—defy her."

"But what if, instead, ye could convince her that I'd guarantee Drummond loyalty?" She laid her hand on his arm and stepped close, her shining gaze almost his undoing. "What if ye and yer clan promised to help me regain what has always been mine? Then we wouldn't have to wed, and Mary would still get what matters most to her."

"Aye, ye and Mary might indeed get what *ye* both desire," he said, clamping down on his renewed swell of pain. "But what would I, in the end, have for my efforts?"

She seemed momentarily taken aback by that question. "Why,

ye'd have served yer queen, ye would," Regan finally replied. "Indeed, we both would have. And isn't that all that matters in the end?"

"Nay, not for me, it isn't."

As she stared at him, comprehension slowly brightened her eyes. Color drained from her face. "Will ye present my plan to the queen nonetheless?"

"And why not just do it yerself?" he ground out bitterly. "Then ye'll know it was delivered properly, with no chance of it being twisted into something ye'd not like it to be. After all, I'm a liar and cut from the same cloth as my father. Why would ye trust me to do this in yer stead?"

Regan had the good grace to blush. "Why else? Mary will receive it more favorably coming from ye. And I could accompany ye to verify my commitment to yer plan. But it must appear as if it were always yer idea."

"I don't like it," Iain muttered. "It smacks too much of a lie."

She glanced up to the ceiling and sighed. "Then what would ye rather say?"

He hadn't even agreed to do this daft thing for her, and already she had him to the point of formulating his presentation to Mary. Still, Iain didn't want Regan to think badly of him, and if this final effort on his part would soften her heart . . .

"How much will ye sacrifice?" Niall's question flashed across his mind. *"I'll sacrifice everything. Everything but my clan, my queen, and my soul . . ."*

Well, Regan wasn't asking for any of those things. All she was asking was for him to relinquish the hope of ever having her love. His mouth quirked wryly. Mayhap, as Niall had said, when it came to this particular woman, he was indeed a fool.

"I'd rather say," Iain replied, his mind made, "that there might be a better way, and then leave the matter up to the queen. *If* ye think ye could finally and forever accept the outcome, whatever it might be."

Misgiving clouded her expression, and Iain could see her thoughts race. At long last, though, Regan nodded. "There's naught more to be done for it, is there, if this plan doesn't work?"

"Nay, it wouldn't appear so."

"Then, aye. I'll accept the outcome. I may not like it, but I'll accept it."

✠

Mary would have none of their plan. Regan had to give Iain his due, though. He tried his best to convince the queen of their alternate idea and, for a time, Regan even began to hope he might succeed. Then Mary asked him point-blank if he no longer wished to wed.

He shot Regan an anguished glance, then looked down, mumbling something about how he didn't care to force her to marry him. The queen apparently saw through his dissembling and reworded her question slightly. "Do you love her?" she asked.

After a long silence, in which Regan hoped as much for an aye as for a nay, Iain looked up, met the queen's gaze, and answered that aye, he did indeed love her.

There was no swaying Mary after that. The marriage would take place in a week's time, she informed them, and she'd honor their union by attending.

✠

Nothing more could be done after that but begin making wedding arrangements. Letters had soon been sent out to both Strathyre House and the Drummond relatives, requesting their presence at the upcoming marriage. And, to Regan's surprise, five days later, William and his wife had arrived and then Walter but two hours ago, just in time for the next day's ceremony.

"What will ye do?" he now asked her as they stood up on the roof walk, gazing at pewter-colored Loch Awe and storm-clouded skies. "Ye surely can't mean to go through with this—this farce of a marriage. Mayhap tonight, when all the castle's fast asleep, we can sneak down to the stables and ride out."

"And go where?" Regan sighed and shook her head. "We couldn't return to Strathyre House. The Campbells would just come after us and likely destroy ye and yer home in the process of retrieving me. The queen has decreed Iain and I must wed, and no one would come to yer aid, Walter. Certainly not my cousin William or anyone else of Clan Drummond. Indeed, it surely suits William verra well to have me back under the control of yet another husband."

"Aye," Walter muttered, "I'm sure it does. But I can't stand by and let ye be wed to that insufferably arrogant, back-shooting coward either. I owe ye—and Roddy—more than that poor bit of loyalty."

"Och, Walter, it'll be all right." Regan turned and laid a hand on his arm. "Somehow, I'll find a way through this. Iain's a fool if he thinks he's won just because he can finally take me to wife. I'll never give up until I discover Roddy's killer. And, living in such close, constant proximity to him as his wife, if Iain truly *is* the killer, I'm certain finally to discover the proof I need to convict him.

"Nay,"—she gave a sharp, resolute shake of her head—"he'll rue the day he wed me, he will."

"Nonetheless, it sickens me to think of ye living with him. He may well bespell ye yet, and then ye'll be helpless clay in his hands. And I'll be too far away to aid ye."

"Och, Walter, Walter." Regan laughed softly, released his arm, and turned back to the view below. "There's no one practicing the black arts in Kilchurn. *That* one worry ye may set aside forever."

"Well, be that as it may, I don't think I can bear to watch ye wed on the morrow. It . . . it'll sicken me, it will!"

"Then who'll stand by me as a representative of my family?"

"William has already offered." Walter scowled. "Indeed, I barely dismounted after arriving here than he was at my side, demanding I tell ye that he, instead, should represent yer family before the queen."

She smiled sweetly. "A bit late to be claiming his strong familial bond and love for me, isn't it? Nay, in this my will's clear. Iain said it was my choice and mine alone. And I want ye, Walter, to be with me. Yer presence will give me the strength and courage I'll need to go through with this."

He took her hand then, lifted it to his lips, and kissed it. "Then, for ye, sweet lass, I'll do it." He paused, gave a harsh laugh. "Who knows? It may well be the chance I've been hoping for to finish off Iain Campbell once and for all. I'll be near enough to take him by surprise before he has opportunity to react. And no one in chapel will be armed, save mayhap me, if I can smuggle in a dagger . . ."

Recoiling from him in horror, Regan jerked her hand away. "Nay! Don't even joke about such a thing! I made the mistake once of allowing ye to risk yer life to avenge Roddy. I won't do so again. There are other ways."

"Aye, there are," he growled, his expression darkening, "but none as swift and satisfying as driving a dagger deep into his gut and watching him scream and writhe in his death agony. He deserves that and more, he does, for what he did to Roddy and what he intends still to do to ye."

Listening to him just then, a chill washed over her. His hatred of Iain, Regan realized, went much deeper than she had previously imagined. Indeed, as he had spoken of her, his voice had thickened, went husky with something akin to possessiveness, even desire. But that was ridiculous. Walter had never, in all their years of being together, shown even the slightest manly interest in her.

She must be so overwrought right now that she was imagining all sorts of strange things, Regan decided. After all, by tomorrow evening, she'd indeed be dealing with another husband's marital overtures. She, who was still a maiden, would have a second husband.

"I can bear it, Walter." Regan forced a smile. "It's no more than any woman must endure when she weds. So dinna fash yerself over me. It's not worth risking yer life for, and certainly no reason to murder someone. We'll get our chance in time. Just keep that ever before ye. Roddy *will* be avenged."

"But ye don't understand . . ." He gripped the top of a merlon and looked down. "It hurts, Regan. It tears at my gut, it does, to let ye go alone into this. Ye're all I've left in this world, and I've missed ye. Och, how I've missed ye! I need ye home. I need ye home so verra badly!"

She had never seen him in such pain. Impulsively, Regan stepped close, wrapped her arms about him, and laid her head on his shoulder. "Och, Walter, I know. I know," she crooned. "It'll all work out. The Lord will see to that."

"N-nay, He won't," her brother-in-law moaned, pulling her tightly to him. "God's surely turned His back on us, to let all these terrible things happen to ye and me. And I don't know what to do anymore. I've failed ye, I have. Ye, the only woman I've ever—"

"Well, isn't this a cozy little scene?"

At the sound of Niall Campbell's sardonic voice, Regan gave a gasp and jerked away from Walter. Though their embrace had been innocent enough, and he was her brother-in-law and hence family, she still couldn't help the hot blood that filled her cheeks. But then, Niall didn't bother to hide his distaste for her these days either.

"Ye could've been polite enough to warn us ye were there," Regan said, in her embarrassment taking the offense. "It isn't courteous to sneak up on folk, ye know."

He eyed her with contempt. "But however would I discover such interesting things then? Like ye and yer brother-in-law in such close, loving intimacy?"

Anger flashed through her. Her fists rose to rest on her hips. "We were in no such thing, Niall Campbell! And shame on ye for yer scurrilous accusations!"

"Och, so that's how it is, is it?" He threw back his head and laughed. "Ye're to be wed to my cousin on the morrow; I find ye in the arms of another man, and now I'm the villain?" Niall's glance narrowed. "Well, spare yer cleverness, madam. It's wasted on me."

He then lifted his dark gaze to Walter. "A word to the wise, Mac-

Laren. Keep yer distance from this woman, or ye'll deal with me. Whether I like it or not, she's soon to be my cousin by marriage, and a Campbell, no less. As clan chief, I protect what's mine. Even," he added with a scornful curl of his lip, "the likes of her."

With that, Niall wheeled about and stalked back to the stairs, leaving Regan standing there, so furious she couldn't find words to fling at his retreating form. One thing was certain. Niall would waste no time running to tell Iain, and likely half the folk in Kilchurn, if he thought it would make any difference. If he thought it would prevent her and Iain's marriage on the morrow.

Which wasn't necessarily, Regan realized with a belated swell of irony, such a very bad thing.

13

"Well, Mither?" Iain asked, spreading his arms wide. "Am I suitably dressed for a grand wedding, with no less than the queen in attendance?"

His mother walked over, straightened the Campbell clan crest fastening the smaller shoulder plaid draped across his chest, left shoulder, and back, tugged up the collar of the fine, white linen shirt beneath his jacket and doublet, then stepped back to critically survey him. "Aye, ye'll do, and no mistake," she finally replied. "Ye always did have handsome legs to fill out trews, just like yer father."

With a wry grin, Iain glanced down at the fitted, long trousers and his simple leather shoes. "I but hope my bride thinks my legs equally as handsome. She is, in the end, the only one I really care to impress."

Mathilda gave a disdainful snort. "That'll be a long time in coming, I'm afraid, if that day *ever* comes." She shook her head and sighed. "For the life of me, I don't know what's come over the lass. I used to think I knew her, and that she loved me as much as I'd come to love her. But not anymore. It's like . . . like some other woman now inhabits her body. And it's most certainly not any woman I care much for, much less want marrying my son!"

"Och, Mither, dinna fash yerself." Iain walked over and took her hands. "The old Regan we knew is still there. We must just give her time to sort it all out."

The blue eyes staring up at him filled with tears. "Och, I only hope ye're right. I've waited so long for ye to find the woman of yer heart, and now . . . n-now ye're to wed a lass who all but hates ye. Och," she cried, the tears now coursing down her cheeks, "I wanted so much more for ye, lad, than to end up in as loveless and unhappy a marriage as I had."

Compassion filled him, and he gathered her into his arms. "Mither, wheesht, wheesht," he murmured, holding her close. "It's in the Lord's hands. It'll all work out, just ye wait and see. I love Regan. In time, I feel certain she'll come again to love me."

"On the contrary, I wonder if she *ever* truly loved ye," Mathilda whispered from the haven of his arms. "Mayhap she truly is the sort Niall worries she is." She leaned back to stare up at him. "He told me, ye know, of her conspiring with that man in Dalmally, and that, just yesterday, he caught her up on the roof walk in the arms of her brother-in-law. Her brother-in-law, no less! I can't think of a more immoral relationship!"

Iain chuckled. "Well, *I* can think of a lot of relationships that are far more immoral. Still, be that as it may, just because Regan and Walter were holding each other doesn't mean there was aught illicit in the act. Though I cannot say I care much for the man, mayhap Regan loves him as a brother. She did all but grow up with him. And they mayhap share a common love—and sorrow—for Roddy."

His mother eyed him with affectionate skepticism. "And *I* say ye're far too trusting at times, lad."

"Och, I wasn't saying I trust Walter MacLaren. I trust Regan. Trust that she'll finally realize that she can depend on—and believe in—me."

"Well, ye can be certain I'll be praying day and night for that to happen." She reached up, tenderly stroked his cheek, then pushed back against his arms.

He released her. "I was hoping ye'd do a bit more than pray, Mither.

I was hoping ye'd warmly welcome Regan as yer new daughter-in-law."

"Indeed?" Mathilda arched a brow. "Warmly? And this for a woman who accused ye of murder and tried to see ye convicted and hanged for it?"

"I don't believe it was personal. The circumstances surrounding her husband's death somewhat implicated me, after all."

"She insulted ye and all ye've ever stood for, she did!"

"Well, I've forgiven her. Can't ye do the same?"

Mathilda scowled. "I don't know if I can."

"Even if I ask it? As a wedding gift to me?"

She snorted. "I'd something more substantial than that in mind for yer wedding gift."

"And what gift would be finer than my wife welcomed into the clan and family?" He smiled. "Think on it, Mither. How else are we to heal the painful rift that has opened between us and Regan? How else is she to begin to see us for what we truly are, rather than what her doubts, fears, and the lies of others have made us out to be? Indeed, if *we* don't first model Christ's love and forgiveness, when will she ever see it?"

"Aye, ye're right about that. She'll certainly not see it from the likes of that unctuous Walter MacLaren, or from that conniving uncle of hers either."

Iain didn't say anything but waited for her to mull it all over in her mind a bit.

Finally, Mathilda sighed. "Fine," she muttered, shooting him a wry glance. "For the Lord's sake, and for yers, I'll try once more to be her friend and to make her feel welcome. But if she betrays ye again . . . well, I don't know what I'll do then."

"We must be patient, and gentle, and understanding. Agreed?"

She released yet another, even deeper, acquiescent breath. "Agreed."

"Good!" Iain took her by one arm, twirled her around to face the door, and proceeded to escort her across the room. "Then let's be on our way. It's time we were attending a wedding!"

His mother laughed. "Ye aren't a wee bit overeager now, are ye, lad?"

He grinned. "Nay, not at all. Not at all."

✠

With a disconcerting sense of déjà vu, Regan went through the wedding ceremony, wedding feast, and the entertainment and dancing afterward like a puppet manipulated by its master. She responded politely with a smile most times when spoken to, followed all requests directed her way without protest, and tried not to think too much about what she had vowed before God and the queen to do.

The wedding night would come soon enough, she well knew. Her glance strayed to Iain sitting to her right at table, talking now with Mary, the obvious guest of honor. He had asked her to dance when the musicians had first broken into a lively jig. She had pleaded that her ankle had begun to ache, what with the day-long rain that had come this morn, and didn't feel up to any dancing. Though he had quietly studied her for a moment, Iain had finally relented and not troubled her about dancing again.

Still, no matter how amenable he had been about accepting her excuse, Regan had no doubt, when it came to consummating their wedding vows later, he'd not be so easily discouraged. And each time the realization managed to creep back into her mind, it filled her with renewed panic. No matter how determined she was to face what was to come with dignity and courage, the longer the evening dragged on, the more upset she became.

Sitting so close to her, Iain must have somehow sensed her rising anxiety. Finally, Regan saw him catch Anne's gaze and motion to her. Niall's wife rose from her seat on the queen's other side and hurried down to him. Because he kept his head carefully angled away, Regan couldn't quite catch what he said to Anne. His intent became crystal clear, however, when Anne next moved to her and bent to speak in her ear.

"Ye look like all the festivities are wearing ye down," her friend said softly. "Come, let's leave and go to yer bedchamber."

Regan looked to Iain, but his head was already turned, once again speaking with Mary. Not that it mattered. She knew what he wanted. He wanted Anne both to calm her and prepare her for his imminent arrival.

"Aye, likely that'd be best." She pushed back her chair and stood. After taking her leave of the queen, Regan followed Anne from the Great Hall.

They walked in silence until they reached the bedchamber door and entered. Jane awaited them, but Anne soon sent her on her way. Then, pulling Regan along, she led her to the two chairs situated by the fire.

"Come, sit," Anne said, indicating one of the chairs. "Most everyone, the queen included, is so into his cups that none will ever know ye're gone. And it helps to have a wee bit of time alone to yerself, after all the commotion and excitement of the day."

"Before Iain arrives, ye mean, to claim his marital rights."

Regan knew there was an edge of bitterness in her voice, but she didn't care. She was fast becoming weary of being pulled and prodded to satisfy everyone else's needs. But Anne was right. As tautly stretched as her nerves were, if she didn't steal a few blessed minutes to herself, she feared she might snap.

Her friend moved close, placed both hands on Regan's shoulders, and pushed her down into her chair. "Ye needn't fear him," she then said after taking her own seat. "He's a good, decent man. He won't force the pace or be rough with ye."

"And how would ye know? Ye've never lain with him, have ye?" Regan cried, regretting her outburst just as soon as the words had left her mouth.

Anne's expression never changed. "Nay. Never. We're friends

and have always been. I just know Iain, and know that he loves ye. That's all, Regan."

Shamed, Regan lowered her gaze to her hands. "Forgive me," she whispered. "I just . . . I just feel like I've betrayed Roddy, marrying a man who may have killed him."

"But ye haven't, dear friend. If ye just meet Iain halfway, ye'll soon see the truth for yerself."

Regan lifted an anguished gaze. "It's not as if I want him to be the killer. But I can't trust my heart, Anne. It might cloud my judgment, blind me to the truth."

"Aye, sometimes it does, indeed," the other woman admitted. "But equally as often, if not more so, it speaks truer than any words ever could. The heart, after all, judges what lies beneath the surface of a man rather than what falls from his lips. The heart's attuned to a silent language, but it's the surest, truest language of all."

"Mayhap." Regan gave a sharp little laugh. "But I've learned not to hear that language, or trust it. Indeed, I trust verra little anymore."

"But ye can learn. Ye can learn again to hear with the ear of yer heart."

"How?" The word was wrenched from the depths of her being. "How, Anne?"

"By letting naught go by without being open to its true meaning. How else do we grow in knowledge and love of God, than by always being open to His voice, His holy Word? And, as we grow in that life, we do so by seeing and meditating on the fruits of our Savior's words and actions. We grow closer by *working* to grow closer each and every day, because we *want* to."

"And that's how I'll also come to know Iain for the man ye claim he truly is? By being open to what his words and actions really mean, and by working to grow closer to him each and every day?"

Anne smiled. "It's a start, isn't it? And it isn't as if ye're a stupid woman, easily led or deceived."

"Nay, I suppose not." Regan sighed. "It means seeing everyone and everything, though, in a different way."

"Is that such a bad thing? Sometimes, when one begins to view everything with a clearer eye and more open heart, one sees reality a lot more easily. And, in the end, isn't that what matters, no matter what that reality actually is?"

Regan knew Anne spoke true. Problem was, it wasn't as easy to change one's way of seeing things as she made it out to be. One's beliefs were built over many years, like rocks piled one atop the other. To risk pulling out one of the lowest ones, one of the ones that all the others were stacked upon, threatened to topple everything. What would be left, if all the rocks upon which she had heretofore built her life came tumbling down? What would she have? What would she be then?

She wasn't like Iain, who wasn't afraid of anything. With the return of her long-term memory, Regan realized that now. She had always been afraid. Afraid of the next blow life would give her. The next loss. The uncertainty of each passing moment. And she didn't know how to change, where to begin, or even if she had the necessary strength and courage.

Because she had no answer, leastwise not right now, Regan chose not to reply to her friend's question. Instead, she rose, deciding it best—or at least easiest—to change the subject.

"Since we sent Jane away," she said, "would ye help me ready myself? I'm sure Iain will be on his way verra soon."

Anne smiled and climbed to her feet. "Aye, I'd wager he will. He's verra happy to take ye to wife, after all." She hesitated, drew in a deep breath, then met Regan's gaze. "I'd ask a boon of ye, if ye would."

Regan cocked her head. "Ask it, and if it's within my power, ye know I'll do it."

The silver-eyed woman looked her straight in the eye. "Be kind to him this night, if ye can. If not for his sake, then for mine."

Be kind to him this night . . . What a thing to ask of a woman who had never lain with a man. But then, Anne didn't know that. And neither did Iain, or leastwise, not yet.

"I'll try," she softly replied. "For yer sake, if not for his, I'll try."

☩

Iain stood outside the bedchamber door, marveling at how rapidly his heart was beating. He was as nervous as some lad, he was, he, who had never felt the least intimidated by any lass, whether she be peasant or queen. But then, this particular woman was now his wife. Whatever transpired between them tonight might well set the tone for their lifelong relationship.

Did she dread his arrival, or was she just resigned to her fate? Iain felt reasonably certain Regan wasn't eagerly anticipating his presence in her bedchamber, no matter what Anne's assurances had been when she had finally returned to inform him his wife was waiting. And no one still present at the wedding festivities had likely thought so either, if the polite smiles and subdued well wishes were any indication.

But none of that mattered anymore. What mattered was Regan and the wedding night to come. He only wanted it to go pleasantly for her. He didn't hope for anything more.

"Help me, Lord," he said softly. "Help me to ease her way this night, and let this be the first step in winning her heart anew."

Then, squaring his shoulders, Iain rapped on the door. There was a long enough pause that he began to wonder if she had even heard him, before a low "Enter" came. He immediately grasped the handle and shoved open the door.

Save for the red-gold light of the hearth fire, the room was swathed in shadow. Iain looked to the bed. Regan wasn't there. He scanned the rest of the room and found her standing at the open window, her back turned to him. Inhaling a deep breath, Iain walked in and closed the door behind him.

She was dressed in a long, white night rail, covered by a sleeveless, green velvet bed robe. Her thick mass of hair was loose and hung down her back almost to her waist. Iain's throat went dry. Standing there, silhouetted by moonlight now that the rain and clouds had passed, she looked beautiful.

So very, very beautiful . . . and his.

He strode over to the low chest placed at the foot of the bed and quickly shed his plaid, jacket, and doublet. Then, clad in trews, shirt, and shoes, Iain crossed the room to stand behind her, placing his hands on her shoulders.

Instantly, Regan tensed, then relaxed. Likely forced herself to relax, he thought grimly. Still, it was evident she was trying, and that heartened him.

They stood there for a time, both gazing out on the star-filled night. Iain considered and quickly discarded several opening gambits, deciding they all sounded either stilted or inane. Finally, though, as his glance caught on a particular constellation, he found himself talking about it.

"That's Ursa Major," he said. "Can ye see it? It looks like some water dipper in the sky."

Regan was silent for a long moment, until Iain began to fear she didn't wish to speak with him.

"Aye," she said of a sudden, "now I see it."

"Do ye know aught of constellations, lass?"

"Verra little."

"Most ancient cultures saw pictures in the stars of the night sky, and many tales as to the origins of those star groupings soon developed. Indeed, by the fifth century before Christ, most of the constellations had come to be associated with myths. The myth of Ursa Major evolved from the tale of Jupiter and his lover, Callisto, whom Jupiter's jealous wife, Juno, changed into a bear. She's the constellation Ursa Major, and her son by Jupiter is the nearby Ursa Minor."

She shot him a quick glance over her shoulder. "Ye sound as if ye've studied the constellations most thoroughly. Stars and roses. Ye never cease to amaze me with the scope of yer knowledge."

"Och," Iain replied with a chuckle, "I only know a verra little about a lot of things. Comes with reading most of the books in Balloch's—and Kilchurn's—libraries."

"I've read everything in Strathyre's library," Regan said. "Unfortunately, that only consisted of about ten books. The MacLarens never had much money for such luxuries, after all."

"Well, they did the best they could, I suppose. And ye won't want for books anymore."

"Nay, I suppose I won't want for a lot of things now, will I?"

Though her words seemed to convey one meaning, the sadness in her voice said something entirely different. His grip tightened on Regan's shoulders. "I didn't mean to imply that material goods are the only route to true happiness, lass. Ye won't lack for love and the warmth of family and friends either. I promise ye that."

"So, ye're all willing to forgive and forget, are ye?"

"Where hurt has been given, aye." Ever so gently, Iain turned Regan around to face him. "As I hope that, someday, ye can do the same. But, more importantly, ye and I begin a new life this day. Can't ye give me a second chance to prove to ye who I really am?"

She sighed and shook her head. "I'm not worth yer time or effort. Truly, I'm not."

"And I don't believe that."

Regan's laugh was strident. "Then don't blame me later, when ye finally do. I tried, after all, to warn ye."

He caught her chin in his fingers and lifted her gaze to meet his. "What did they do to ye all those years," he demanded hoarsely, "to make ye think so poorly of yerself? By all that's holy, if I knew who had done this, and if they still lived, I vow I'd soon make them pay for their cruelty!"

"It's too late." She wrenched her chin away. "And it's over and done with. What matters is now, this night, and what *ye* plan to do to *me*."

Her abrupt change of topic took Iain by surprise. But then, on closer consideration, he supposed what she had said was true. The past, however unpleasant it may have been, was tucked away, safe and sound, while tonight still loomed before her.

Iain smiled down at her. "I had hoped we might lie together as man and wife. If ye don't think that'd be too distasteful for ye."

"I suppose I can stand aught, as long as it's not verra painful, and soon done with."

There was something about her reply that gave Iain pause. "And why wouldn't ye know exactly how it'd be? I'm not yer first husband, after all."

"Aye, but ye're—" She flushed crimson. "Ye're the first . . ."

"The first what, lass?" he asked, after patiently waiting for her to continue. Then realization dawned. "Are ye yet a maiden?"

"A-aye."

"But how? Ye were wed."

"How else?" Her sharp, short laugh shattered the silence. "On our wedding night, Roddy was too drunk to be gentle with me, and I fought him. The next thing I knew, he'd passed out. I ran off and hid from him after that. And when he couldn't find me later, he rode away with his men to reive yer cattle." She dragged in a shuddering breath. "He returned to me on a plaid carried by his men. Returned dead."

Iain choked back his incredulity. Could it be true? But then, what purpose would it serve for her to lie?

"I'm sorry. I didn't know."

He reached up to stroke her cheek. The skin was smooth, flawless. Almost of its own accord, his finger wended its way to her mouth, which he then gently circled.

"Ye still haven't answered my question." The look she shot him was wary and anger bright.

Iain frowned. "What question?"

"Will ye be quick about it, and not make it painful?"

"I won't force ye, if that's what ye're asking. I love ye, lass, and I don't wish for our marriage to begin with pain or fear or disgust.

Indeed, if ye desire, we can wait a time to consummate our vows. Until ye're more of a mind to do it, I mean."

"I just want ye to be done with it!"

She was so afraid. He could see it in her eyes, hear it in her voice. "That's not how a husband and wife love each other, lass. Not in some hurried, furtive, shamefaced way. Our union's blessed by God, and blessed in every way. What we share between us in the marriage bed is equally blessed—and beautiful."

"I-I wouldn't know." Regan clenched shut her eyes. "In truth, I don't think I *want* to know."

He took her in his arms then, because he couldn't think of anything else to do to ease her fears. As Iain pulled her close, however, her eyes snapped open, and she stared up at him with wide, wary eyes.

"Would ye at least let me kiss ye, lass?" he asked, gentling his voice as best as he could. "That's not such a horrible thing, is it?"

The terrified light in her eyes seemed to dim a bit. "Nay, I suppose not."

Iain slid his hand up her back to cradle her head in one hand. Then, ever so slowly, he lowered his mouth toward hers. When their lips were but a hair's breadth apart, Regan closed her eyes.

He kissed her with consummate care, tenderly caressing her slightly parted lips, neither rushing nor overwhelming her. After a surprisingly short time, she began to relax. Her hands came up to entwine about his neck. She arched against him.

A sweet, savage joy exploded within Iain. He felt his tightly held control slip a bit and forced himself to pull back, end the kiss.

Regan stared up at him with a sated, glazed expression. She was more ready and willing, Iain realized, than she was even aware of, or leastwise, able to admit. For the first time this eve, he thought there might be hope.

"Will ye trust me that the rest of our coupling will go just as pleasantly?" he asked, his voice gone husky and deep with a barely contained emotion. "All I ask is ye give me a chance, lass. Just one chance."

She eyed him skeptically. "Ye sound verra sure of yerself."

He chuckled. "Only on the surface, to be sure. Inside, I'm shaking."

"Nay, not ye." A wobbly little smile tipped one corner of her mouth. "Not the great Iain Campbell."

"But ye don't understand, wife," he said, his own smile slowly stretching into a grin. "It only matters that *ye* imagine me great. Ye are, after all, the only woman I must please from here on out."

As if considering his statement, Regan's brow furrowed in thought. Then, seemingly having made up her mind, she nodded. "Aye, I suppose ye're right about that. And, since just this day I did make those holy vows, I likely owe ye at least one chance."

Iain laughed and, grasping her beneath her legs, swung her in his arms. "But one chance, and just one chance, only?"

His suddenness in picking her up must have set all the old terrors into motion again. Regan clenched shut her eyes for an instant, then inhaled a deep breath and opened them.

"Pray, let's take this one step at a time, shall we?" she finally asked. "I am a maiden, after all."

"Aye," Iain replied as he turned on his heel and made his way to the bed. "But only for a verra short time more. A *verra* short time, indeed."

14

Regan woke the next morn to sunlight streaming in the window, a gentle breeze tugging at the heavy velvet bed draperies, and a sense of immense relaxation and satisfaction. She yawned, stretched, and momentarily reveled in the play of muscles and sinew working out all her body's nocturnal kinks.

Then remembrance of the past night came flooding back. She froze. Iain . . . their wedding night . . . She looked to her left and found the expanse of bed empty. The imprint of another body, however, was plain on the sheets and second pillow. It hadn't been a dream.

Yet, as her thoughts flew back, recalling him and his loving, the memories did indeed possess a dreamlike quality. A soft smile touched Regan's lips. Iain had been true to his word. What they had shared had been blessed—and beautiful.

He was tender, gentle, and exquisitely patient, and she soon thrilled to his kisses, the touch of his hands. Afterward, it seemed the most natural thing in the world to snuggle close to him, lay her head upon his broad, hair-roughened chest, and fall asleep in the protective clasp of his arm. She would've almost, she thought with a giggle, had imagined herself some wanton woman, if not for the fact that she was wed. She never imagined herself capable of such an ardent response.

Some woman's instinct told her, though, it was the man who

elicited such a response in a woman, playing her like some beloved clarsach, his fingers plucking the strings with such care until the harp—and the woman—sang with the most stirring, heartfelt music. And not just any or every man either. Regan knew that now.

Even if Roddy hadn't come to her that night in a drunken state, she wondered now if he could've ever loved her like Iain had last night. Though she had loved him like a brother, Regan also knew Roddy's heart. He had never, ever, possessed the depth and breadth and richness of character that she had glimpsed in Iain in but a few short months.

Yet Roddy at least had always been forthright with her. Though she suspected he hid one of his motives for wedding her—to prevent her from making any Drummond leadership claims—Regan knew he had done it to spare her feelings, to keep her safe. In his own way, Roddy had truly and deeply loved her.

Iain, on the other hand, she wasn't entirely sure about. It still made no sense for him to want to take her as wife. True, the queen had commanded it, but Regan felt reasonably certain if Iain had truly wanted to protest that decree, Mary would've relented. It was more than evident the queen had a soft spot for Iain in her heart. A very soft spot, indeed.

Regan pushed up in bed and wrapped her arms about her drawn-up knees. Did Iain perhaps hope, by wedding her, to silence once and for all the suspicion she had cast upon him for Roddy's murder? But then, it would suit Mary's needs as well to silence the accusations—accusations that couldn't conclusively be proven one way or another—made against one of her most loyal supporters.

She sighed and rested her chin on her knees. *Why does it always come back to this?* Regan wondered. Even after last night and all the truly astonishing pleasure she had experienced in Iain's arms, her old, inherently mistrustful nature inevitably regained its hold. Why *couldn't* she listen more with her heart, like Anne had suggested she should? What did she really have to lose, when all she had ever loved had either ridden away, never to return, or never wanted her to begin with?

Regan shivered and clenched shut her eyes. Och, she well knew what she risked losing. Iain was the most magnificent of men. He touched her to the deepest parts of her being with his kindness, his humor, his love of learning, and his openhearted, generous nature. And, after last night, he had touched her on yet another level. Now, she was as physically drawn to him as she was emotionally and intellectually.

Someday, though, he'd leave her—or she'd have to leave him. Her deepest fear was that, either way, she couldn't endure that devastating sort of loss again. Yet what choice was left her but to continue on the path she had begun just yesterday, when she had made her marriage vows before God? More than the queen's command led her now. She had made her promise to the Lord. That vow bound her more surely than any ever made to man.

Her hands came together in a prayerful clasp. Regan lifted her thoughts heavenward. *Dear Lord, the road that lies before me is hidden, and I'm so afraid. I obeyed the queen and married Iain, never once considering if it was Yer will that I do so. If that was wrong, forgive me. Show me what I must next do. And if it was right, give me the strength to face what lies ahead with courage and love.*

Father Henry spoke true, after all, that day he took me to task for agreeing to Walter's plan. I did stand on a threshold and could never turn back. That day, though I couldn't see it then, I began a new path, a path I've yet to comprehend verra clearly. I only pray that I've chosen the true path.

The path that, in the end, will lead me where Ye've always meant for me to go.

✛

Though he would've far preferred remaining with Regan this morn, Iain couldn't risk William Drummond leaving Kilchurn before he'd had a chance to talk with him. And, as luck would have it, Iain met the man and his wife walking from the Great Hall just after they finished their breakfast.

He wasted no time in striding over to them. After a brief nod of greeting to William's wife, Iain looked directly at the other man. "If ye please, I'd like a word with ye in private."

William arched a bushy gray-blond brow. "And aren't ye up rather early on the morn after yer wedding? I'd have thought ye would've far preferred spending it in the arms of yer bonny wife than with the likes of me."

Iain smiled thinly. "It's *because* of my bonny wife that I need to spend this time with ye, Drummond." He stepped aside, half turned, and indicated the library. "This won't take long, I assure ye."

The other man shrugged, then glanced at his wife. "Well, Clara, if ye can see to the final preparations for our journey, I'll soon rejoin ye."

She eyed him uncertainly, then nodded and hurried away.

As soon as they were within the library's secluded confines, Iain motioned for William to take one of the chairs at the head of the table. Iain seated himself in one of the others.

"Since I see ye're eager to begin yer journey home," he then began, "I won't waste either yer time or mine. Through Regan, Clan Drummond's now aligned by bonds of marriage with Clan Campbell. Which means, of course, that ye've gained some verra powerful allies."

"Allies," the other man replied smoothly, "Clan Drummond's greatly pleased to have."

"Such an alliance, however, comes with a few requirements." Iain leaned forward. "But then, ye're a practical man, aren't ye, Drummond? Ye knew that such a privilege was a two-edged sword."

The meager smile on William's lips faded. "What do ye wish of me, Campbell?"

"There's been some concern of late over yer political leanings. Rumor has it ye prefer the lords who support the Earl of Moray over his sister."

"Mary has made a fool of herself with her marriage to Darnley!" William's mouth tautened to a hard-edged smirk. "And worst of all, she'll never renounce her papist loyalties. Ye know that as well as I, ye who belong to a clan who follows the Reformed Kirk."

"Not all of Clan Campbell follows the Reformed Kirk," Iain growled. "Still, be that as it may, this branch of Clan Campbell has chosen to cast their lot with the queen. And we expect that same loyalty from all our family, be they of blood ties or marital ones." Iain leaned back. "Do I make myself clear, Drummond?"

The other man's gaze narrowed to fiery, furious slits. "Aye, ye're plain enough. And what am I to gain for turning my back on Moray and his friends? Because I'll need more than just the assurance of yer continued friendship, I will."

Iain well knew what Drummond wanted. Still, he wished to hear it from the man's own lips. "What exactly did ye have in mind?"

"What else?" He shrugged. "I'd like the same agreement I made with Roddy MacLaren, before I gave him leave to wed Regan. That ye'll promise not to allow her ever to make a claim for the Drummond chieftainship." William smiled. "Keep her, instead, occupied with matters of yer home and lands. Keep her busy bearing ye the bairns I'm sure ye need to secure yer succession. It should be a pleasant enough task, after all. Regan's a bonny, well-formed lass. And Roddy certainly saw no difficulties with our plan."

"But Roddy MacLaren," Iain said silkily, "is now dead. And I don't care much for yer offer."

Drummond's face turned red, but he wisely held on to his temper. "And what good would it do ye, Campbell, to see yer wife as clan chief? Ye're tanist. Ye might one day be chief. Ye don't need our meager wealth or men."

"Nay, I don't, whether I always remain clan tanist or one day become chief. Truth is, though, ye're in no position to bargain with me. Just do as I suggest in regards to Mary, and that'll suffice."

"So, ye mean to use Regan to gain control of Clan Drummond, do ye?"

Iain eyed the other man who, if his stiff shoulders, fisted hands, and murderous glare were any gauge, appeared as if he were about to leap across the table and attack him. "Nay, I didn't say that. I've no need—leastwise no personal need—to acquire control of yer clan."

William sagged back in his chair. "So ye'll not permit Regan—"

"I'll not *encourage* Regan," Iain was swift to correct him. "I won't, however, *discourage* her if she one day expresses a wish to seek control of her clan. Still, if ye're verra fortunate, mayhap she'll never wish to do so. Personally, I can't see why she would. Attempting such an undertaking, after all, would be like wading into a nest of vipers."

He shoved back his chair and stood. "So, are we now of a common understanding and commitment, Drummond?"

William shot him a mutinous glance, then quickly looked down. "Aye, since it seems I've little other choice," he replied with a sullen edge to his voice, "I suppose we are."

"Good. Then I wish ye a pleasant journey home."

Iain pushed in his chair and gave the other man a curt nod. Then, without another word, he strode across the library and out the door.

✠

Mary and her entourage departed for Edinburgh the next day—according to Anne, *most* reluctantly. Plans were made, as well, for Iain and his group to return to Balloch the day after. It was past time, he informed Regan, to get back, considering the harvest was all but over and had, of necessity, gone on without his oversight as was the usual custom.

She knew she was to blame for the extended stay at Kilchurn but was grateful nonetheless that neither he nor Mathilda made an issue of it. Still, it was difficult saying her farewells the next morn, especially to Anne, as Niall kept his distance save for a curt but polite kiss on the cheek and proffered wishes for a safe journey home.

"Come back and visit us soon," Kilchurn's lady whispered as she gave Regan one final hug. "We're cousins by marriage now, as well as sisters of the heart."

Regan's eyes misted with tears. "Aye, that we are. I can't thank ye enough for yer continued friendship and trust in me, even when things looked their bleakest. Mayhap, in time, ye can come and visit us at Balloch." The thought gave her momentary pause, and she laughed. "It still sounds strange, speaking of Balloch like that. As if I now truly belong there, that it's my home."

Anne chuckled. "Aye, it was that way for me as well, once Niall and I wed. That I was truly lady of such a grand place as Kilchurn. But ye'll get used to it soon enough, ye will."

"Aye, I suppose . . ." At Iain's smiling approach, Regan's voice faded.

Both women turned to him. His attention, however, was riveted on Regan, his gaze so intent and loving that she couldn't help but blush with sudden shyness. Even now, three days since their wedding, the fierce-burning fire in his eyes whenever he looked at her made her heart leap with a giddy happiness.

"It's time we were going, lass," he said in that wonderful, deep voice of his. "We've a long three days' journey back to Balloch, after all."

"And what of me?" Anne demanded just then with a laugh. "Have ye totally forgotten about me, Iain Campbell, now that ye've finally found yer lady love?"

"Och, of course not, lass," he replied, wrenching his glance from Regan with what could only be described as a great effort. He stepped over and took Anne into his arms. "Ye'd not allow me to do so, even if I tried. Not that I ever would, mind ye. I love ye, lass."

"But only as a sister," Anne said with a mischievous grin.

"Aye, of course." Iain grinned back. "Niall would sever my head from my neck if I attempted aught else, and well ye know it." He gave her a kiss on the cheek, then released her and stepped back. "Fare ye well, lass. I'll miss ye and that pigheaded lout of a husband of yers."

"A pigheaded lout, am I?" Niall asked, choosing that moment to join them. He sidled up to his wife and slipped a hand about her rapidly thickening waist. Their gazes met, and some silent and very warm and personal message arced between them.

Regan envied them their deep comfort and closeness with each other. She supposed, over time, she and Iain might eventually share such an intimate relationship as well. If she could ever come to trust him and, even more importantly, trust herself.

A touch on her arm drew her attention away from Niall and his wife. Regan turned to Iain.

"Come, lass. We must be going."

She nodded, then paused for an instant more to look to Anne and Niall. "Farewell. And thank ye again for yer most wonderful hospitality."

Anne smiled. Her husband met her glance with a stern look, the merest tightening of his lips, and brusquely nodded in reply. Then Iain escorted her over to the horses, where he helped her mount. A few minutes more, and they were riding from Kilchurn.

The morning sun glinted off the waters of Loch Awe, reflecting shards of light in all directions. In the distance, Ben Cruachan was dusted with a fresh coating of snow. A chill breeze whipped down, setting hair and cloaks to fluttering. The trees, adorned in gold, rusts, and browns, were already beginning to shed their leaves. Winter wouldn't be long in coming to the Highlands.

But this year, Regan realized as their party soon left behind the great stone fortress of Kilchurn Castle, she'd spend the frigid winter months far from all that she had known and loved. She'd spend it as the wife of a man she'd have never, in a hundred thousand years, imagined now to be calling husband. Yet the consideration, as much as she strove to deny it, wasn't all that unpleasant.

Nay, not that unpleasant at all.

✠

After three days of rain alternating with sleet, they finally arrived at Balloch Castle. At Iain's insistence, the three women immediately entered the keep to get out of the inclement weather, while he and the rest of the men unloaded their belongings and put up the horses. Regan and Mathilda had no sooner removed their damp cloaks and handed them to Jane, however, than Margaret, the head cook, hurried over to greet them.

"Och, yer timing couldn't be better, m'lady," Margaret said, halting before Mathilda. "I've a pig roasting on the spit, in the hopes ye'd be here this eve, but there's still the accompanying dishes to prepare. Would ye prefer cullen skink with some chunks of smoked haddock or yesterday's Scotch broth for the soup? And would stovies and cabbage do for the vegetables, besides a nice raisin and spiced bread pudding for 'afters'?"

Iain's mother opened her mouth to reply, then paused. "Of course ye wouldn't know this as yet, Margaret, but Regan and Iain were wed just a week ago at Kilchurn. So ye really must now defer to her in all household matters."

As the cook murmured her congratulations, Regan turned a shocked gaze on Mathilda. True enough, as Iain's wife, she did now outrank his mother as lady of Balloch. But she hadn't thought Mathilda would care to relinquish her authority, much less do so quite so quickly.

"Ye needn't do this," she said in a low voice. "It doesn't seem right, much less fair to ye."

"And do ye imagine yerself unsuited to take on these tasks, child?" Mathilda arched a brow. "Because if ye do, ye must soon learn them at any rate. Whether ye wish it so or not, it's the proper way of things."

"Well, over the years, I've pretty much taken charge of Strathyre's household when I lived there," Regan said. "Balloch, however, is far larger, and I'm sure the running of it's also more complex. I'd appreciate any advice ye might be able to offer."

"Even in deciding what we're to have for the supper meal?"

Struck by the ridiculousness of that minor undertaking, Regan laughed. "Och, nay, I suppose I am up to that particular task." She met Margaret's considering stare. "Save yerself the extra work. Yesterday's Scotch broth will be even tastier today, so let's have that for the soup. And all the rest of yer suggestions are most appropriate too." She paused. "Is there aught more ye'd ask of me, Margaret?"

The woman shook her head. "Nay, m-m'lady. That'll do nicely." With that the head cook backed off a few paces, then bobbed a curtsy and hurried away.

Jane, still clutching the cloaks, sidled over. "Er, excuse me, m'lady," she said, glancing from Regan to Mathilda and then back to Regan. "Now that we're home, would ye both be wishing for me to continue to wait on ye, or would m'lady Regan prefer some other serving maid?"

Regan wasn't sure how to answer her. She looked to Mathilda.

Iain's mother smiled. "Likely Regan will need her own serving maid, but until we can talk over her needs in the next day or so, ye can continue to serve us both." She glanced at Regan. "If that's to yer liking, of course, child?"

"Aye." She nodded. "That's most satisfactory."

As the men finally walked in with the bags of belongings, Jane curtsied and left with the cloaks. "We need to sit down and work through the details of both our new roles here, don't we?" Regan asked her companion.

Mathilda nodded. "Aye. It'd help the transition and lessen the staff confusion, it would." She watched the men carry the bags up the stairs to the bedchambers, then turned back to Regan. "Why don't I have one of the kitchen help prepare us both a nice mug of hot cider and bring it up to yer bedchamber in about a half hour? That'd give us about an hour or so to discuss the basics before the supper meal. Then, on the morrow, we can continue with the details."

Relief flooded Regan. Though Mathilda had been most courteous since Regan and Iain's wedding day and had warmly welcomed her into the family, Regan had still felt a certain reserve from Iain's mother. Despite that continuing reserve, it appeared the older woman was willing to help rather than hinder her transition into her married life at Balloch. It was more than she had dared hope for.

She smiled. "That'd be most appreciated, m'lady."

"Mither."

Regan frowned in puzzlement. "I beg pardon?"

"If ye would, I'd like ye to call me Mither. If ye'd feel comfortable doing so, of course. If not, Mathilda will do. But I'm not above ye now, child. If aught, I'm below ye."

"Nay!" She flushed. "Never, never, think that. It's I who feel the usurper, and a most undeserving one in the bargain."

"Yet ye're now my son's wife, and he *is* lord of Balloch Castle."

Unable to meet Mathilda's steady gaze, much less comprehend why the other woman would offer her such kindness, Regan looked down. She felt shamed and humbled. No matter the pain *she* had caused the son—and she had, no matter how justified she had felt in doing so—the mother still treated her with fairness and courtesy. Regan knew she could do no less.

"Will ye help me, Mither?" she asked at last, meeting Mathilda's now piercing appraisal. "To be a fit wife and mistress of Balloch? I'd try to do so, but I fear I cannot do it half so well as ye without yer support and assistance."

"For Iain's sake, aye, I'll do so and gladly."

So, the barriers were still there, Regan realized. But at least Mathilda was willing to try. It was a beginning, and it was more than enough.

"Thank ye, Mither." With a nod, Regan turned and made her way up the stairs to her bedchamber.

✠

As Iain's wife, Regan soon discovered she was no longer permitted to use the old chamber she had been given when she first arrived at Balloch. Or, leastwise, she learned that just as soon as Iain finished seeing to the unloading and care of the horses and found her in her old bedchamber.

Luckily, Mathilda had the sense to figure out where she had gone and met Regan there a half hour after they last parted. They discussed castle affairs until time for the supper meal. Afterwards, she joined Iain and Regan for a short while and sat before the fire in the Great Hall. She soon, however, pleaded exhaustion and retired. Not long thereafter, Regan's lids began to droop.

"Time for bed, is it?" her husband asked, amusement in his voice.

Regan was instantly awake. "Och, nay. I'm good for another two or three hours, I am."

Iain chuckled. "Well, be that as it may, I'm not." He rose from his chair and extended a hand.

She looked from it back up to him. "Aye? Must I go to bed because ye wish to?"

"Normally, nay. But once I leave, there'll be no one to carry ye up to bed when ye fall asleep. Which ye and I both know ye'll soon do. So, best ye come with me now."

There was no point in arguing, she supposed. And she was weary. Regan just didn't know if she was ready for another physical encounter with her husband. Between the onset of her women's courses the day after their wedding and the lack of privacy on the journey home, she and Iain hadn't lain together since that first night. But they were safe and soundly home now, and her courses had ceased. There was no further excuse possible for avoiding him.

Not that she in truth wished to avoid him, Regan admitted to herself as she took his hand, rose, and made her way across the Great Hall. Not out of fear or loathing at any rate. Well, not out of fear of *him*. What she feared were emotions, emotions that threatened to seize her heart and send her careening down a similar path to renewed loss and pain.

With each passing day, it became harder and harder to remain closed to Iain, to maintain her objectivity. Since their wedding night, he had seemed to relax around her, become again the man she had come to know during those early days and weeks together. He laughed again, was ever solicitous of any and all of her needs, and his love for her shone unashamedly in his eyes.

She wanted, och, how she wanted, to bask in that love, to return it with an equally ardent response. But Regan knew if she did, she must finally and forever surrender her need for justice for Roddy. If she couldn't keep an open mind to *all* possible suspects, then she risked missing the truth, however hard and painful it might be.

Yet who else, she thought of a sudden, had she truly considered besides Iain? Because a pistol had killed Roddy, Regan realized she hadn't given much thought to anyone else. No one else that night could afford pistols, could they? There were others that night, though, who possessed possible motives for killing Roddy. And one man above all came to mind.

Walter.

Though she hated to consider him and indeed had all but put it from her thoughts, Regan knew the time had come to do so. He stood to gain much if his older brother died. And then there were possibilities among the MacLaren clansmen who had accompanied Roddy that night. Roddy could frequently be a strict, even brutal leader. Perhaps one of the men nursed a secret grudge.

Pistols could be stolen or taken from dead men and secreted away until the proper opportunity presented itself. The proper opportunity of a dark night, with fighting and confusion. But she had stubbornly—aye, even unjustly—clung all this time to the likelihood of Iain being Roddy's murderer.

As they climbed the stairs together, hand in hand, Regan shot her husband a quick glance. Apparently catching the movement, Iain turned his head and smiled. His expression was so open and unabashedly affectionate, she couldn't help but smile back.

Dear Lord, she thought, *don't let him be the killer. Once again, I fear I'm losing my heart to him. Still, I can't help but think if I do, I'm turning my back on Roddy. I just want to do what's right. I only fear that doing what's right may be a different path than the one that may well bring me the happiness I've long been seeking.*

And then they were heading down the corridor and soon standing at their bedchamber door. Iain wasted no time in opening it and drawing her inside. Barely had he pushed the door shut behind them than he took her in his arms and kissed her.

His mouth slanted over hers with hungry ardor, but it was at the same time gentle and tender. After an instant of breathless surprise, Regan pressed close, wrapped her arms about his neck, and kissed him in return. She was, she realized, just as hungry and needful of him as he seemed to be of her.

Finally Iain pulled back, gazing down at her with bemusement. "Ye seem particularly eager, ye do, wife, now that we're in the privacy of our bedchamber."

Embarrassment flooded Regan. "I . . . I was just trying to act like I thought ye'd wish for me to act. But if my behavior offends ye . . ."

He caught her chin as she turned her head and began to look down, and brought her gaze back to meet his. "Och, and did ye imagine I found offense in an eager wife?" Iain grinned. "On the contrary. I was but marveling at my good fortune."

She didn't know whether to be pleased or aggravated by that statement. But then, of late, she was so confused and tugged in one direction then the other that she frequently found herself indecisive. This time, though, Regan decided to take Iain's statement at face value.

"Well, all right then," she muttered. "Just don't let it puff up that fine opinion of yerself any more than it already has. I haven't fully made up my mind about ye, ye know."

"I know that, sweet lass." He bent down and kissed her again, this time lightly. "I'm just grateful ye're willing to give me—give us—a chance. And that ye at least like kissing me."

She eyed him with thinly veiled amusement. "I'm thinking I could like doing some other things with ye too. If our wedding night was any indication, that is."

At that, Iain threw back his head and gave a shout of laughter. "Och, it was and more, lass. And, by yer leave, I'll begin straightaway to show ye."

15

Two months later, after finally overcoming the mild nausea she had been feeling upon awakening for the past two weeks, Regan sought out Mathilda one morn. Iain's mother was already busily engaged for the day, consulting with the castle weaver over the colors of wool to be used in the fine plaid the woman was currently setting up to weave. At Regan's arrival, she looked up.

"Good morrow, child." Mathilda paused to eye her closely. "Are ye ill? Ye look a wee bit pale, ye do."

Regan managed a halfhearted smile. "Aye, mayhap. Could I speak with ye?"

The older woman nodded. "Shall we take a short walk in the garden? It's a bit brisk outside, but the fresh air might do ye good."

"Aye. I'll but need to fetch my cloak."

Mathilda nodded. "Good. I'll meet ye near the back door in ten minutes' time then." She turned back to the weaver. "Yer suggestion of scarlet, dark green, and fawn sounds like a most pleasing combination. But are ye certain ye've enough crotal and heath for the scarlet and dark green? The birch bark for the fawn's available all the time, but this late in the fall, there's not much chance of finding any of the other two plants . . ."

Regan didn't hear the weaver's reply as she walked toward the door. It didn't matter, though. The loom work was Mathilda's bailiwick, and she took great pleasure in it. Besides, there were plenty of other duties nowadays to keep Regan more than occupied. Well, leastwise, before this strange malady had struck, forcing her to keep to bed for half the morn or risk vomiting out her guts. Well, mayhap not quite so strange, she corrected herself. She had an inkling of what might be wrong with her. She had seen similar symptoms in Anne Campbell, after all.

Ten minutes later, Iain's mother joined her at the back door, and they set out on their stroll through the garden. Few plants had survived the hard frosts that, even this early in November, had begun coming in close succession. Regan thought she missed the roses most of all. At least there was hope now, though, that she'd be here to see them bloom again.

"So what did ye wish to talk with me about, child?" Mathilda asked after a time. "Since it was apparent ye wished to speak in private."

"I've been ill most morns for the past two weeks," Regan said, deciding there was no point in prevaricating. "It's also been over nine weeks since my last woman's courses."

Iain's mother stopped short and stared at her.

Regan halted with her. She didn't know if the other woman was shocked speechless with joy or dismay. One way or another, it was too late to do aught about it, *if* either of them had wished to.

"So," Mathilda all but whispered, "are ye trying to tell me ye're with child?"

"It'd seem the most likely cause, wouldn't it?"

"Aye, it would." Mathilda cocked her head, studying Regan closely. "And if ye were, how would ye be feeling about it?"

"Verra happy," Regan quickly replied, smiling. "I've always wanted bairns of my own. Indeed, at one point, they seemed to me the only good reason to wed. Well, leastwise," she quickly amended, realizing how that might sound, "the only good reason when I knew I was about to wed Roddy. I loved him as a brother, but the thought of sharing the marriage bed with him—or any man—didn't please me."

"And is it the same now, with Iain? Sharing the marriage bed?"

Regan's eyes grew wide. Was it proper for her husband's mother to be asking such a private question? But then, perhaps Mathilda still had her doubts about the stability of their marriage.

"Nay, it's not the same," Regan replied, blushing fiercely and not quite able to meet Mathilda's gaze. "But then, I long since ceased to see Iain as a brother." She looked up. "And everything's so much better between us. Surely ye've seen that, Mither."

"I've seen that my son's verra happy, and ye appear to grow happier with each passing day, but ye still hold a lot close. There's yet a wariness about ye, as if ye're not entirely certain this isn't some dream that'll soon pass and ye'll once more be that poor girl who first came to us, not quite sure who she really was or that she deserved the fate that had befallen her."

"And now, still full of doubts as to my commitment to yer son," Regan said, "I've just told ye I'm to bear him a child and heir. An heir that'll only complicate this unexpectedly happy but uneasy union we've made."

"A union, to my son's potential sorrow, that's only unexpectedly happy but uneasy for ye."

Sadness filled Regan. "So, after all this time, ye still fear I've not relinquished my desire to see Iain convicted of killing Roddy, is that it?"

Fire flashed in her companion's eyes. "Ye tell me. Have ye?"

Regan squatted before a rosebush. Save for one brown, withered bloom and a few dry, scraggly leaves, the plant was now bare. She plucked the flower from its stem and stood. Not looking up, she began, one by one, to pluck and discard the desiccated petals.

"Aye," she replied at last, "I do believe I've relinquished that desire. Anne advised me on my wedding night to give Iain a chance, to try being open to what his words and actions really meant. To work to grow closer to him each and every day. And I've attempted to do that, to view him as dispassionately as possible and discern the real man beneath his most charming exterior.

"Try as I might, though,"—Regan lifted her gaze now to meet Mathilda's—"I've failed to separate the two. Iain *is* as he appears to be—a good, kind, generous man. A man not capable of cold-blooded murder."

The older woman smiled. "Have ye told Iain yet that ye're with child?"

"Nay. Besides some remedy for my poor stomach, I wanted to ask ye when the best time was for such an admission. Should I wait a while longer, in case I'm wrong about this, or should I inform him now?"

"What do yer woman's instincts tell ye?"

Regan thought a moment on that, and had her answer. "I want to tell him now. I think the news will make him verra happy."

Mathilda chuckled. "Och, it will indeed, and no mistake. But not half as much as it makes me." She exhaled a wondering breath. "At long last, I'm going to be a grandmither. A grandmither!"

"And I'm to be a mither."

In silent, joyous contemplation, the two women turned and resumed their walk in the garden.

✠

That afternoon, waiting for Iain to finish some last-minute instructions on a repair of the granary roof that lay just inside Balloch's inner walls, Regan couldn't help fidgeting with the clasp of one of the two cloaks she held. Though she suspected her husband would take the news of her pregnancy very well, she still felt a certain nervous anticipation. More than anything she had ever wanted, Regan wanted to make Iain happy.

Watching him as, with bent head and intent expression, he spoke with Charlie, she couldn't help a thrill of pride. He was such a braw man, he was, tall, broad-shouldered, and strong. And he was hers. This good, wonderful, caring man was *her* husband.

She didn't know how she had ever come to deserve him. She was past caring why. He was God's gift to her and, for however long she would have him, she was learning to accept it and be content. To do otherwise was the height of ingratitude and no small amount of cowardice. Regan refused to live her life in fear anymore.

But then, how could anyone live life in half measures when one was so blessed? A good home. A magnificent, loving husband. A wee babe growing in her womb. What more could any woman want? Och, but she was so verra, verra happy!

Iain glanced up just then, caught her staring at him, and grinned. He turned back to Charlie for a minute more, then nodded and began to walk toward her.

"Ye must really cease the hungry looks ye send my way," he said by way of greeting. "It's becoming quite the talk of Balloch, it is."

Regan knew him too well now to permit him to unsettle her. "Och, and ye love it, and don't even try to deny it." She laid a hand on his arm. "It's a fine day for a stroll. Can ye spare a short time away from all yer duties to accompany me?"

"Aye, but only if ye agree to go to a special spot I've been meaning to show ye and gaze at me adoringly all the while. I'm not a man who soon tires, after all, of his wife's doting attentions."

"Well," Regan replied, pretending to give his request some intensive thought, "I suppose it's a small price to pay for yer company. But just this once."

He nodded solemnly, though a smile twitched at one corner of his mouth. "Of course. Just this once."

She handed his cloak to him. "Then we're off?"

"Aye." Iain swung his cloak over his shirt, trews, and jacket, fastened the neck closed, then helped Regan don her cloak.

The land was frost-edged and glinted in the late morning sun. It was a cold day, but no breezes blew. The snowcapped peak of massive Ben Lawers reflected sharp and clear in the waters of long, narrow Loch Tay. The dark, bare, ascendant arms of the myriad oaks, ashes, and elms on the valley floor contrasted with the long, drooping branches of the willows growing at the lake's edge. Mixed woodlands of birch, rowan, pine, and juniper dotted the higher elevations before giving way above the tree line to upland heath dominated by what was now snow-covered heather and blaeberry bushes.

At Regan's insistence, their walk was leisurely. The cold, however, soon turned their cheeks and noses pink, and they expelled white clouds with each breath they took. At last, though, they arrived at a spot on Loch Tay where a wooden, straw-thatched roundhouse on stilts, connected to the shore by a timber walkway, stood about twenty feet out in the water. It was obviously no longer inhabited and looked to be slowly falling in on itself. Still, Regan found it a fascinating sight.

"This is a crannog, isn't it?" she asked, striding up to the beginning of the crumbling causeway. "I've heard of these man-made islands, though this particular one isn't built on a pile of rocks like the ones I've read about."

"Nay, it isn't." Iain ambled over. "It's just one variation, I suppose. Not that cutting all that wood to build such a structure would've been much easier than dragging tons of rocks out into the loch to form a small island would be. They're all verra ancient, or at least the original crannogs were anyway. Some of them have been modified and reused over the centuries as farmers' homesteads, or refuges during times of trouble, or for hunting or fishing stations. Likely their original use was as individual family homesteads, which housed not only the people but their livestock."

Regan studied the dwelling with renewed interest. "How old do ye imagine these places to be?"

Iain shrugged. "It's hard to say. Some of them may date back to well before the birth of Christ. Some of the tales about them, anyway, go that far back."

"Do ye think those folk were verra different than we? I know their lives must have been much harder, of course, but do ye imagine they had the same sort of hopes and dreams as we do, fell in love, wed, and were just as happy raising their families and working toward a future together?"

He moved to stand at her side and slipped an arm about her waist. "Even that far back, I think they were just like us, lass. Just trying their best to live their lives with honor and to make a safe, happy home for themselves and their loved ones."

"And some of them may well be yer ancestors." Regan leaned her head against his shoulder. "Just like, someday if the good Lord is willing, we'll be ancestors of folk who'll mayhap look back on the ruins of Balloch Castle and wonder what sort of people we were."

"Ye're certainly in a thoughtful mood." He kissed the top of her head. "Wondering about legacies, ancestors, and children."

"Aye, that I am." She straightened and regarded him with tender consideration. "I love ye, Iain Campbell. Love ye with all my heart."

Joy flared in his deep blue eyes. "Do ye now?"

"Aye," Regan replied with a firm little nod, "I do."

"And I love ye, lass."

"I know."

"Do ye now?" He gave a sharp bark of laughter. "Well, I suppose I'm not one for hiding what I truly feel."

She chuckled. "Nay, ye're not, or leastwise, not with me. I like that, though. Indeed, I needed it even when the time came when I couldn't understand why ye'd ever care for someone like me. Even when I dared not accept or even trust yer love."

"But now ye do."

"Aye, I do." She sighed and laid her head back against his shoulder. "And in just enough time too, I'd say. Our bairn will need both parents loving it and each other. Bairns require, after all, quite a lot of work and patience."

Iain's hand tightened on her waist. "Are ye trying to tell me, in yer own roundabout and especially unnerving way," he asked hoarsely, "that ye're with child?"

"So it seems." Regan grinned. "Does that please ye?"

He sighed and nodded. "Aye. It pleases me greatly. And what of ye? Are ye equally pleased?"

"Aye. I am."

"When's the bairn to be born?"

"In early July, from yer mither's calculations."

"My mither!" Iain released her, turned, then took her by both arms and searched her face. "My mither knows, and ye're just now telling me?"

"I saw no point in telling ye until I was certain. And who else would be able to advise me but another woman?" She smiled up at him. "Mathilda was verra happy, she was, to know she'll finally be a grandmither."

He gave a snort of laughter. "I can well imagine she was. Many were the times when I'm sure she despaired ever of seeing me wed, much less gifting her with grandchildren. She'll be forever in yer debt now, lass."

"No more so than I'll always be in hers."

"Och, lass, lass!" Iain pulled her to him and held her tight. "I'm to be a father. Indeed, Niall and I'll both soon be fathers. Won't Anne and Niall be happy to hear this news! I'll have to write them this verra day."

"Don't ye think we should wait a time, like Niall and Anne did, to make certain all's well with the wee one?"

"And how long would that be?" Iain asked, holding her from him now so he could see her face.

"Well, I'll be over three months along by Christmastide. Wouldn't that be a most wonderful Christmas gift to send them? And we could tell all of Balloch the news at the same time."

"Christmastide, eh?"

She nodded.

"Another three weeks, eh?"

"Aye."

Iain smiled, and, standing in the wake of his smile's breathtaking beauty, Regan thought she might melt right there at his feet. Och, how she loved this man! How good the Lord had been to the both of them!

"Well, if it pleases ye to wait, lass, then I'll do it," he finally replied. "But I warn ye they may all suspect something's afoot anyway, seeing as how I'll constantly be grinning from ear to ear and strutting about like some banty rooster."

"Then our secret's safe enough, it is," she said with a chuckle.

He frowned in puzzlement. "Indeed? Why so?"

"Because, dearest husband, grinning and strutting are yer usual behaviors." She smiled up at him sweetly. "Ye did know that, didn't ye?"

Iain arched a dark blond brow. "Nay, I didn't."

"Well, it's true enough. Or, leastwise, true since ye brought me home as yer wife."

"Och, lass," he said, pulling her back into the strong, warm haven of his arms. "Ye speak true. Indeed, what man wouldn't strut and grin with a bonny wife such as ye?"

She snuggled up against him, so happy and content she thought her heart would burst with the sheer joy of it. "Aye," Regan whispered, "and what woman wouldn't feel the same, with a bonny husband such as ye?"

✠

Two months later, Walter brushed the snow from his thick leather jacket and plaid as he waited for William Drummond to be notified of his arrival. It had been a miserable journey here, through a driving snowstorm and near blizzard conditions, but he knew better than to keep William Drummond waiting. Especially when the man's terse letter had suggested a joint plan to return Regan to MacLaren control.

William's manservant finally returned. "M'lord's otherwise engaged for at least another fifteen minutes. He said for ye to take yer ease in his study closet. There's a fire to warm yerself there, and I'll soon fetch ye a hot drink. Have ye any preferences?"

"I took a fancy to yer fine ale last time I was here. Would a pitcher of hot King's Cup be too much trouble to prepare?"

"Nay, m'lord. It'd be my greatest pleasure." The man bowed and hurried away.

Quite a change in his reception since his last visit, Walter thought, watching William's manservant depart. It could only mean one thing. Drummond was very upset about something and desperately needed his help.

A smile on his lips, he headed across the entry area to the small room William used as his study. The room was indeed warm from the hearth fire. Walter was soon settled in a high-backed chair with his feet propped on a stool. It didn't take long for him to thaw his frozen limbs and, indeed, even begin to doze a bit. The manservant, however, soon returned with a small pewter pitcher and two mugs on a tray.

Walter lost no time in pouring out some of the hot brandy and strong Scotch ale drink, then swallowing half the mug's contents. It was a most pleasing mixture, with the slightly sweetened, liquid fire of brandy and ale, passing tang of lemon, and rich flavors of cinnamon, cloves, ginger, and nutmeg. As the King's Cup slid down his throat, a satisfying warmth spread from his gullet out to fill his whole chest. He sighed deeply, closed his eyes, and savored the delicious sensation.

With a resounding thud, the door behind him slammed open. Mug in hand, Walter wheeled around. William, hands on his hips, stood there in the open doorway, grinning back at him.

"Rather fond of the grand entrances, aren't ye?" Walter asked before rising from his chair. He lifted his mug. "Care for a wee swallow of King's Cup? It's verra tasty, it is."

"Don't mind if I do." His host grabbed the door and pushed it shut, then strode over to the fire. He took the mug Walter offered and, throwing back his head, proceeded to drain its entire contents.

Walter watched him with no small amount of irritation. If William thought to intimidate him by all this showmanship, he'd soon learn otherwise. *He* already knew all that he needed. William needed his help. *He*, for a change, held the upper hand.

After a refill, the Drummond chief finally settled in the other chair facing the fire. Walter was content to wait for him to make the first move. He sipped his spiced ale and brandy and pretended interest in watching the fire.

Finally, William cleared his throat. "So, have ye heard from Regan of late?"

"Aye. About Christmastide, she wrote me a verra cheery letter, informing me how happy she was and that her and Campbell's first bairn is due in July." He gave a disparaging snort. "I wonder who coerced her into writing that drivel, leastwise the part about how happy she was."

"And I say ye delude yerself if ye imagine she isn't settling nicely into life at Balloch." Walter's host paused to take a deep swallow of his mug. "The lass has aught she wishes, and wants for naught. She's happy, and no mistake."

Walter's irritation simmered into anger. "It's but a charade she plays to lull that preening peacock of a husband into betraying his cold-blooded, murdering side. Give her time, and ye'll see."

"Well, time's not a luxury I can spare." William eyed him over the top of his mug. "Despite his assurances to the contrary, I feel certain Iain Campbell plans to manipulate Regan to seek the Drummond chieftainship. And ye know as well as I that, with Campbell forces to back them up, I've no chance of keeping my position."

Ah, at last we get to the heart of the matter, Walter thought. "Aye, neither of our clans can hope to defeat any Campbell attack, be it separately or united."

"Regan should've stayed where she belonged—at Strathyre House. Curse Roddy for going off that night, to reive Campbell cattle, no less! He was daft, he was!"

"It was ill-advised, to be sure." Walter shrugged. "Even now, I frequently revisit that ill-fated night and wonder what I could've done to prevent the tragedy. But Roddy never was one to listen to reason."

"Well, ye certainly profited from that ill-fated night." As William took another drink of his mug, his gaze never left Walter's. "Ye're now laird of Strathyre and its lands. One would almost wonder if ye didn't have a hand in yer brother's death."

Walter knew there had been talk among Clan MacLaren about that very possibility. But he also knew there was no proof, and without proof no one could be convicted. Iain Campbell's exoneration, by the queen, no less, was ample evidence of that.

He smiled. "Just because a man stands to profit by the unfortunate death of his kin doesn't mean he had a hand in that death."

"Nay, to be sure." The other man's glance narrowed. "We'll both profit, however, if Iain Campbell dies."

Walter wasn't about to appear overeager, though he had thought long and hard about ways to murder the Campbell tanist. Even the thought of him touching Regan made his blood boil. Indeed, when he had first read of Regan's pregnancy, he had thought he'd choke on his upsurge of rage and envy. But William didn't need to know that. Such knowledge would only give him the upper hand.

"I'd like Regan back at Strathyre where she belongs," he said. "That's true enough. But to kill to get it . . ."

"Well, I've no scruples about seeing Campbell dead," William muttered darkly. "He thinks he can blackmail me to support the queen, he does. I won't permit anyone to do that. Not even a Campbell!"

"And is he mayhap using the threat of Regan returning to claim the Drummond chieftainship as his inducement?"

William shot him a furious look. "What else *could* he use against me? The conniving, viperous worm!"

"More like an abortive, rooting hog, to my mind of it."

"Aye, and a foul lump of deformity," William countered, his voice beginning to slur a bit. "Deep, hollow, treacherous, and full of guile to boot."

From the sound of him, Walter decided the man had been in his cups long before he had arrived. It was likely past time to get this matter settled, before William slipped into a drunken stupor.

"Well, be that as it may," he said, "ye've yet to tell me yer plan."

"Plan?" His host glanced up from the mug he had just emptied, a slightly befuddled expression on his face.

"Aye," Walter patiently reiterated. "Yer plan to rid us both of the scourge of Iain Campbell."

"Och, aye." He nodded. "My plan. It's simple enough, it is. We need to keep in close contact as to Campbell's whereabouts, and mayhap even lure him to Strathyre for a wee visit. I'm sure ye could convince Regan to pay a visit home, couldn't ye?"

"In time, aye. She dotes on my wee sister." Walter smiled. "And Campbell's apparently so besotted with Regan, it might be an easy enough undertaking to get him to come along. Once I get him to Strathyre, however, what do ye propose I do with him?"

"Naught save inform me when ye know their departure date. Then I'll bring my men, all dressed as outlaws, to lie in ambush. Since ye'll also apprise me of the number of men accompanying Campbell home—and his route—it'll be an easy enough thing to send a sufficient number of my lads to overpower them, as well as to set up the perfect ambush along the way."

"And naught about that attack will incriminate me?"

William grinned. "Naught will incriminate either of us, my friend. Otherwise, the plan's ultimately a failure, isn't it?"

"Aye, I suppose it is." Walter paused. "And what of Regan?"

His host gave an offhand shrug. "What of her? It matters not to me if she dies in the attack. Indeed, her death's of even greater personal advantage than Campbell's."

"Well, it matters to me." Walter leaned forward, dangling his now empty mug between his legs. "In truth, ye must give me yer word Regan won't be harmed, or I'll not help ye in this."

"So, ye still want her, do ye? Another man's leavings? Carrying *his* child?"

A grim, cold resolve filled Walter. "It's true. I don't think I could stomach Campbell's child hanging about. But bairns die all the time of a variety of illnesses and accidents."

"It matters not to me what ye do with the brat. Just as long as ye hold to our earlier bargain and keep Regan at Strathyre, I'll be content."

"Aye, I'll keep her so safe and sound she'll never set foot off MacLaren lands again." Walter cocked his head. "Ye also still intend to honor yer offer of a yearly stipend for her upkeep, don't ye?"

William's mug clattered to the stone floor. "Aye, to be sure, MacLaren," he muttered thickly. "I'm an honorable man. I keep my word . . ."

With that, the Drummond chief fell back in his chair. His eyes slid shut, his mouth fell open, and a soft snore emanated from the back of his throat. Walter watched him for a time, considering all the possible ways he could turn this windfall to his best interests. Finally, though, he rose and left the room, his purpose to find William's manservant.

He needed food and a place to sleep for the night. The morrow was soon enough to confirm their agreement before heading back to Strathyre. Then, all that remained was to await the perfect opportunity. After all, even if William tended toward a reckless impatience, he didn't.

He had all the time in the world. All the time in the world to win back his lady fair.

16

Iain lay there in the darkness, suddenly awake though he didn't know why or how he had come to be so. All was silent in Balloch, the thick stone walls and window shuttered against the late winter cold an effective deterrent against the usual household sounds.

Beside him, Regan slept peacefully, curled on her side facing him. They had only retired an hour or so earlier, so the hearth fire still dimly illuminated the room, casting her features into soft, shadowed relief.

He smiled tenderly. Och, but she was so dear to him, his beautiful, loving wife! His gaze lowered to her belly. Though she had carried their child for five months now, it was barely rounding beneath her night rail. Indeed, only this night had she finally felt the bairn's first movements deep within.

In a little over four months, he'd hold that child in his arms. His and Regan's child. Iain longed for that day with all his heart. And he vowed he'd be the father to it that *he* had never had.

His mouth twisted wryly. Strange that the longer he was wed to Regan, the less and less he thought about his father. Perhaps that bitter time was finally behind him.

Already, he felt he had surpassed the man Duncan Campbell had been. He had a wife whom he loved and who loved him, the first child of what he hoped would be several on the way, and a castle and lands that, under his diligent management, were far more prosperous than they had ever been in his father's time. And he was tanist of Clan Campbell based on his own merits, not as a result of treachery and subterfuge.

He was also a man of God. He loved the Lord and strove always to do His will. To treat others with kindness and a fair hand. And he was blessed, och, so very blessed in turn. In truth, he felt as if the Lord led him, and His right hand held him up.

Outside, the stout wooden gate of Balloch's outer wall squealed open. Iain slid from bed and hurried to the window. Shoving aside the thick woolen curtains, he unfastened the latch and pushed open the shutters. Down below, in the inner courtyard, twenty riders were just pulling up.

He closed the shutters, latched them shut, then pulled the curtains to. Next, Iain made his way to the clothes chest and quickly began to dress.

As quietly as he attempted to do so, however, his actions must have wakened Regan. She sat up in bed.

"What are ye doing?"

"Some men just rode in." He hopped around as he tried to don his soft leather brogues. Finally, giving up the attempt, Iain sat on the side of the bed. "I need to go down and see who they are."

Regan tossed aside the comforter and climbed from bed. "Well, then so must I. They may need something to eat and most definitely a place to sleep for the night."

Iain was tempted to tell her to stay abed and he'd take care of their needs, but he knew such an order wouldn't sit well with his wife. She took great pride in fulfilling her duties as lady of Balloch. "Well, dress warmly then," he said, donning his shirt and tucking it into his trews. "Ye know how chill it gets once they bank the fire in the Great Hall for the night."

She grinned. "I will." Regan angled her head, eyeing him up and down. "Ye look verra fetching, ye do. I look forward to snuggling with ye, once we return to bed."

"Do ye now? Then let me be on my way. The sooner I deal with our nocturnal visitors, the sooner we'll be back abed."

He left her then to finish her dressing and was soon striding down the long corridor to the stairs leading to the entry hall. As Iain reached the head of the stairs, the front door opened and Niall and five of his men were let in by Charlie.

Iain's heart commenced a furious pounding. Anne had been due to deliver in the past few days or so. And Niall would never leave her side until she had, unless . . .

His throat constricted. *Please, Lord Jesus. Don't let aught ill have happened to Anne.*

As Iain forced himself to descend the stairs, Niall caught sight of him. The Campbell chief grinned. Relief swamped Iain. He smiled back.

"And what of Anne and yer bairn?" he asked just as soon as he drew up before Niall. "Has she delivered?"

His dark-haired cousin nodded, his eyes gleaming with pride and satisfaction. "Aye, but a week ago. We've a son, a strong, braw lad with Annie's eyes and my hair."

"And is she well?"

"Her childbearing was difficult, but, aye, she's well. Despite everyone's admonitions to stay abed, Anne's already up and about."

Iain gripped his cousin by the arm. "Och, I'm so glad. Congratulations, Niall. Ye finally have the son and heir ye've so long desired."

A movement at the head of the stairs apparently caught Niall's eye. His smile dimmed. Iain knew it had to be Regan.

"And what of yer wife?" the Campbell asked. "Is all well with her and yer wee bairn?"

"Aye." Iain nodded. "All's well with her—and with us. We're verra happy."

Niall wrenched his gaze back to Iain. "Then I'm verra happy for the both of ye."

Despite his words, Iain knew his cousin still had his misgivings about Regan. There was naught to be done for it, though, save allow time to smooth over that rift. Which it would soon enough, Iain knew. Niall only had his best interests at heart. When Niall finally accepted that all was truly well between him and Regan, Iain felt certain he'd put his misgivings about her aside for good.

"So, I was expecting word from ye once Anne delivered," Iain said with a grin, "but I didn't anticipate the proud father being the one to deliver the message."

Niall's smile turned grim. "Och, to be sure that wasn't my plan either. If the queen wasn't in such dire straits, ye'd have to pry me away from Annie with a stout iron lever. But Mary needs us, she does, and we must attend her posthaste."

Regan drew up at that moment, just in time to have overheard Niall's disturbing declaration. "Welcome to our home, m'lord," she said with a quick curtsy. "And what's happened with Mary?"

He returned her salutation with a brusque nod. "Her husband's been murdered, and she and Lord Bothwell, among others, are being implicated in the death."

She put a hand to her throat. "When?" she whispered hoarsely. "Where, and how?"

Iain moved to her side and slipped an arm around her waist to steady her.

"Darnley was residing outside Edinburgh at Kirk o'Fields, apparently recuperating from the pox. Two hours after midnight on the morn of February 10, an explosion rocked the city, destroying Kirk o'Fields. Darnley, however, was found outside in his nightshirt, strangled along with his manservant."

Regan swayed against Iain. He tightened his grip and pulled her close.

"Two days later, Mary sent off a messenger, requesting that Iain and I join her in Edinburgh." Niall looked to Iain. "Even then, she seems to have feared there'd be some sort of public—and political—hue and cry raised against her because of the suspicious circumstances surrounding Darnley's death. Will ye come with me, cousin?"

Iain looked to Regan. Understanding gleamed in her eyes. But there was an equally strong reluctance burning there as well. He had to admit to similar feelings.

Still, there was naught to be done but obey Mary's summons. He turned back to Niall. "Aye, ye know I will. I'm yer tanist, after all."

"Good. Then we depart at first light. As it is, what with the snow and road conditions, it'll be nearly two weeks since Darnley's death before we finally gain Edinburgh."

"So soon?" Regan's voice came out in a dismayed squeak. "Must ye leave so soon?"

When Niall glanced back at her, his hard expression had softened. "Aye. There's no telling what's come about in the meanwhile. If we don't make haste, we might not make it in time to be of any use to the queen. If there's aught we can do at any rate."

Puzzlement clouded her gaze. "I don't understand."

"Mary's marriage to Henry Darnley was likely the most ill-considered, politically destructive thing she ever could've done," Iain interjected, looking down at her. "In the doing, she likely permanently alienated the Earl of Moray and Maitland, her secretary of state, not to mention the lords Mar, Kirkcaldy, Atholl, and others." He sighed. "Though we'll go to her, I'm not certain it'll do any good."

"Not with Bothwell so increasingly glued to her side, it won't," Niall muttered. "He's no better for Mary than Darnley was, and it hasn't been for want of trying on my part to convince her otherwise."

"Then if ye truly feel the queen's bent on her own downfall," Regan asked, "why continue to support her? Likely she'll only bring ye down along with her."

Niall and Iain exchanged troubled glances.

"Because, sweet lass, we've given our word to be Mary's true and loyal servants, that's why," Iain said. "And there's yet hope, especially now with Darnley's death, that Mary may finally see the error of her ways. There's yet hope that Bothwell might finally dig himself a hole from which he cannot extricate himself."

"In Darnley's murder, ye mean?"

He nodded. "Aye."

"And if she persists in standing by Bothwell, what then?"

Once again, Iain and Niall looked at each other. They didn't need to say a word. He and Niall had already spent countless hours debating their options if such a calamity were actually to occur. In the end, both had arrived at the same conclusion. The welfare of Clan Campbell would come before Mary's crown. It had to, if she persisted in not listening to reason and instead continued to follow her heart rather than good Scottish sense. Unfortunately, for a queen at any rate, sometimes following one's heart wasn't always a good thing.

"We'll address that problem if and when it becomes one," Niall firmly said. "Now," he added, glancing around, "my men and I haven't eaten since midday, and we're sore weary. Would it be possible—"

"Och, aye." Regan pushed free of Iain's clasp. "I beg pardon, m'lord." She glanced at her husband. "Iain, why don't ye take Niall and his men into the Great Hall? I'll soon have Cook and the others up and preparing a meal. And then I'll see to the preparation of several bedchambers."

"Aye, that sounds like a fine plan." Iain turned to Niall. "I'll see to yer needs. Then, if ye will, I'll excuse myself to begin arrangements for the morrow's journey."

Niall nodded. "Aye, best ye do. It's been a long day, and a few hours' rest will be most appreciated, it will. We've likely got a good five days' journey ahead of us. And then, there's no way of knowing what awaits us in Edinburgh."

"Whatever awaits us," Iain muttered, filled with foreboding, "I fear it may be the beginning of the end for the queen."

"Aye, I fear that as well." His cousin heaved a great sigh. "I but pray to God that there's still a chance left us. I don't like the thought of what might become of Mary if we fail."

✠

News of Darnley's murder reached Walter at nearly the same time Niall and Iain set out for Edinburgh. He knew that, for the spy he had sent to Balloch Castle returned with a report of the two Campbells' departure on the same day William Drummond arrived for a visit.

"Past time, I'm thinking," the big Drummond chief said, "to be enticing my wee cousin to Strathyre for a visit. Iain Campbell, once he returns from Edinburgh, will then lose no time racing to be at his wife's side."

"Getting a bit queasy over all the political upheaval, are ye?"

William gave a snort of disgust. "The Campbells are fools to remain loyal to Mary. Mark my words, this is the beginning of the end for her. And, of all times, I don't need Iain Campbell forcing me to join with them to support the queen!"

Walter motioned to the chairs before the fire. It was a bitterly cold day, the wind seeking out every chink in Strathyre's crumbling mortar walls to whistle down the frigid corridors and into the rooms, until the only place of warmth was directly before the hearth fires. There were nights when he actually slept there, wrapped in woolen blankets, waking only to stoke the fire to keep it burning.

What he needed, if the truth be told, was to rebuild Strathyre from the ground up. If he had the money, which he never would unless he obtained it from somewhere outside Clan MacLaren. Clan Drummond had sufficient coin, if only Walter could find some way to finagle it from them. And the only way to do that was to convince Regan not only to return here but ultimately to wed him.

"Aye, I must agree with ye on that," Walter said as he settled in the chair opposite William. "And I'll gladly do what I can to aid ye in not pledging fealty to the queen. I must, however, have some pretext

227

for luring Regan from Balloch at this time of year. Otherwise, she'll just put me off, and Iain will likely become suspicious."

Drummond leaned forward expectantly in his chair.

It was time to wheedle some money from the man, Walter decided. Not as much as he'd eventually demand, but at least some token of William's commitment. What possible pretext could he use, though?

"Regan's verra devoted to my wee sister, Molly," he finally said. "Indeed, she's been all but a mither to her."

When he paused, his guest's impatience quickly got the better of him. "Aye? And how do ye plan to use that to lure Regan here?"

"Well, Molly's birthday is March 14. Mayhap, if I could scratch up the funds, I could throw a grand party for the lass and invite Regan to attend. If she knew it was a verra special occasion, she might be willing to come, even being with child and all. She won't be that far along in another three weeks or so, after all. From what I've heard, she'll be but six months along."

Walter paused again, then sighed. "Unfortunately, I've barely the funds for a simple birthday gift, much less a fine party. There are just too many repairs needed for such an old house as this."

William shot him a relieved look. "Och, if that's all that's keeping ye from persuading Regan to come here, that's no problem at all. I can cover the costs of a birthday celebration." He reached down to unfasten a leather pouch hanging from his belt. "How much do ye need?"

Eyeing the size of the pouch, Walter named an amount that soon emptied half of William's coin. If he had dared, he'd have asked for most of what the other man carried. But Walter didn't want to appear greedy. Once William had implicated himself in Iain Campbell's murder, it'd be a simple enough thing to extract periodic payments from him. And that, on top of Regan's annual support stipend, should cover his needs very nicely.

"I thank ye for yer generous donation to my sister's birthday celebration," he said as he rose and placed the coins in a small, carved wooden box sitting on the mantel.

"Just see that Regan attends and stays here until her husband comes to fetch her," Drummond growled, "and it'll be money well spent."

"I'll do what I can." Walter turned from the mantel. "Just pray that Iain doesn't linger overlong in Edinburgh. If the queen's problems aren't soon solved, we may have a bigger problem on our hands."

"And that problem would be?"

"Any use of force to keep Regan at Strathyre wouldn't sit well with her husband. And, her devotion to Molly notwithstanding, I can only keep her here for a finite amount of time."

✠

"Are ye certain this is such a good idea?" Mathilda asked two weeks later as Regan prepared to mount her horse. "I know it's yer foster sister's birthday and all, but what if Iain returns while ye're gone? He'll not be pleased to discover ye've ridden off to visit Strathyre in the middle of yer pregnancy."

Regan laughed. "And what's so terrible about a half day's journey in the middle of a pregnancy? Most peasant women work until the day they deliver, and sometimes that's in the fields where they've gone to assist their husbands in the harvest or planting. In light of that, I'm thinking I can endure a wee ride." At her mother-in-law's worried expression, she relented at last. "Fine. How about if I ride in a pony cart instead of upon a horse? Would that ease yer concerns?"

"Aye, it would. It's just that I wish . . . wish ye'd stay safe and sound here, that's all." Mathilda lifted her gaze. "And what am I to tell Iain? He'll blame me, he will."

"Tell him to come fetch me posthaste. I've been wanting to pay Strathyre a visit for a time now. I miss Molly. She's only seven, going on eight, after all. She doesn't understand why I've been so long away from her."

"Then mayhap ye could bring her back with ye for an extended visit. Surely Walter MacLaren wouldn't mind, would he? What little I saw of him at yer wedding, I wasn't taken with him or his surly nature. Indeed, the wee lass would likely do better at Balloch for a time than moldering away with that unpleasant man for a brother."

It was true Walter rarely had time for his sister. But he was also a man beset with myriad problems, the very least of which was where sufficient funds would next come to keep Strathyre going, much less see to the endless repairs the old tower house needed. Still, Regan had to admit Mathilda's suggestion was a most pleasant consideration.

Molly would definitely accept the offer, and Regan felt certain she could convince Walter to do so as well. After all, it'd be one less mouth to feed for a time, and he could let the nurse who cared for Molly go while the little girl was at Balloch. That, too, would save him money.

"Yer idea has merit," Regan replied. "Despite what ye may think, though, Walter does love his sister. Nonetheless, I might well be able to convince him to allow her an extended visit. Mayhap, if we're verra fortunate, even through the summer."

Iain's mother clapped her hands together. "Och, and wouldn't that be a wonderful time! She'd be here for the bairn's birth, she would. And she and I could go for walks in the garden, and I could read her stories, and ye and I could see her in some new gowns. Och, I can't wait!"

Regan grinned. From wearing a long face and almost begging her not to leave, Mathilda had changed to nearly shooing her from the castle. It was evident the older woman loved children and wished for more of them at Balloch. Her and Iain's children would certainly be blessed with a doting, loving grandmother.

"We'll be off then," she said, reining in her horse. "After all, the sooner I get there and celebrate Molly's birthday, the sooner I can return with the wee lass."

Mathilda nodded and stepped back. "Aye, best ye do. Indeed, if all goes well, mayhap ye'll even be back before Iain returns."

"Aye, mayhap I will." With that, Regan strode off to find Charlie and commandeer a pony and cart.

✛

On a fine, late April afternoon, Iain finally returned home. As he reined in his horse in the inner courtyard, he gave a great, contented sigh.

"I know we've been gone barely two months," he said, glancing at his cousin, "but it feels like two years."

Niall grinned, then swung down from his mount. "Aye, it does. But that, my friend, comes with being in love and counting the days until ye can return to yer beloved. It's a most unsettling problem, to be sure."

"A problem, of course, from which *ye've* never suffered."

"Och, never, of course." Niall's grin faded. "I can't believe my son's now over two months old, and I've missed all those early, precious days with him. And then, there's Annie . . ."

"Aye, there's Annie." Iain dismounted. "Well, it won't be but another few days and ye'll be with her again. As for me, I can't wait to see Regan. Do ye think her belly will be huge by now?"

His cousin chuckled. "That's unlikely, with over two more months to go. Ye haven't much pleasant time left with her, though. She'll soon become verra weary of her childbearing, what with her back aching all the time, and her inability to get out of bed or chairs without help, and her sleepless nights. By the time she finally delivers, ye'll almost feel as if ye've borne the bairn with her."

"Will I now?" Iain laughed, then handed his horse's reins to one of the stable lads who ran up. "Now, that's a most pleasant consideration."

"Well, mayhap I exaggerate a bit. It's hard, though, to see the

231

woman ye love so miserable. Especially during the actual birthing." Niall dragged in an unsteady breath. "It nearly tears yer heart out."

"Aye." Iain sobered. "I fear it as any man would. Still, it's the woman who must suffer the pains and risk the dangers. I want to be there for Regan, though. I won't let her go through it alone."

"Be prepared, then, to fight yer way past the midwife, maidservants, and, for ye, yer mither. They seem to think a man's place isn't in the birthing chamber."

"Mayhap." Iain indicated they should head for the keep, where his mother was just now exiting. "But if Regan wants me there, there I'll be, and no one will tell me otherwise."

As they approached Mathilda, Iain glanced around for sign of his wife. Strange that she hadn't been one of the first to greet them. Unless she was perhaps ill, or something—a chill coursed through him—had happened to her and their bairn.

"Where's Regan?" he immediately asked, forgoing the usual greetings. "Is she all right?"

His mother smiled and laid a hand on his arm. "Aye, she's fine. And it's most pleasant to see ye again too."

Relief almost making his knees weak, Iain took her into his arms and gave her a hug. "I've missed ye, Mither, and I'm so verra glad to be home!" He loosened his grip on her to lean back and gaze down into her face. "Now, where's Regan? If she's fine, why hasn't she come out to greet us? Surely she's not angry with me? I know we've been gone far longer than we'd hoped, but there was naught to be done for it."

"Well, we can talk about the queen over the supper meal," Mathilda said briskly. "And the reason Regan hasn't come out to greet ye is because she isn't here."

Iain went very still. "Where has she gone then, and why?"

"About a week into March, she received an invitation from that foster brother of hers. Seems he was having a special birthday celebration for his sister, Molly, and Regan, being so close to the wee lass, wanted desperately to attend. I saw no harm in it. The lass, after all, was pining after ye something fierce. I thought a short visit to her old home would do her good. So she left with an escort of ten of yer men, and, save for a few letters in the first weeks, I haven't heard from her since."

Iain frowned, released his mother, and took a step back. "And the lads ye sent along with her? Are they still at Strathyre House as well?"

"Well, nay. Regan soon sent all but one of them back, claiming their board was too great a drain on Walter's meager funds. The plan was to send the one lad back to Balloch to fetch a sufficient escort when she was ready to return."

"And don't ye think it strange she's been there close to six weeks now, with no further communication or having sent our man back with a request to fetch her?"

Mathilda looked chagrined. "Aye, of course I was beginning to wonder. But I kept hoping ye'd return any time and see to the matter yerself. Not that *ye* were overly conscientious in keeping me apprised of the goings-on at Court or yer plans either!"

Niall chose that moment to intervene. Taking Mathilda's hand, he tucked her arm in his. "There was little time to be writing, if we'd even dared tell ye of what was going on," he said. "And, one way or another, Iain's now home and can soon fetch his wife."

He shot Iain a look over the top of his mother's head. "Seems like we'll both be heading out again on the morrow. And a wee detour to MacLaren lands won't put me all that late in getting back to Kilchurn."

"My thanks," Iain replied. If Walter MacLaren thought to play some game with him, the added presence of Clan Campbell's chief and his men would soon give him pause. Not that *he* wasn't up to confronting the other man himself. Indeed, he'd ride to the gates of hell and back for his wife and unborn child.

Nonetheless, a sense of foreboding filled Iain. "Aye, we'll indeed head out at first light," he muttered. "There's something not right about this overlong visit. Whether Walter MacLaren likes it or not, I mean to bring Regan home posthaste."

17

"Regan, I'm *so* bored! Could we go for a walk?"

Glancing up from the tiny set of stockings she was knitting, Regan looked over at Molly. The little girl had long ago given up on the simple scarf she had been trying to knit and had taken up a spot on the bench beneath the bedchamber window. She looked back now, though, with a pleading expression in her bright blue eyes.

Regan smiled and set aside her own knitting. "Aye, that'd be a nice change from all this hard work, wouldn't it?" She rose, walked to where Molly sat, and extended her hand. "And where would ye like to go?"

Molly jumped down from the bench and took her hand. "Let's walk down to the loch. It's warm enough, isn't it, for me to go wading?"

"Hardly," Regan replied with a chuckle. "Though it's next to the last day of April and the springtide flowers are blooming, the loch is still sure to be verra cold." At the girl's crestfallen expression, she laughed. "But mayhap we can pick a pretty bouquet of flowers instead. For the dining table in the Great Hall. It'll look so nice there for the supper meal, don't ye think?"

"Och, aye!" Molly's expression brightened, and she tugged on Regan's hand. "Let's go. Come on, Regan!"

It was a mild, sunny afternoon, and they were soon strolling down the narrow, winding dirt path from Strathyre House to Loch Voil. Eventually, a little burn joined up to run alongside the path, its banks covered in yellow-petaled marsh marigolds interspersed with red and white tulips. In the shade of nearby oak and rowan woods, colorful primroses grew. White heather bloomed on the sun-kissed hillsides, and marsh violets peeked through the sprouting grass beneath the newly budded birch and willow trees perched on the very edge of the shore.

They must have spent a good three-quarters of an hour walking along, picking flowers, when Molly paused to glance up the hill toward Strathyre House. She stood there, her hand shading her eyes, for so long that Regan finally turned to see what she was looking at.

A large group of men on horses—she guessed it to be thirty or more—had drawn up before the old tower house. Even from a good quarter of a mile down the hill, Regan thought she could make out Campbell colors. Her heart gave a great lurch. Iain! Could it possibly be him?

"Come, Molly." She extended her hand to the little girl. "We've visitors. It's only proper we go up to greet them."

Molly paused only long enough to shift all the flowers she had been picking into her other hand, then took Regan's hand and fell into step alongside her. "Do ye think it's yer folk, come finally to fetch us?"

"Mayhap."

Regan certainly hoped so. After a month visiting Walter and Molly, she had thought it time to send David Campbell, the only one of her escort she had kept behind, back to Balloch to request additional riders to accompany her home. But that had been over two weeks ago. Even with the repeated bouts of spring rains, it had begun to seem overlong for the men's return. Walter's decided lack of enthusiasm for sending one of his own men to discern what the problem might be had additionally been troubling.

Now, though, there might well be no further cause for concern.

Even if Iain wasn't with the other men, perhaps David had at last returned with the others to fetch her. One way or another, she'd be glad to return to Balloch. It was, after all, her home now.

Just then one of the riders turned, appeared to catch sight of her and Molly, and swung off his horse. He started down the path to the loch, his long, ground-eating strides carrying him swiftly to them. His tall, broad-shouldered form and blond hair soon gave him away. It was Iain.

Regan gave a low cry and attempted to quicken her pace, but the extra weight of the child she carried soon slowed her once again. It didn't matter, though. Iain broke into a run.

In a matter of seconds, he slid to a halt before her. Regan inhaled a deep breath. "Well, it's about time ye were coming for yer wife," she said, her heart pounding so hard she imagined he could hear it. "I was beginning to think the wonders of Court and all its fine ladies had dazzled ye into forgetting about me."

Iain's deep blue eyes sparkled with amusement. "As if there were any other woman for me but ye, lass." He moved close, took her hand, and lifted it to his lips. "Och, I confess I counted the days until I could return to ye, I did," he said hoarsely when he had finally lowered her hand to clutch it over his heart. "Court and all its allure hold no appeal for me anymore. Not when I've a wife I love, a bairn on the way, and the finest home in all of Scotland to return to."

It was all Regan needed to hear. With a joyous sound, she flung her arms about Iain's neck, lifted on tiptoe, and kissed him. Pulling her to him, he returned her kiss with an equally ardent one of his own.

Regan didn't know how long they would've stood there like that if Molly hadn't finally tugged on her skirt.

"It's not polite to ignore a body," she said rather grumpily. "And it's even more impolite not to introduce us. Ye taught me that yerself, ye did."

With an amused snort, Regan hastily disengaged herself from

Iain. "Och, Molly, I'm so sorry." She looked from the little girl to Iain. "M'lord, I'd like to introduce ye to Molly MacLaren, Walter's sister. And Molly, this is my husband, Iain Campbell."

Her cheeks dimpling with a shy smile, Molly curtsied prettily. "M'lord, I'm verra pleased to meet ye."

Iain dropped to one knee before her. Taking her hand, he brought it to his lips in a gallant kiss. "And I'm verra pleased to meet ye at last, m'lady."

Molly examined him with solemn interest. For a fleeting instant, Regan feared she had taken a sudden dislike to Iain. But then, as if finally making up her mind, the little girl nodded.

"I like ye," she said. "And ye're verra bonny, ye are."

"Am I now?" Iain chuckled, released her hand, and shoved to his feet. "Have a care, lass, or ye're sure to turn my head."

"Aye," Regan added, shooting her husband a wry look. "He's already quite insufferable as it is, what with all the lasses swooning at the mere sight of him. It's up to us, I fear, to keep his head from exploding with conceit."

"Och, and wouldn't that make a mess!" Molly wrinkled her nose and stared at Iain's head as if watching it for signs of a sudden size increase. "Still, as bonny as ye are," she next said, suddenly changing the course of the conversation, "ye're not half as bonny as my brother Roddy was. That's why Regan married him first, ye know."

Regan couldn't help a small inhalation of breath. She looked to Iain.

Thankfully, he didn't seem the least offended by the little girl's remark. Instead, he gave a thoughtful nod.

"Aye, but I love Regan so much that I was happy she'd have me anyway."

Molly twisted her mouth. It could only mean one thing. She was struggling with something really difficult and confusing. Regan moved close and laid a hand on her shoulder.

"Ye marrying her." The child gazed up at him, her eyes suddenly tear bright. "Ye took her away from us, me and Walter. It's verra mean, ye know."

Iain looked to Regan, entreaty now gleaming in his eyes. She smiled, then squatted beside Molly. "And have ye already forgotten that Walter gave ye leave to visit us the entire summer?" She shot Iain a quick, pleading glance. He smiled and nodded. "So ye see, we're all but neighbors now, and can visit back and forth whenever we wish."

"I'd like it better," the girl muttered, "if ye still lived with us."

"Yet ye also know that when women wed, they usually move away from their childhood homes. As ye'll surely do someday, when ye find a braw man to wed."

"Nay." Molly shook her head with firm resolve. "I don't want ever to leave Strathyre House. And I don't want ever to wed."

Regan chuckled softly and stood. "Well, that may be for now, but let's see how ye feel in another ten years or so." She looked up the hill to where everyone still waited. "Now, I think it best we finish our walk back to Strathyre. It also isn't polite to keep guests waiting."

As they turned back to the path, Molly grabbed Regan's hand and held it tightly. Iain joined Regan on her other side, and they were soon striding up the hill together.

Walter and Niall awaited them before the steps leading to Strathyre's main door. Their escort, which consisted of Niall's as well Iain's men, remained mounted. Regan, still holding Molly's hand, and Iain finally drew up before the two men.

The Campbell chief gave Regan a long, considering look, then rendered her a curt nod. "Ye look well, madam," he said. "Like my Annie, ye appear to carry bairns with little difficulty."

"My health is good, m'lord," she replied, still able to manage a half curtsy without losing her balance. "And, now that Iain's returned, I'm certain it'll improve all the more."

"Well, leastwise yer mood's bound to improve," Walter offered, smiling. "Ye must admit ye've grown a bit testy these past few weeks."

Regan arched a slender brow. "Indeed? I hadn't noticed."

Walter laughed then. "Be that as it may, I'll wager yer husband soon will." He paused and looked around the group. "But forgive my poor manners. Please, come inside so I may offer ye something to drink. And the meager hospitality of my house is also yers for as long as ye wish to remain."

Niall glanced at Iain. "Ye've found Regan hale and hearty. Have ye further need of me?"

Iain shook his head. "Nay. Ye wish to be heading on out then, do ye? Back to Annie and yer wee bairn?"

His cousin grinned. "Aye. Now that ye've returned to yer lady, I've a great need to do the same."

"Then go, with my deepest gratitude for all ye've done." Iain extended his arm, and they clasped, hand to elbow.

"Send me word then, when yer bairn comes."

"Aye." Iain looked deep into Niall's eyes. "Ye can be certain of it."

They stepped back from each other then, and after another perfunctory nod to Regan, the Campbell chief turned and strode over to where his men and horses awaited. In one lithe move, he swung up onto his mount, reined it in, then paused to wave his farewell. Iain and Regan waved back. An instant later, Niall signaled his horse forward. Followed by his men, he rode away.

Iain was the first to turn back to Regan and Walter. "The day draws on, lass. It's best we, too, were on our way."

"Och, nay." Walter held up a hand in apparent protest. "There's no need for ye to depart so soon. Indeed, I was hopeful ye might stay on for a wee visit. In a sense, we're family now, Regan being a MacLaren fosterling. Though ye and I've had a few tense moments in the past, I'm all for setting old disagreements aside and starting anew." He offered Iain his hand. "If ye can find it in yer heart, that is, to do so."

Iain's eyes narrowed, and his mouth tightened. Regan sensed her husband wasn't predisposed to lower his guard against Walter. Why there was such animosity between the two men, she didn't know, but whatever it was, it was past time to do as Walter suggested and set it aside.

"He makes a fair request," she said, meeting Iain's gaze. "Not to mention, it'd please me greatly."

"And exactly how long a visit would it take to please ye, lass?" Iain asked.

He was still reluctant, but at least he was willing to concede, and that was the first step. "Och, but a few days would suffice," she said. "We can always return at a later date for a longer stay." She turned to Walter. "Would that suffice for ye as well?"

"Aye. Three days should be a most pleasant length for our first visit." He bent down and picked up Molly, holding her close. "Now, my stablemen will see to the care of yer horses, then help yer men find adequate lodging. And tonight we'll have a grand feast in the Great Hall in yer honor," he added, meeting Iain's gaze.

Iain nodded, his expression inscrutable. "I thank ye for yer hospitality."

"Och, think naught of it," Walter said as he turned and headed over to the steps. "The pleasure's all mine."

✠

"Would ye mind telling me why ye've taken such a dislike to Walter?" Regan asked later that evening after they had retired to bed.

Iain turned on his side to face her. For an instant, she was distracted at the most pleasing sight of her husband's broad chest and muscled arms. She didn't think she'd ever tire of looking at him or fail to experience a thrill at the thought of being his wife.

"It was that apparent, was it?" he asked, his deep voice wrenching her back to the matter at hand. "My dislike for Walter?"

Regan rolled her eyes. "Aye, and well ye know it."

He reached over, took up a lock of hair that had tumbled over her shoulder, and twisted it about his finger. "I'd much prefer," he replied huskily, his gaze fixed on the candlelit strands in his hand, "spending our first night back together discussing more pleasant matters and, even more so, engaging in them."

"And why's that? Are ye afraid ye'll anger me by speaking ill of my foster brother?"

Iain finally glanced up. "The thought had crossed my mind. Yer continuing affection for him is quite apparent."

"And do ye fear it's stronger than my affection for ye then?"

"When I finally returned to Balloch and found ye'd come here," he said, his gaze now locked with hers, "and that ye'd been gone for nearly six weeks, I wondered at yer reasons. Especially when ye'd originally planned to attend Molly's birthday celebration, then return home after a week or so."

Regan sighed. "Aye, that was my original plan. But Molly begged me to stay on for a time more, and then once I sent David back to Balloch to fetch my escort, a few more weeks passed before ye and—"

"What do ye mean, ye sent David back?" Iain shoved to one elbow. "He wasn't at Balloch when I arrived home, and Mither never made mention of his return. Indeed, she was wondering when he *would* return."

Apprehension twisted her gut. "But I sent David back two weeks ago, Iain. What happened to him?"

Her husband's expression darkened. "Whatever happened, I doubt the lad lived to tell about it." He sat up in bed. "This doesn't bode well, lass. Something foul's afoot here."

"Outlaws could've set upon him." Regan blinked back a sudden swell of tears. "Och, he could've been wounded and lain there all alone until he died, and no one would've known to come to his aid!"

"It's strange no one found his body."

She jerked her gaze back up to him. "What are ye implying?"

He opened his mouth, then clamped it shut again. "Naught. Leastwise, not yet. I've no proof, only suspicions."

Anger filled her. "Suspicions that Walter's involved in David's inexplicable disappearance? Is that what ye mean?"

"Och, lass, leave it be." Iain sighed and leaned against the bed's wooden headboard. "It's true enough I think little of Walter Mac-

Laren. But I'm here, am I not, and willing, for yer sake, to give him another chance."

Regan crossed her arms over her night-rail-clad body. She didn't like Iain having such a poor opinion of Walter. True, Walter was a very private sort and could have a bit of ruthlessness about him at times. And she *had* had her passing doubts about his possible involvement in Roddy's death, but that had soon dissipated once she was back at Strathyre. Walter had changed in the time they had been apart. He was now calmer, more patient and secure, as if becoming laird had brought with it the self-fulfillment he had always needed. Their friendship had bloomed as well. Regan knew now he had never had anything but her best interests and welfare at heart.

Yet she also knew Iain loved her and would do anything for her. Surely two good men could eventually be brought to find peace with each other.

"Fine." Regan sighed her acquiescence. "I'll not ask ye to make Walter yer bosom friend. It's enough for now that ye're willing to give him a chance." She paused, shooting him an impish grin. "Ye needn't worry, though, that Walter will ever steal my heart. It's hopelessly, and eternally, yers."

"Indeed?" He cocked his head, smiled, and she could tell he was pleased. "Well, it's the least I'd expect, ye know. Ye being the queen's most obedient subject, and her having commanded ye to wed me and all."

Iain's mention of Mary reminded Regan she had yet to hear the outcome of his and Niall's journey to Edinburgh. "How is she, by the way?" Regan asked. "And whatever came of Darnley's death? Did they ever discover his killer?"

"Nay, though there are many who suspect it was Lord Bothwell and several other conspirators who had a hand in that unpleasant affair. And there are just as many who also suspect Mary."

"Mary? Why?"

"Because it's long been evident she was unhappy in her marriage to

Darnley, because Bothwell's always been her loyal and devoted servant, and because she couldn't have pulled off her husband's murder on her own. And, now that all charges have been dropped against Bothwell, there are new rumors he means to take her as his wife."

"But Bothwell's already wed!"

Iain's mouth went taut and grim. "Not for much longer, I'd wager. The man's riding high after the failed attempt by Darnley's father to bring him to trial. Lennox was afraid to face him, what with four thousand of Bothwell's supporters roaming Edinburgh the day of the trial. So, in the absence of an accuser, Bothwell was declared innocent. After that, the rumors of his intent to seek Mary's hand began."

"Och, poor, poor Mary." Regan shook her head, so overcome with a sense of impending disaster that she found, for a moment, she couldn't speak.

"Aye, poor, poor Mary," her husband muttered. "It was then that Niall and I decided it was past time to take our leave of Court and Edinburgh. Mary had her chance to repudiate Bothwell and distance herself from him, but she didn't. She listens only to him now, and apparently has no further need of us."

"She may just be lost and confused right now, Iain. So much misfortune has befallen her in the past year or so. Mayhap if ye just give her some time, then approach her again . . ."

He sighed. "Aye, mayhap. We'll see what the next few months bring."

There was such sadness, such a sense of defeat in his voice and words that Regan's heart went out to him. He and Niall had worked so hard to aid the queen, as friends, advisors, and loyal subjects, remaining true to her when many of their own clan had begun to distance themselves from Mary. Yet now it seemed as if all they had done had been for naught.

She scooted close and laid her head on his shoulder. "Ye've done the best ye could," she whispered. "It's time to place it all in the Lord's hands."

"Aye, mayhap it is." Iain kissed the top of her head. "And it's time, as well, to see to what's truly the most important things in my life—ye, our bairn, and Balloch."

Regan looked up and smiled. "I find no fault in that, m'lord."

"And neither do I, m'lady. Neither do I," he said, his voice going thick with longing as he pulled her down with him onto the bed.

✠

Just a few more days, Walter repeated over and over as he paced the confines of his bedchamber late that night. The message had been sent to William Drummond, alerting him to bring his men for the long-awaited ambush. Just a few more days, and Iain Campbell would never again strut off to bed with Regan on his arm. Just a few more days, and Campbell would be dead and she'd be his at last. If only he could endure the torment just a few more days.

There were plans of his own to make while he waited on Drummond's men's arrival. A site had to be chosen for the attack, one that positioned Campbell and his meager escort to their greatest disadvantage. Precautions also had to be clarified to ensure Regan survived unscathed.

One thing was certain in that regard. He intended to set himself and his own men at some secret but advantageous spot to oversee the whole affair. He didn't trust William Drummond not to "accidentally" have Regan killed in the ensuing chaos. Her death, after all, would remove all threat of her ever laying claim to his chieftainship. And it would also absolve him of any future support payments on her behalf, monies Walter would always desperately need.

Additionally, something had to be done to prevent Molly from accompanying them, despite both Regan's and his sister's expectations to the contrary. Perhaps some unpleasant but innocuous herbal concoction from the local healer would do the trick. All he needed, after all, was to make Molly temporarily too ill to travel.

It was bad enough Regan had to endure the horrors of the slaughter. She at least, though, was an adult. As much as he hated making his sister sick, it would be far worse to subject sweet, innocent little Molly to the sight of what was sure to be some ghastly butchery.

A sudden thought assailed Walter, and he drew up short. Indeed, such a traumatic event might be enough also to send Regan into premature labor. If it did, she'd surely lose the child.

Walter couldn't help but smile at the consideration. In one short, expedient act, he could well be free not only of the father but also the child. Regan—and he—would be able to begin anew, unencumbered by anything that bound her to her former life with Iain Campbell.

The more he thought on it, the more convinced he became that this was the most perfect of all plans. The warlock would finally lose his hold on Regan, and she'd finally open her eyes to the truth. The truth that he, her lifelong friend, was the real man of her dreams.

And he and Drummond had already agreed the attackers would all be men Regan had never met, dressed as outlaws and broken men. There'd be no way to trace the killers back to them. And, not long after the ambush was over and the outlaws had all ridden away, Walter and his own men would come riding up on the pretense of trying to catch the Campbell party to deliver some item Regan had left behind. Riding up to find her there among the dead and rescue her, to bring her back to the safe, familiar home she had always known and loved.

After that, it would be a simple thing to play the stalwart comforter to the grieving widow. He was certain he could win her back to him, once the effects of Campbell's spells waned with his death. And if perchance the shock of the massacre didn't cause her to lose the bairn, there were other ways to see the child gone soon enough.

Aye, Walter thought as he once more began to pace. There were many plans yet to be made, the details refined to unerring perfection. Just a few more days and he'd have everything he had ever wanted, ever dreamed of.

All he had to do was remain busy. All he had to do was keep his mind off the revolting image of Iain Campbell lying in bed just down the hall, holding Regan in his arms.

18

Two days later just after breakfast, Iain and Regan bade Walter farewell and headed out on the half-day's journey back to Balloch. Though Iain knew Regan was disappointed at having to leave Molly behind, there was nothing to be done for it. The little girl had begun vomiting last night and was now too ill to travel. Regan seemed somewhat mollified, however, when Walter had promised personally to bring Molly to Balloch when she was fully recovered.

Not that Iain was overly thrilled at the thought of having to take Walter MacLaren into his house for even one night, he admitted as he rode along, Regan at his side and his men lined up behind them. But he was resigned to the possibility. Highland hospitality demanded it, if not just for the fact the man was all but Regan's kin.

Try as he might, though, Iain found little to change his opinion of Walter MacLaren as a grasping, untrustworthy, shallow-hearted man. And he didn't care much, either, for Walter's proprietary, calculating air around Regan. If he hadn't been her foster brother and dear to her, Iain would've gladly taken the man aside and set him straight about several things, the least of which was who was and who wasn't Regan's husband.

And he might still do so, if the man dared put on airs when he came to Balloch. Still, *that* day was likely at least a week or more away, if little Molly's appearance this morn was any indication.

The poor lass looked very sick, with a pasty complexion and dark circles beneath her eyes, and was so weak she could barely sit up in bed. Thankfully, though, she was finally taking a bit of broth, or he feared Regan would've refused to leave at all.

They rode for a time in silence, the horses all going at a walk to keep pace with the pony cart wherein Regan rode. Iain glanced at her every so often as well, attempting to gauge her toleration of the ride. She looked none the worse for it, he supposed, but still he worried.

Eight more weeks, and he'd at last be a father. Even now, all these months since Regan had first revealed her pregnancy to him, Iain still experienced the same excitement and eager anticipation each time he thought of his impending fatherhood. The Lord was so good. At long last, he had everything he had ever wanted.

"Ye look verra pleased with yerself," Regan said just then.

He looked over at her. Och, but she was so beautiful. Soft color bloomed in her cheeks, her striking brown eyes sparkled, and she looked voluptuously healthy in her childbearing.

"Can ye think of any reason why I shouldn't be pleased, sweet lass?" he asked as the trail began to dip down into a narrow glen, its steep hillsides covered in dense forest. "It's springtime in the Highlands, we're going home, and I'm so verra much in love with ye. What man wouldn't be pleased?"

She smiled and colored most becomingly. "Yer pleasure's all that matters to me, husband."

Iain chuckled. "As well it should, wife. Still, I wish for ye always to find equal pleasure in—"

From somewhere above them in the trees, a horse snorted and Iain caught the faint clink of metal upon metal. All his warrior's instincts sprang immediately to the forefront. He turned, glanced back at Thomas Campbell, one of his most trusted clansmen, and signaled for him to join him. Before the man could even nudge his mount forward, however, a crossbow quarrel hissed through the air and struck the man square in the chest.

Thomas gave a sharp cry and toppled from his horse. An instant later the air was thick with quarrels, all arching down toward them. Iain tore free the targ fastened to the back of his saddle and tossed the round, leather-bound shield to Regan.

"Cover yerself and hold on!" he cried as he next grabbed her pony's reins and kicked his own mount in the side.

Both animals leaped into a gallop, and they raced down the glen. Behind him, Iain heard his men follow his lead, what men were still with him. As he had set out, he had heard additional quarrels strike home.

There was naught to be done for them. To tarry a second more in that narrow little glen would've surely been the end of them all. Their only hope lay in their getting out of crossbow range. Even if their attackers were mounted, it would be a difficult if not impossible task to reload a crossbow while in pursuit.

The glen, however, was longer than he had bargained for, especially at the slower pace the pony and its cart set. Two quarrels sunk deep into the targ Regan held up before her. Then one, burning like fire, pierced his left shoulder.

Iain ground his teeth at the pain, reached up to wrench the quarrel free and toss it aside, then forged on. For a few dizzying seconds, the world spun around him. Behind Iain, another man cried out and fell, striking the ground hard.

Fury boiled up and seared through him, clearing the dizziness like a cold splash of water. The cowardly knaves! Let them come out and face them like men! He'd gladly give them a wee taste of his claymore.

The end of the glen rose before him like some blessed entrance to sanctuary. Once they were out in the open, there was hope they could outrace their attackers to safety. Iain didn't dare look to Regan. It was enough she managed to hold on, stay in the cart, and shield herself with the targ.

And then, men on horseback were suddenly there at the mouth of the glen. Armed men, men whose myriad colors of plaids bespoke of no specific clan or family loyalty. Outlaws, broken men who stood as a human barrier three or four ranks deep, between Iain and freedom.

He reined in his horse. Regan's pony halted on his right. His remaining men drew up on his left.

One had a quarrel in his thigh. The other was yet unscathed. Two men left out of nine, to face at least twenty men.

"Och, Iain," Regan cried softly just then. "Ye're hurt!"

As he turned to her, panic swelled. Even with just his two remaining men, he'd have gladly, even eagerly, rode to do battle against such overwhelming odds. But this time it wasn't as simple or easy as that—he had Regan and their unborn child to think of. How could he protect her and still fight these men?

Help me, Lord. Help us all, Iain thought, lifting a quick, desperate prayer as he scanned the terrain around them. There were scant defensible spots where Regan would be sufficiently out of harm's way. A pile of boulders and several fallen trees about twenty yards back down the glen looked the best place.

He pulled his claymore free of its sheath on his back and pointed with it toward the boulders. "There, lads," he growled. "We'll make our stand there."

Urging his horse on, Iain sent the animal racing toward the boulders, pulling Regan's pony along with him. His two men followed close behind. Yet even then the outlaws were racing toward them.

They barely made the boulders. Immediately, Iain leaped down, thrust his claymore several inches into the earth, and pulled Regan from the cart.

"Go," he cried, pushing her in the direction of the boulders. "Take shelter behind those rocks and trees!"

She opened her mouth as if to protest, then apparently thought better of it. Instead, Regan tossed his targ to him before hurrying to do as he commanded. She made cover none too soon. The first rank of outlaws attacked, slamming into the defensive barrier Iain's men had made to protect him.

He swung up onto his horse, grabbed first one pistol and fired it, then the other. Both shots at such close range hit their targets, and two outlaws fell, mortally wounded. Then there was no time left but to fight. He drew free his short sword, a far more effective weapon on horseback than the huge claymore. With a targ on the other arm, Iain moved into position beside his men.

Sheer desperation, and likely greater skill, served them well for a time. One outlaw after another fell. Eventually, however, some in the back were able to reload their crossbows and began again to fire. Richard Gordon died, his throat transected by a quarrel. Then Willie Campbell's horse took a bolt in its chest.

The animal screamed, reared, its front legs flailing the air, before toppling over sideways, taking Willie with him. He was immediately set on by three assailants.

"Cruachan!" Iain roared and reined his horse around, kneeing the beast into the thick of the battle for Willie's life.

He used the sharply pointed tip in the middle of his targ to spear one man, and then his sword to all but slice off the hand of another. Both fell back, screaming in agony, but there were always more to take their place. There was nothing, though, he could do to help free Willie from beneath his fallen horse. To dismount now would've been the end of them both.

Hacking, slashing, stabbing, Iain fought on and on. There were times he held them all at bay, and then times when they surged forward like an uncontrollable floodtide, and he could barely defend himself. His sword arm grew heavy. His lungs heaved for air. Blood trickled from the hole in his shoulder, weakening him until it became increasingly difficult to lift his targ. Sweat poured into his eyes until he could barely see.

The wounds began to come more frequently now—slices to his arms and legs, small, passing jabs that pierced his skin more and more deeply before Iain could parry them away. And then the volley of quarrels flew again.

One struck him in the thigh, penetrating to the bone. Two more he barely defended against with his targ. Another three found his horse.

With a grunt, the mortally wounded animal sank to his knees and began to roll to its side. Iain leaped free, pivoted to run back to his claymore, when the quarrel tip in his thigh ground against bone.

Sharp, brilliant bits of light exploded in his brain, and he nearly cried out from the excruciating pain. He staggered, went down on one knee. A blade plunged into his back, then withdrew and plunged again. He thought he'd black out from the searing agony.

With the last bit of strength left him, Iain swung around on his good leg and thrust his sword into his attacker's chest. The man plummeted to the ground.

And then Regan was there, catching him in her arms as he swayed then toppled over backward. Catching him to ever so gently lower him to the ground.

The tears streaming down her cheeks, she reached around to try and pull his sword from his hand. Iain gripped it all the tighter.

"Nay, lass," he groaned.

"Let me have it," she pleaded. "Ye fought for me. Now let me fight for ye."

"N-nay." His voice sounded curiously distant now, and only a superhuman effort brought him back through the encroaching mists. "If ye fight . . . they may kill ye. And, no matter what happens to me, ye must live . . . live for yerself . . . for the sake of our b-bairn."

"I-I don't want to live without ye, Iain," Regan sobbed, holding him close. "I haven't the courage, the strength!"

"Aye . . . but ye do." He tried to smile, but he even seemed to be losing control of his lips. "Ye do . . ."

Something from the corner of his vision caught Iain's attention. He turned his head. A man stood there, black rage in his eyes and a sword raised overhead.

He meant to strike, and strike a killing blow. But the man's gaze wasn't fixed on him, Iain realized fuzzily. It was directed to another. It was directed at Regan.

"Nay!" he cried and, with the last bit of strength left in him, threw himself in front of Regan.

Almost simultaneously, a shot rang out. The man hesitated; a befuddled look spread across his face. His sword tumbled from his hand. He took one, then two, staggering steps backward and toppled over.

It was the last sight Iain saw. Like a heavy curtain falling before his eyes, everything went black.

✠

Regan had but a split second to glance up after the shot rang out and killed her assailant—a man she knew had meant to murder her. Her gaze flew past him to another man mounted on a horse but thirty feet away. A man who, until this moment, hadn't been part of the outlaw band. In his hand, he held a smoking dagg. It was Walter.

She gave a sharp cry of recognition. Then Iain slumped, went limp in her arms. Suddenly, Walter's unexpected arrival meant nothing. All that mattered was her beloved husband.

"Och, Iain!" The words barely made it past a constricted throat. "Don't die. I beg ye. Don't die!"

He looked so pale now, his mouth slack, his beautiful eyes closed, and there was blood, so much blood! Regan stared down at him in wordless anguish. He was dying. Iain, her joy, her good, kind, loving husband, was dying, and she could do naught to save him.

Pulling him tightly to her, Regan clenched shut her eyes and prayed. *Spare him, Lord,* she cried out in her silent agony. *He doesn't deserve this, not now, not when he's so close to seeing the child he wants with all his heart. He's one of Yer most devoted servants. And I love him! Och, how I love him!*

As she rocked Iain to and fro, sobs began to wrack her body. She tried to will all her strength and life into him. But, no matter how hard Regan tried, he lay there limp and unmoving.

A wren called from a nearby tree. A gentle breeze kissed her cheek. The scent of crushed, new grass enveloped her. Strange, she thought, that at a time like this she was so acutely aware of everything around her. It seemed as if she were in some dream, hovering between heaven and hell.

Then a hand settled on her shoulder, and a familiar voice filled her ears.

"Come away, lass," Walter said. "It's too late. He's gone."

She opened her eyes, saw him squatting beside her. For an instant her head spun. Walter was here. But how? And why?

Then it didn't matter anymore. All that mattered was Iain. Iain . . .

"N-nay," Regan whispered. "He's not dead. He's not! Help him, Walter. Help him!"

He sighed and shook his head. "Come away, lass." He began to pull her hands free of her hold on Iain. "It's not safe for ye here. Though a bit of coin has managed to convince these men to spare yer life, they're an undependable lot and might soon change their mind. Come away while ye still can."

There was real concern in his voice. Some instinct told her he was likely right. "Aye, I'll come away," she said. "But bring Iain. Please, Walter. Bring Iain."

She let him move Iain aside and help her to her feet. When he slipped a hand about her waist and tried to walk her away, though, Regan dug in her heels. "Bring Iain, Walter. Please!"

A taut, grim expression tightened his features. "Not now, lass," he growled. "They only gave me leave to take ye away. We daren't press our luck."

"Nay!" Hysteria finally gained a stranglehold on her. She twisted wildly in his grip, struggling to turn back to Iain. "Nay!"

"We'll come back for him later." Walter fought to maintain his hold on her. "Later."

A scream rose to her lips. "Nay!"

And then a pain came, deep in her belly, twisting and coiling so hard and tight that it took her breath away. She gasped, doubled over, and clutched at her swollen abdomen.

The pain came again, and Regan recognized it now for what

it was—a birthing pang. Fear swamped her. The child! She was losing the child!

She screamed. Her knees buckled, and only Walter's quick response in catching her and swinging her up into his arms saved her from falling. For a fleeting moment, Regan felt his jarring motions as he carried her away. Then another pain came, sending her over the brink of consciousness and into a blessed place where nothing mattered.

✠

"Och, my poor, sweet child. It'll be all right. Just ye wait and see."

The soothing voice—Cook's voice—rose from the graying mists, accompanied by a cool, damp cloth sliding down the side of her face. Regan groaned, pushed it away, and rolled over to face in the opposite direction. For her efforts, she was rewarded with another belly cramp. This one, though, was far less intense.

Her eyes snapped open. Her bairn! Was it all right? It *must* be all right!

On the heels of that thought came the memory of Iain, of holding him in her arms as he lay dying. Freshened grief flooded her. Once again, all Regan saw was the blood, and his dear, waxen face. She heard his beloved voice speaking to her for the last time. And all she felt was helpless, empty anguish.

She wept, but the tears didn't wash away any of the searing pain. How could they? Iain was gone, and he had been everything to her. Everything!

"There, there, child. Don't cry so. Yer weeping may yet harm yer bairn, and ye might lose it."

Cook laid a hand on her shoulder and patted it. It was a big, broad, work-roughened hand, but the woman's touch comforted Regan nonetheless. She rolled back to face her.

"My bairn? Ye mean I haven't already lost it?"

"Och, nay." Cook smiled and shook her head. "Ye were bleeding a wee bit when Walter first brought ye back home, but once I got

254

ye into bed and bathed ye, it came no more. We may well have to keep ye in bed until it's yer true time for birthing, but I think there's yet a chance we can save yer wee one."

Yet a chance we can save yer wee one . . . The consideration that she might still carry Iain's child to a safe birth was a bittersweet one. Though Regan knew it was what Iain had died trying to protect—her life and that of his unborn child—she found scant solace in the realization. She wanted Iain. Without him, life—the future—seemed nothing but a bleak, endless torment. More than anything she had ever wanted, Regan wanted to be with him, even if it meant following him in death.

But two things held her here. It was a sin to take one's life. She'd then never be with Iain in heaven, a place Regan was certain a man such as her husband would go. And there was the bairn. She'd soon be a mother. That bore with it a responsibility to care for her child. Her child . . . and Iain's.

"I'm glad for that at least," she managed to choke out at last. "That there's still a chance for our bairn. But what of Iain? His b-body . . . It needs to be taken back to Balloch and his mither."

"I don't know aught about that, child." Cook paused to pour a cup of water, then slid her hand behind Regan's head and lifted it. "Here, take a sip. Ye need to drink something. Later, I'll bring ye up a fortifying broth and a nice, soft bannock or some fresh-baked bread."

Though she obediently drank a few swallows of water, Regan shook her head once Cook had lowered her back to the bed. "I'm not hungry. Dinna fash yerself."

"Well, if ye won't eat for yerself, then eat for the bairn."

Regan sighed. "Aye, well I know that. And mayhap in time I'll eat, but not just now. I need to speak with Walter. Will ye fetch him for me?"

For some reason, the older woman didn't look at all happy about that request. "Can't it wait for a time? Ye need yer rest. And it isn't wise to be upsetting yerself unnecessarily just now."

"Then the sooner ye fetch Walter, the less upset I'll be," Regan said stubbornly. "Until I know my husband's body has been retrieved and is on its way to Balloch, I assure ye I cannot rest."

"Fine." Cook rolled her eyes and shook her head. "Have it yer way. Ye always do in the end."

Remorse filled Regan. "Och, I'm sorry, Cook. I didn't mean that to sound so unkind. There's just naught else I can do for Iain, and I want—I n-need—to do what little is left me. Please try to understand."

Compassion filled the other woman's eyes. "I do, child. He was a good man, yer husband was. Even the short time he was here, I could see that, and see, as well, how happy he made ye. But now he's gone, and I've got ye to worry over."

"Then help me with this, Cook. Please."

"I will." She hesitated. "I'll fetch Walter now, I will, if ye promise me one thing."

Regan arched a brow. "Aye, and that one thing is?"

"Stay in bed, for yer bairn's sake if not for yer own."

Her bairn. It was all she had left of Iain. "Aye, I promise." Then, as a freshened surge of tears filled her eyes, Regan closed them and turned away.

✠

An hour later, Walter crumbled the letter Regan had written to Iain Campbell's mother and tossed it into his bedchamber's hearth fire. The parchment smoldered but a few seconds, then burst into flame, its remains soon wafting up the chimney as large flecks of ash. That task completed, he took to his chair to contemplate his next steps.

Regan had begged him to return to the glen where her husband's body still lay, to bring it back to Strathyre so it could be prepared, before she accompanied the corpse to Balloch Castle for its proper burial. Walter had soon dissuaded her from her plan to return to Balloch. The continuation of her pregnancy was in jeopardy, and well she knew it. Though he half hoped she'd lose the bairn and be done with it, Walter also knew that keeping her abed for a time better served his purposes.

And, as far as the retrieval of Iain's body went, if he'd had his druthers, he'd never return it to Balloch. Let the fool's corpse lie there until it either rotted or became carrion for the vultures or wild beasts. Only later, much later, when the flesh was stripped from the bones along with those of the rest of Campbell's men, might he visit the massacre site, pick out an appropriately sized skeleton, and send it to Balloch. Indeed, the thought of Clan Campbell burying someone other than Iain Campbell in his grave amused Walter greatly . . .

Still, all pleasant thoughts of such things aside, Walter knew it was in his best interests just to get the unpleasant deed over and done with. He couldn't dare risk, after all, the suspicion sure to be raised if he failed promptly to carry through with the delivery of Iain Campbell and his men's bodies back to Balloch. One way or another, though, he'd then immediately return to Regan's side to help her through the worst of her mourning and the crucial remaining months of her childbearing.

A day or two more in seeing to a distasteful task, he comforted himself, and he could finally turn to more important things. Things besides Regan's welfare, such as paying William Drummond a wee visit. The man owed him money, he did, and it was past time, now that Regan was back at Strathyre and Iain Campbell was dead, that the recompense begin.

Next, fortified with some badly needed funds, Walter intended on returning home for a very long stay. He needed time with Regan, lots of time, in which to evolve, leastwise in her mind, from the concerned, comforting brother to a cherished friend whom Regan both cared for and depended upon. From there, it was a simple enough leap to her falling in love with him.

In entirely different but equally effective ways, he had removed the two men who had come to stand between him and Regan. At long last, the way was clear to devote himself to winning her heart. And he would. He was certain of it.

All he needed was time and an absence of distractions. And there was but one distraction left standing in his way. Still, there was hope Regan might yet prematurely shed herself of the bairn. If not, a wee babe was an easy enough obstacle to overcome. Indeed, with its untimely and most unfortunate death, an additional opportunity to play the devoted, compassionate friend presented itself.

Thinking over it all, Walter couldn't believe how everything—*everything*—was falling into place. If he had been one of those true and devoted followers of God, he'd have almost thanked Him for His most generous assistance.

19

As the days, then weeks, began to pass, the enforced bed rest appeared to work its calming effects—leastwise on Regan's body. She experienced no further birthing pangs or bleeding. It was the only blessing, however. With little to keep her mind occupied, Regan endlessly relived the events surrounding Iain's death, finding no relief save in slumber.

Even now, it seemed as if that horrific day had occurred but yesterday. She examined it from every angle, seeking to discover the answer that would yet save Iain's life. If strength of will and intensity of desire could've turned back the clock to that fateful morn, Regan would've gladly prevented them from leaving Strathyre. If only they hadn't set out that day, perhaps the outlaws wouldn't have been at the glen when they had finally come that way.

Yet, even as she dwelt on the possibilities, another consideration crept into her mind. The outlaws had not only been at the glen at the correct time but also apparently had been waiting for them. As if . . . as if they had known the exact day and time of their departure. As if someone had told them, and even sent them to that place for their murderous purpose.

But who would wish to do such a thing? True, Clan Campbell had its share of enemies. All Highland clans did. But how had they discovered Iain's whereabouts so easily, not to mention knew when they were to depart for Balloch?

Or was the outlaws' intent, instead, to murder her, and Iain and his men were but unfortunate impediments to that purpose? At the thought, a shiver coursed through Regan. Who would want her dead? Certainly not Walter—though, if her husband's and his continuing enmity were any indication, his motives could well be suspect when it came to Iain's death. Still, Walter *had* possessed the information as to their departure date and time.

When it came to folk who wished *her* dead, there was only one possibility, and it fell at the feet of her own clan. Her relatives, William Drummond most of all, were the most likely suspects. With her gone, there'd be one less obstacle to their continued infighting over the clan chieftainship. Aye, and William, who now was titular head of Clan Drummond, would wish her gone most of all.

There had certainly been no love lost between them when he had attended her and Iain's wedding. Though his responses to her, the rare times they had talked, had been courteous, there had always been an icy layer just beneath the surface.

William hated her. There was no doubt of that. And, for some additional reason she had yet to fathom, he hated Iain equally as much. She had seen that in his eyes the morn he and his wife had departed Kilchurn. Seen hatred and a most appalling fury.

There was nothing she could do, though, about any of it just yet. Her first responsibility was to her unborn child. And, once it was born, she must have a care to its continued safety. Not only was the child Iain's heir, but through her, it was also true heir to Clan Drummond. There were those who'd be equally upset over that, as there were those who knew the bairn to be a Campbell.

Clan Campbell, however, would be apprised of her suspicions just as soon as she delivered and had recovered from her childbearing. It was a hard thing, it was, not to be able to act immediately to seek out and punish Iain's murderers. But there was yet time. And, just as she had diligently attempted to discover Roddy's killer, she'd do the same now for Iain.

Two husbands, both murdered. That such a thing could happen to the same woman in less than the space of a year was all but inconceivable. Was she cursed somehow? Had God turned His face—and His love—from her?

The thought terrified Regan. Under Iain's gentle tutelage, she had come to see the Lord as a benevolent, merciful Father, and His Son as a lover and friend. She had come to see herself, as well, as a good person worthy of all the love and tender care Iain and his family had showered on her. But now . . . now she wondered.

Almost everyone Regan had ever truly and deeply loved had ultimately left her. They had all died. Was she somehow tainted, a cursed person who could only bring tragedy and death? It had been her secret fear for a long while, and now it seemed to have been amply justified. But why? What had she ever done to deserve this? And would this child she bore be relegated to the same fate?

"No matter what happens to me, ye must live . . . live for yerself . . . for the sake of our bairn."

Those had been some of Iain's last words. Yet despite his insistence that she possessed the strength and courage to go on without him, if she also lost her child, Regan wasn't certain she could survive that atop all the other losses she had endured. Nor, if the truth be told, would she want to.

Aye, there were always Molly and Walter. Molly did her best to try and cheer her up, spending hours each day playing games with Regan and telling her stories. And cool, distant Walter had become a most surprisingly solicitous friend, a solid presence who patiently listened to her endless outpourings of grief. But Molly was just a little girl, and after all these years of guarded friendship with Walter, trust and a true affection for him would surely be slow to come.

The disturbing lack of communication between her and Balloch also nagged at Regan. Though she had sent off her letter to Mathilda over three weeks ago along with Iain's body, Regan had yet to hear back from her. She had hoped against hope that, once Iain was buried, his mother and perhaps even Niall and Anne Campbell would come to Strathyre to visit her. But instead it seemed that with Iain's death, Clan Campbell had all but washed their hands of her.

A sudden thought assailed her, sending an icy chill through her veins. What if they suspected she had a hand in Iain's death? Regan wouldn't put it past Niall to harbor such a suspicion. She had long ago despaired of winning his friendship or trust.

But surely Anne and Mathilda . . . She heaved a great sigh. With Iain gone, the two women who loved him almost as much as she had would surely be so grief-stricken it wouldn't take much to turn them against her. Especially when the one doing the convincing was someone as persuasive as the Campbell clan chief.

Despair seized Regan. She buried her face in her hands. Would it never stop, the seemingly limitless repercussions of Iain's death? Instead of Iain, it should have been her who had died that day. Her death would have been mourned by few, her influence soon forgotten. True, their bairn would have died with her, but they would have soon been safe and eternally happy in heaven.

And Iain . . . Iain could have easily found himself another wife. A wife far, far worthier of him.

But instead, the Lord had chosen *her* to be his wife. Even now, Regan didn't understand that. But He had, and she must see it through to the end, whatever end God had in mind for her. She couldn't conceive how she could have chosen any other path than the one she had. Everything she had done had been done in the name of human decency or justice. If she had been wrong, then she had done so in good faith. She had chosen the way she truly thought she had been meant to go.

And that path had, in the end, led to her healing and happiness. She had done nothing wrong; she had tried to do the right thing. And she had experienced, if only for a brief time, the most astounding, heartbreakingly beautiful love. No matter what came next, she would always, always have that.

"If only Ye hadn't asked for such a terrible purchase price," Regan whispered hoarsely, the tears falling anew. "I'll try to be strong and courageous, Lord, but och, I want Iain back. How I want him back!"

She wrapped her arms about herself and pulled up her legs as far as her swollen belly would allow. There, in the gathering twilight of yet another day without Iain, Regan lay there weeping, until she finally drifted off into an exhausted slumber.

✠

Barely a month later, deep, contracting pains woke Regan in the middle of the night. Jolted awake, she lay there gasping at the sheer, breath-grabbing intensity of them, her hands clenched in the bedsheets, her back arching from the mattress. The pains went on for what seemed an eternity, then gradually abated.

Regan lay there in the darkness, taut and perspiring, terrified of what the pains might mean. Her thoughts raced. It was June 19, if the night had already turned to the next day. Two weeks until her calculated birthing date.

A short time later, the pains came, just as intense as before. Regan couldn't be positive, but there seemed barely five minutes between this one and the last. She gritted her teeth and rode the ever-worsening wave of contractions. Suddenly, she felt a gush of warm fluid between her legs.

"C-Cook!" Shoving up in bed, Regan glanced toward the little pallet set across the room. "Cook! I need ye!"

The older woman all but leaped from her bed. Since Regan's arrival back at Strathyre, Cook had insisted on sleeping close by in case Regan required anything. Though Regan had thought her efforts went far beyond what was necessary, tonight she was glad the woman was near.

"What is it, child?" Cook drew up beside her with a candle she had hurriedly lit. She held out the candle until it illuminated Regan's face.

"My waters have broken," Regan replied. "And in the short time since I woke, I've had two verra strong birthing pangs."

"Have ye now? Well, let me examine ye and see what I find."

With that, Cook quickly checked Regan. "Aye, I'd wager yer confinement's begun," she finally said. "But don't fear. Yer bairn's grown sufficiently now to survive."

Regan clasped her hand tightly. "What should we do?"

"Well, first I'll help ye from this sodden bed, wash ye, and dress ye in a fresh night rail. Then ye can sit in a chair and wait while I send a servant to fetch the midwife."

Excitement and a happy anticipation coursed through Regan. "But what if the babe comes while ye're gone? What shall I do then?"

The older woman chuckled. "If only we gave birth so quickly, leastwise when it's the first time." She patted her on the cheek. "Fear not, child. Naught will happen in the short time I'm gone. And then, when I return, I promise not to leave ye again until the wee one's born."

As Cook attempted to help her then from bed, another contraction came. Regan sat on the side of the bed, refusing to move further until that pain subsided. Then she undressed, Cook quickly washed her, and she donned another night rail.

An hour later, the midwife arrived. By then Regan's birthing pangs were coming regularly, with increasing intensity and frequency. An hour later, she was in hard labor.

She tried not to cry out or complain. Most times she succeeded. But she had never before known such agony. Though a large part of it was physical, Regan was overcome as well by an overpowering need to have Iain at her side. He had dreamed of this moment for so long and had promised he'd be there for her when the birthing came.

And he still was, Regan repeatedly reassured herself as she lay there limp and exhausted after yet another contraction had passed. Iain was here in spirit, looking down at her from heaven. Even though in this life he'd never hold his child in his arms, he'd know, nonetheless, that he'd soon be a father. She had to believe that. She just had to.

The birthing seemed to drag on forever, until Regan thought she'd go mad from the pain. Finally, however, an uncontrollable urge to push came, and the pain was suddenly made bearable by a fiercely satisfying sense of purpose. Just as the sun peeked over the mountains, Regan delivered of a fine, healthy baby boy. His strong cries soon rang through the air.

Seeing him for the first time, Regan felt herself fill with pride and a deep, abiding joy. She watched impatiently as the midwife bathed her son in salt water and performed all the traditional rituals. At long last, the woman carried her babe over and laid him in her arms.

As she gazed down at her perfect child, her heart swelled with satisfaction. She had succeeded. She had carried Iain's son and safely delivered of him. She had done what she'd had to do, and done it well.

For ye, my beloved, Regan silently thought. *My parting gift to ye, as is my vow to raise him well with full knowledge and love for his magnificent father.* She leaned over and tenderly kissed her son.

"We fetched the priest, we did," Cook offered just then. "In case ye'd like him baptized straightaway."

"Aye," Regan said, "I'd like that verra much."

Cook turned and left the room, soon returning with the old cleric. He set out his bottles and linens, then faced Regan.

"We need a name for the wee lad, we do. What would ye be calling him?"

A soft smile lifted her lips. "Colin. I'll be calling him Colin. It was his father's wish that he bear the name of his great-grandfather, and so it shall be. Colin Campbell."

✠

Walter was becoming increasingly irritated, and when he was irritated, it became difficult to keep his temper in check. He was making headway in Regan's affections, however, and didn't dare risk upsetting her. Therefore, he saw no other alternative than to vent his anger on the servants.

"It's been two weeks now since the bairn was born," he snarled at Cook one warm, early July morn. "Why haven't ye moved him to the nursery?"

The older woman glanced up from the cooked chicken she was slicing with a sizable knife and sent him an exasperated look. "It's really quite simple, m'lord. Regan refuses to let the child out of her sight for even a minute. And, since she sees no need for Colin to sleep apart from her in some nursery, neither do I."

Walter eyed her with ill-disguised displeasure. The woman was becoming far too impertinent these days. No matter her twenty-some years of service, he had half a mind to let her go this very instant.

Unfortunately, Regan loved Cook and trusted her like she trusted no other at Strathyre. He'd not endear himself to her if he sent Cook away. But later, Walter vowed, once Regan was his, he'd find some excuse to send this interfering woman packing. She had always been a stumbling block to his influence over Regan, and she always would be. He intended that to change, though, and soon.

"Well, Regan won't regain her strength if she doesn't get some sleep at night," he said. "And if ye're unable to convince her of the wisdom of a nursery, I won't be."

"Suit yerself." Cook returned to the chicken, chopping it into parts with what seemed a particularly vicious enthusiasm. "Ye've met yer match, though, I'd wager, in going up against a mother she-wolf."

Walter snorted in disdain. "Well, we'll just see about that, won't we?"

"Aye, we most certainly will," came the woman's cheeky reply as he turned to leave.

It was fortunate the walk from the kitchen to the second-floor bedchambers took several minutes. Walter needed that time and a bit more to choke down the foul mood Cook had so unwisely stirred. Still, the consideration of seeing Regan helped immeasurably. She had always, after all, been the brightest spot in his life.

That realization cheered him as he drew up finally before her bedchamber door. He knocked, was answered by a request to enter, and, with a broad smile on his face, immediately opened the door and walked in.

Regan glanced up from her seat before the open window, Campbell's spawn wrapped in a light blanket and lying in her arms. At sight of the child, it was all Walter could do to keep from grimacing. Then, when Regan saw that it was him and smiled, all thoughts of that unwanted child fled.

"Och, it's ye," she said. "Come over, Walter, and sit with me. I was just thinking about ye, I was."

Happiness filled him. She had been thinking of him? He was indeed the most fortunate of men! He closed the door and hurried over.

"And were yer thoughts of me pleasant ones?" he asked as he took his seat in the chair facing her.

Regan laughed, and the merry sound washed over him like a soothing caress. "Of course they were. Ye've been so verra kind to me these past weeks. Indeed, I don't know what I would've done without ye."

"Ye're family, lass." He couldn't help the husky catch in his voice. "I was happy to do whatever I could for ye."

"Aye, as I'd always do the same for ye. But I'm nearly recovered from my childbearing now, and think it's time I make plans to return to Balloch."

She couldn't have stunned him more if she had reared back just then and struck him full across the face. "R-return to Balloch? But why? Ye've had not a word or visitor from there since ye lost yer husband. Cruel as it must be to consider, it's evident the Campbells wish naught more to do with ye."

Regan sighed and turned her gaze toward the window. "Aye,

so it'd seem, but mayhap if I return with Iain's son in my arms, Mathilda at the verra least will welcome me for his sake. And Colin *is* Iain's only heir. Whether Mathilda likes it or not, Balloch is now his."

Walter's mind raced. Now, more than ever, he had to find some way to put an end to that child. He was Regan's last link to Balloch Castle and the Campbells. Once *he* was gone, she'd have no reason ever to want to leave Strathyre . . . leave him. He knew she was all but falling in love with him. He could tell by the joy in her eyes whenever she saw him these days. All he needed was just a little more time.

"Balloch Castle's indeed wee Colin's birthright," Walter forced himself to agree in a reasonable tone of voice. "But there's no hurry, is there, to return to a place and people who now seem to bear ye such ill will? Everyone there knows ye carried Iain's child. Let the wee bairn, instead, grow up for a time in a happy place."

She turned back from the window. "Ye're most kind to worry so about my son. And, even if things eventually improve for us at Balloch, ye can be certain we'll gladly spend a generous amount of time at Strathyre each year. I want Colin, after all, to know his MacLaren side of the family equally as well."

"Well, we can speak of this later." Walter felt his nails dig into his palms, and he had to will his hands to unclench. "There's no need—"

Regan inhaled a deep breath. "Aye, there *is* a need. I wish to return to Balloch the day after the morrow, Walter. Will ye please make arrangements for a party of clansmen to escort me home?"

Once again he stared at her, dumbfounded. How could she do this, be so heartless and cruel, after all he had done for her? His gaze narrowed as she looked down at the child. Her lips curved in a tender smile, and she lifted a finger to stroke the bairn's cheek.

Hatred welled, as caustic and hurtful as some bitter gall. It was bad enough that Iain Campbell had stolen her heart. Now the child, in its own way, had cast his spell over her. But why should that surprise him? It was in the bairn's blood, this ability to ensorcel. He was, after all, his father's son.

Even in death, it seemed, the warlock mocked him.

Walter had thought he had freed Regan from all enchantment when Iain Campbell died. He had apparently been wrong. Regan was yet bound, even if by the slenderest of threads, by the dead father's aura of magic through his son. But not for long. If he had to tear the child from her arms to kill it, he would.

There was yet time, though. He must just come up with some pretext temporarily to separate Regan from her son. He didn't need very long with the bairn. Just long enough to end its life without any sign of foul play. Just long enough to smother it.

"Well, if yer mind's made to travel back to Balloch, I suggest ye begin taking some short rides to strengthen yerself," he said, seizing on a plan. "It's a long half-day's journey, and ye've hardly left yer room in the past few months, not to mention you've recently endured the strain of childbirth."

She appeared to consider that for a moment, then nodded. "Aye, I suppose ye're right. And I'd dearly love to get out and see some of the countryside." Her brow furrowed. "I must, though, devise some sort of sling to carry Colin in when I go riding."

Walter choked back a sharp surge of anger. "For the short while we'll be gone, I'm sure the child will be quite safe in his cradle." He began to reform his plan. While they were gone, he'd now have to get someone else to kill the child . . .

"Nay." Regan shook her head. "I won't go anywhere without Colin."

"And why's that?" he demanded, his patience shredding. "Don't ye trust him to be safe in Strathyre?"

She looked away suddenly—and most suspiciously—unable to meet his gaze. "He's precious to me. He's all I have of Iain."

Walter threw up his hands. "Well, if ye won't even meet me halfway on this, then I see no reason to allow ye to risk yer health by attempting to leave prematurely."

Regan jerked her head around, her eyes gone wide. "What are ye saying, Walter? Are ye threatening to keep me here against my will?"

There was a strange light in her eyes. Almost as if . . . as if she suddenly feared him. As if she doubted him and his motives. As if she *suspected* him. But that was ridiculous. There was no way Regan could link him to her husband's murder.

Still, the realization that a chasm had unexpectedly opened between them sealed his resolve.

He indeed needed more time to win her heart. And if that required he keep her here for her own good, he would. He had, after all, the perfect bait in her child to dangle over her head, to coerce her into obedience.

"I'm only doing what's best for ye, lass," he replied at last. "Ye've been through so much of late that I don't think ye're seeing things verra clearly. Ye lack sufficient health for a journey back to Balloch just now, not to mention the strength of mind to endure the cruelties ye're certain to face once ye're back amongst the Campbells. And then there's yer unreasoning distrustfulness." He sighed and shook his head. "Nay, ye're in no condition to be going anywhere just yet."

She rose to her feet, her eyes blazing. "What are ye about, Walter? I know ye. I can tell when ye're up to something."

He smiled and stood. "It'll be all right, lass. Just ye wait and see. I'll take care of ye, I will."

With that, he turned on his heel and strode across the room and out the door.

✠

Regan didn't have to follow him and try the door to know she was now a virtual prisoner. She had heard Walter give orders to some man just outside—orders that she wasn't, under any circumstances, to leave her room. She was trapped here now, and well she knew it.

But what was Walter's true intent in keeping her here? Did he realize she suspected he had played some part in Iain's death? He should.

She hadn't dared let herself dwell overlong on that issue during the last weeks of her pregnancy, fearing what the mental anguish over such doubts might do to her and the babe. Still, just as she had tried mightily not to think overlong about Iain either, the questions had returned anew once she had delivered. How had Walter known to arrive just in time to save her from being killed? Had he mayhap been there all along, hiding, and only the threat to her life had brought him out from cover? And where had he gotten the dagg he had used to kill the outlaw?

Perhaps he imagined she hadn't seen it, but she had. And it wasn't one of Iain's pistols picked up from the ground where he had tossed them once they were spent. Regan well knew those two ornately decorated silver daggs, and the one Walter had fired was of far lesser quality.

A sudden, terrifying thought assailed her. What if Walter owned that pistol and always had? How he could afford to come by one was beside the point. But what if . . . what if he'd had that dagg the night Roddy died? And what if, instead of Roddy dying by one of Iain's pistols, he had been shot in the back by his own brother?

Daggs needed to be fired at close range to have any chance of accuracy. And who'd be any closer than Walter, riding at Roddy's side? It was a dark night. Both Iain and Walter had attested to that. It would've been easy enough for Walter to drop back from Roddy a bit, pull his dagg from his plaid, and fire it in all the confusion.

But why would Walter kill Roddy? Did he covet Strathyre and its lands that desperately? And why had he helped in Iain's murder, if he really had? True, it was evident there was no love lost between the two men, but enough to kill?

The enormity of her plight struck Regan with shattering force. If Walter had indeed killed or been actively involved in the murder of both her husbands, she was in the gravest of dangers. He was either a murderously vengeful man who sought to punish any who crossed him, or he had purposely killed anyone who came between him and whatever he wanted. And perhaps she was at least some small part of what he had always wanted.

Colin stirred in her arms, opened his sweetly curved little mouth in a wide yawn, then settled back to sleep. Gazing down at him, Regan's heart swelled with love. She'd do anything to protect her child. Indeed, some instinct had made her insist on keeping him always at her side. An instinct that was now becoming a genuine fear for his safety.

And, as much as she hated to do so, for the time being it seemed his continuing safety was best secured in pretending to acquiesce to Walter's demand that she remain at Strathyre. Why he wished it so, she could only surmise.

As he had informed her he was keeping her here for her own good, though, Regan had seen something spark in his eyes. Something that unsettled her greatly. Something wild and irrational. Something almost insane.

Aye, she'd pretend to acquiesce for a time more. But then, even if she had to set out on foot, she meant to flee Strathyre. It was becoming increasingly likely Walter had had a hand in the deaths of the two men she had taken to husband.

Regan had no intention of losing her son at his hands as well.

20

The next day dawned rainy and cool. Thick mists rose from the land, swirling, curling, and spreading ever outward like some huge, white serpent devouring everything in its path. All sight and sound seemed swallowed in the insatiable maw of the vaporous beast, until the world disappeared into nothingness.

As Regan gazed out the window of the bedchamber that had now become her prison cell, her mood mirrored that of the dreary, almost foreboding day. An eerie feeling hung heavy in the air, presaging some unknown events to come. Events that promised ill for some and perhaps, God willing, good for others.

Regan shivered, then hastily closed the shutters and drew the thick curtains against the damp chill. Lifting her thoughts heavenward, she prayed to the Lord that, whatever happened, no ill would come to her son. He was innocent of all the foolishness and misguided acts that had brought them to this wretched moment in time. His life still spread out before him, pure, unscathed, and full of potential. And he deserved, oh, how he deserved, a chance to make something better of his life than she had of hers.

She had spent a sleepless night considering all possible ways to approach Walter. She knew she must find some way to win his trust. It was the only chance to get him to lower his guard long enough for her to escape with Colin. And something told Regan, for Colin's sake at the very least, she must make her escape soon. Very, very soon.

A sound—was it a man's shout?—rose from somewhere outside. Regan hurried to the window, threw aside the curtains, and swung open the shutters. Just then, out of the gray fog, riders appeared, three or four abreast, emerging as dark forms swathed in their plaids. Armed men in a seemingly endless file, until the open space before Strathyre House was filled with them.

Excitement and a wild hope rose in her. She leaned out from the window, straining to ascertain from which clan the small army had come. At nearly the same time, her bedchamber door violently crashed open, striking the wall with a resounding thud.

Regan jumped back, her heart slamming against her breast. She turned, caught sight of Walter's enraged countenance, and glanced immediately toward Colin asleep in his cradle near the hearth. As if drawn by her glance, Walter's gaze followed.

With a snarl, he set out toward the cradle. Regan gave a dismayed cry and ran in the same direction. Walter, however, had the advantage and covered the shorter distance before she was even halfway there. Grabbing up Colin, he handed him to Fergus MacLaren, who had followed Walter into the room.

In the next instant, Regan was there, fighting to get around Walter to reach her son. "Nay!" she cried. "What are ye doing, Walter? Give me back my bairn. Give him back!"

"Wheesht, lass," her foster brother said, taking a firm hold on her. "No harm will come to the lad. He's but assurance that ye'll cooperate. And ye will, won't ye?"

She didn't like the wolfish look about him. He had the appearance of some cornered animal, with his panicky gaze, sweat sheening his upper lip, and nervous laugh. She swallowed hard, willing her rising apprehension to ease. Something was afoot. She needed to think and act calmly, or all could be lost.

"Of course I'll cooperate," Regan replied, pretending surprise.

"Whyever would ye think otherwise? What's happening, Walter? And who are those men who just arrived?"

His grip tightened on her arms. "They're Campbells, and Niall Campbell leads them."

Wild hope sprang anew, but Regan feigned only a look of puzzlement. "Aye, and what does he want with us?"

"He demands to see ye and the child. He won't say why."

Regan gave a careless shrug. "Well, that seems a simple enough thing. Mayhap he's finally decided to fetch us both back to Balloch."

"Aye, mayhap," Walter muttered, his expression clouding in sudden anger. "But ye cannot leave me. Ye see that, don't ye? I've worked too hard to get ye, struck down too many, to lose ye now."

So, Regan thought, it was as she had feared. Walter had fashioned some bizarre fantasy about the two of them, and the consideration of what he had done to achieve it filled her with revulsion. This wasn't the time, though, to disabuse him of that crazed notion.

"He has a verra large army with him, Walter," Regan began, carefully choosing her words. "It might be dangerous to refuse him."

"Aye." He nodded his head sharply in agreement. "That's why I need yer help. Ye must tell him the child's ill and ye'll not be parading him just now for all to see. And then ye must tell him ye don't wish to leave here, that Strathyre's now yer home."

Frantically, Regan tried to work out some way to keep her child with her. If she could just get the bairn into Niall's presence, she knew Colin would finally be safe. Even if that ultimately required that she give him into Niall's custody and remain behind, at least Iain's son would be safe.

"Mayhap it'd be better just to bring Colin along," she finally said. "I could still tell Niall that I wish to stay here at Strathyre, but I'd wager he won't be satisfied until he sees the babe. And we don't wish to make him suspicious, do we?"

For an instant, it appeared as if Walter were considering her plan. Then his gaze shuttered. He shook his head.

"Nay. The bairn will stay with Fergus, hidden where Niall cannot find him. It's the only way I can be certain ye'll say what needs to be said."

He grinned of a sudden, and the smile was cold, icy cold. "It's up to ye now, lass, whether the child lives or dies. Because Fergus has orders to smother the lad unless *I* come for him. And I'll die first before I lose ye."

Once again the crazed look flared in his eyes, and Regan knew he spoke true. Even if Niall killed him in the attempt to force Walter to reveal where Colin was hidden, Niall's efforts were doomed. It was indeed up to her to convince Niall that all was well and to depart Strathyre. The reward for her lies, after all, was the life of her son.

Despair filled her. Niall had always suspected her. He was also not a stupid man and wouldn't easily be deceived. No matter what Walter demanded, no matter how hard she tried, she might still fail. No matter how hard she tried, Colin might well die.

Regan closed her eyes, sucked in a deep breath, and prayed. Prayed for guidance in the ordeal to come, that she'd say the right words necessary to convince Niall, even though they might all be lies, and prayed, most of all, for her son. Then, opening her eyes and lifting her chin, she nodded.

"It's past time we went down to greet Niall," she said softly. "To tarry overlong will only increase his suspicions. And we don't want to do that."

He regarded her with a piercing intensity, then nodded in turn. "Aye, we don't want to do that." Walter released her and offered her his arm.

Taking it, Regan spared one final glance at Colin, held now in the arms of a man who'd stop at nothing, even the murder of an innocent child, to serve his master. She prayed it wasn't the last time she'd see her son alive.

Then Walter was leading her away, and Regan forced her thoughts to the task ahead. They descended the turnpike stairs to the second floor and the Great Hall, where Niall Campbell, scowling like some storm rising over the mountains, awaited them with at least a score of his men. Though a few still had their heads covered by the excess length of their plaids, most had thrown aside the damp wool and tucked it back in their belts.

All, Regan noted, bore short swords and dirks and looked to be spoiling for a fight. Which shouldn't surprise her. Not only were they true sons of the Highlands, but there was the wee matter of Iain's death that still needed avenging.

With Walter at her side, she walked up to stand before the Campbell clan chief. For a long moment, he ignored Strathyre's laird and fixed his intense gaze on her. Regan stoically returned it with a steady one of her own.

"Ye look none the worse for the wear, considering the events of the past few months," he said at last.

"I had Iain's son to think of," Regan replied, her glance never wavering. "At times, it was all that kept me alive." As she spoke, from the corner of her vision, she saw one of Niall's men slip off to descend the turnpike stairs to the lower level. For an instant, she thought to call him back, then discarded that idea. What did it matter to her anymore what happened in Strathyre?

Niall's eyes narrowed, and some indefinable light flickered there. "Indeed? Despite yer words to the contrary, ye don't look much the grieving widow to me."

Anger, fueled by a deep anguish, welled up and bubbled forth before she could stop it. "And why would I bare my feelings to the likes of ye?" she asked, her voice vibrating with fury. "Ye never believed the truth of my love for Iain. Never!"

Beside her, Walter gave an unsteady laugh. "Wheesht, lass! That's no way to welcome our guest. And the past is past. In Christian charity, ye need to lay aside yer animosity and forgive."

Regan jerked around to stare at her foster brother, astounded at his shameless, blatant hypocrisy. An impulse to berate him rose to her lips, and only the hope of saving Colin quashed it.

"Aye, ye're right," she murmured, lowering her gaze and turning back to Niall. "I beg pardon, m'lord."

"Dinna fash yerself," his deep voice rumbled above her. "As Mac-Laren said, the past is past. What matters now is that Iain's son be taken home to Balloch. Where is the wee lad?"

She steeled herself for what she knew was to come. "He's ill." Once again, Regan locked gazes with Niall. "And I'll not be bringing him down for all of ye dirty-handed men to touch and make even sicker."

The Campbell chief shrugged. "Suit yerself. But, whether ye wish to accompany him or not, the lad's leaving with me."

"And who are ye to determine where *my* son is to live?" she demanded. "He may well be fatherless, but he most certainly still has a mither!"

A muscle began to tick in Niall's jaw. "And *I* said ye could return with him to Balloch. Despite my personal opinion of ye, I'll not deny the bairn his mither."

"Well, I don't wish to return to Balloch. In all the weeks since Iain's body was carried back home, not one of ye has bothered to visit to see how I was faring, much less ever answered my letters."

Niall frowned. "What letters? And no one from Strathyre ever attempted to return Iain's body." Almost in unison, both he and Regan riveted their attention on Walter.

The blood drained from Walter's face. "I-I can't say what happened to the letters ye had me send, lass, but I sent them. I swear it."

"And Iain's body?" Regan prodded softly, her blood going cold. "Ye said ye returned his body the verra next day after he was killed. What of that?"

For a long moment, Walter couldn't seem to meet her gaze. "Truth was, I couldn't find it. Some animal must have dragged it away, and, though I and my men searched for it for a time, we never found it. But I couldn't tell ye that. Ye were already in such pain, and there was still great danger that ye'd lose yer wee one . . ."

As much as she hated to admit it, Walter spoke true. As distraught as she had been, if she had learned that Iain's body had been devoured by wild animals, she may well have lost all control, if not have finally gone mad.

"Nonetheless," Regan said, "ye could've told me after Colin was born."

"Aye, but it was past, and I hadn't the heart to steal the first glimmers of joy ye'd had in such a long time." Walter took her hand. "Can ye forgive me, lass?"

Regan stared at him, struck speechless. He had all but admitted he had killed or assisted in the killing of both her husbands and was even now threatening the life of her son, and he could still stand here and pretend to have acted compassionately in her behalf. It was almost . . . almost as if there were two distinct parts to this man, and neither were influenced, leastwise in any moral way, by the other. Two parts, and she hadn't ever known either one.

"Aye, I suppose I can forgive ye that," Regan mumbled, so appalled by all the lies and deception that she thought, for a moment, she might be physically ill. She wrapped her arms about her and lowered her head. "Och, Iain . . . Iain. Now I don't even have the consolation of yer grave to visit."

"Well, as touching as this all is," Niall chose just then to interject, "it's all beside the point. As Colin's mither, ye're welcome at Balloch, and as Iain's only heir, Colin's proper place is there as well."

It was too much, Regan thought. All she'd ever be was a pawn between Niall Campbell and Walter, each one tugging her first one way and then the other, and neither had her best interests at heart. Only Iain had truly cared for and about her, and he was gone.

Grief pressed down on her with such a heavy weight that she couldn't speak, much less think coherently. Regan felt as if she were falling into some abyss that she'd never be able to escape. An abyss from which no one, not even her sweet little child, would be able to call her back.

Her hand went to the silver cross she always wore, and she

clutched it to her. The silver cross . . . her mother's parting gift that sad day she and Regan's father had departed for Edinburgh, never to return. Regan had not forgotten the brief prayer her mother had written and enclosed in that precious piece of jewelry. *Dear Lord Jesus, be ever near my beloved daughter . . .*

A freshened swell of anguish surged up, threatening to smother her. Regan closed her eyes, fighting with all her strength not to be overcome. Yet, even as she considered the darkness promising an end to the pain, a sudden, blessed assurance filled her. A sense of a Presence, speaking in a soft, quiet voice deep within her heart.

No matter how far she tried to flee or how deeply she fell, there would always be One who would pursue her, who, indeed, would always be there for her. He was her strength and her courage when she had none of her own. He was all the love she'd ever need, even when there seemed no love left her in this world.

All she had to do was reach out and take His hand, the voice whispered, and He would surely lead her, hold her up. Take her and bear her on the wings of morning until, someday, all would be healed and she'd once again find the happiness she had always sought.

But, until that day, there was more than just her happiness and welfare to think on, Regan realized, the reality of the moment flooding back. There was Colin.

She looked up and, through the tears, met Niall's puzzled glance. "Aye, Colin's proper place is at Balloch." She then turned to Walter. "Let Niall take my child, and I give ye my word I'll stay with ye.

"Please, Walter." Regan laid a hand on his arm. "It's what ye've always wanted, after all."

He stared back at her, his eyes darting nervously in his disbelief. Then, with a quick nod, he appeared to accept her offer. "Aye, mayhap that's for the best, lass. The lad will be with his kind, and ye'll remain with—"

"Not so fast, MacLaren!"

Regan wheeled around. From the turnpike stairs behind them,

a tall man, his head still covered with his plaid, slowly descended. Behind him was Cook, looking inordinately pleased with herself. One of Niall's men, as well as Cook, had slipped up the stairs while they talked. But why?

The answer came when something in the man's arms moved, and a lusty cry rose from the bundle he carried. Terror seized Regan. It was Colin! The man had Colin!

She cried out and took a step forward. Walter grabbed her arm. "Let them have him," he said in a low voice. "It's better this way."

Her tears nearly blinded her. "Aye," she whispered, "but I'll at least hold my son one last time, and no man here had dare try and stop me!"

Behind her, Niall Campbell chuckled. "I'd say ye'd better let her go, MacLaren. It's over for ye, at any rate."

As Walter turned back to the Campbell chief, his grip on her momentarily loosened. It was all the opportunity Regan needed. She twisted free and ran, drawing up only a few feet from the foot of the stairs.

The tall man, his face shadowed in the depths of his plaid, halted before her. She held out her hands. "Give me my son."

"Aye, that I will, lass."

Regan froze. There was something about that voice . . . *Och, dear Lord above,* she thought, *I'm losing my mind!* Her knees buckled. If not for the man's swift move to take her arm, she knew she would've fallen.

"Have a care," he said, his deep, rich voice setting all her senses tingling. "With our son in my arms, I'm hard-pressed to hold ye up as well."

It wasn't possible. It was surely a vision conjured by her over-wrought mind, or leastwise all just some dream. Whatever it truly was, Regan meant to see it through to its end. Because she needed it and had so long been bereft.

Reaching up, she took hold of the plaid and slid it back. Iain's beloved face came into view, pale and thinner than when she had last seen him, but, from the dark blond, wavy hair, eyes as deep blue as some bottomless loch, and the well-molded mouth, it was him. Aye, she thought, and he was just as she had always remembered him . . . and always would.

Then he smiled, and the smile was just as dazzling and warm and open as it had always been. And she remembered how it always spread all the way to his beautiful eyes. And, like all the other times, she was undone.

"Och, Iain . . . Iain," Regan whispered achingly. Though she knew she risked destroying her beautiful vision by doing so, she couldn't help herself. She reached up, touched his face, hoping, praying for a fleeting instant where reality melded with the dream, and she could feel him—*really* feel him—one last time.

The face she touched, however, was warm and substantial. It didn't disappear as her fingers stroked his cheek. Regan blinked hard, sending her tears coursing down her face, and saw that he remained. Once more her knees buckled, and the clasp on her arm tightened. She glanced down at the long, strong fingers holding her, then back up again.

"Aye, lass," he said. "I'm not a dream. I'm alive."

With a moan, Regan went to him then, sliding her arms about his waist, burying her face in the damp wool of his plaid. The tears seemed to break the floodgates about her tightly guarded heart. She wept, sobbing until she had nothing left to give. And all the while, Iain held her, crooning to her as he rocked her gently to and fro.

"Nay!"

From a distant place, Walter's outraged cry wrenched Regan back to the present moment. She released Iain and turned, hastily wiping away her tears.

Even then, Strathyre's laird had withdrawn his dirk and was heading toward them. He had barely taken three steps, however, before Niall and two other men sprang forward, taking him down and wrestling the dirk from his hand. Finally subdued, Walter struggled to his feet.

"Ye gave me yer word ye'd stay with me if I let them have the child!" he screamed, his face purpling with fury as he fought to escape the men restraining him. "And the devil now has his spawn, so come back. Come back to me!"

Before Regan could reply, Iain stepped between her and Walter. "The only devil here is ye, MacLaren," he growled. "I saw ye there that day. Indeed, ye were the only man among them all that I recognized. And ye'll pay, and pay dearly, for the lads I lost, as well as for the attempt on my life."

Walter stopped struggling. As if a sudden comprehension had at last penetrated his enraged mind, the blood drained from his face. "I . . . I but happened by," he stammered. "It was but a coincidence that I came upon those outlaws, and fortunate it was that I did, or Regan would've surely died."

"Coincidence, was it?" Iain gave a disbelieving snort. "Ye knew those men. How much did ye pay them to try and kill me, MacLaren? And, even better, where did the likes of ye even get the money?"

"It wasn't me!" His countenance going positively waxen now, Walter vehemently shook his head. "I-I but did William Drummond's bidding. It was all his idea. He didn't fancy ye telling him where he must cast his allegiance. And he meant to kill Regan as well. Ye saw that. But I suspected he might try, so I watched in a secret place. And I saved ye, Regan. I saved ye!"

Iain shook his head in disgust. "Get him out of my sight," he said, looking to Niall. "Throw the dog into his own dungeon until we decide what to do with him."

Niall grinned. "I was wondering how long it'd take ye to sicken of him. Come on, lads," he said, looking to his men. "Let's see to clamping the laird in his own irons."

Regan watched them drag Walter away. It was over then. Walter would finally receive his long-delayed punishment, and William Drummond's wouldn't be far behind. She could only feel pity for the both of them.

Iain slipped an arm about her waist and pulled her close once more. "Och, but I'm the happiest of men, with my wife in one arm and son in the other!"

She laid her head on him and stood there for a time, content now just to feel his chest rise and fall and hear the steady beat of his heart.

"H-how?" she finally asked, lifting her head to gaze up at him. "How did ye survive?"

"A tinker passed in the opposite direction soon after the outlaws and ye and Walter must have departed. Or so he told me. I was still unconscious at any rate. In checking all the bodies, he found that I was the only one still alive. So he bound up my wounds and took me back to the town he had just quit. In time, I was able to tell them who I was, and someone was sent to Balloch to inform them."

"But how did ye get to Colin? Fergus had hidden him away at Walter's bidding to ensure my cooperation. How did ye find and rescue him before Fergus could kill him?"

"I knew to seek out Cook to aid me and, as luck would have it, she'd followed Walter and Fergus upstairs when they came to ye. Then, when she saw Fergus skulk off with Colin, she followed him to the attic where he hid with the bairn." Iain smiled in grim satisfaction. "I lowered myself down on a rope from the roof and entered a window behind the man while Cook came up the stairs to distract him. It was a simple enough thing to overcome him."

"Yet, all this time, ye never returned for us until now." Though this one last question hung like a pall between them, Regan had to ask, had to know the reason. "Indeed, it's been nearly two months since the day of the attack. Why did ye wait so long?"

"Because I took an infection, and for a time it was feared I might not recover. And then I was so verra weak that I lacked the strength to ride until but a week or so ago." At the disbelieving look she sent him, he paused, then inhaled a deep breath. "That's hardly enough a reason, though, for my tardiness in coming after ye, is it?"

"Nay, it isn't."

He sighed and looked away. "Until just a short while ago, I also doubted ye and yer loyalty to me. It was evident the men who ambushed us were waiting for us. And ye, of us all, survived unscathed to return to Strathyre. To return in the arms of the man who had apparently arrived at just the right time to rescue ye."

Regan's hand fell from his face. "If ye'd known what I suffered, thinking ye dead and that I'd lost the love of my life, ye never would've doubted me." Freshened pain slashed through her. "Och, Iain, I thought we were finally past the suspicion and recriminations!"

All the joy she had experienced at finding him alive faded in the face of the searing admission of his mistrust. Suddenly, Regan couldn't bear to be close to him. She twisted and fought to break free of his clasp.

Iain refused to let her go. "Forgive me, lass. Och, please forgive me! I know I betrayed ye, betrayed our love in doubting ye. But it's a weakness, a thorn in my side, that, with the Lord's help and Niall's wise counsel, if ye can believe it, I think I've finally overcome. And then, it was yet reaffirmed again today when I saw ye walking down the stairs with Walter. I saw the truth in yer eyes, and I knew. I knew!"

The sincerity of his words was mirrored in his beautiful eyes, resonated in his deep voice. But the blade of his suspicions had struck her hard. After all she had gone through for him, how could Iain think such things about her? And how could she ever forgive him?

But how could she not, after all the times he had forgiven her for doubting him? He had forgiven her even when others remained convinced of her duplicity; he had seen past it all to the person she truly was. He had seen and trusted that the goodness, sometimes buried beneath all the pain and feelings of unworthiness, was genuine and deserved a chance to shine.

He had seen, trusted, and loved until, just once, mired in his own pain and battling for his life, he had faltered for but a brief time. Faltered but had never given up.

She'd never have such a man again, and she wasn't fool enough to lose him. With a shuddering breath, Regan turned back to Iain. Standing on tiptoe, she grabbed hold of his shirt and plaid and kissed him full on the mouth.

For an instant, as if uncertain what next to do, he stood there. Then, with a husky groan, Iain pulled Regan to him and hungrily deepened their kiss. A great, spiraling gladness filled her until she thought her heart would burst.

For in that kiss was enough love—and forgiveness—to last a lifetime.

Kathleen Morgan has authored numerous novels for the general market and now focuses her writing on inspirational books. She has won many awards for her romance writing, including the 2002 Rose Award for Best Inspirational Romance.

Other books by Kathleen Morgan

Brides of Culdee Creek Series
Daughter of Joy
Woman of Grace
Lady of Light
Child of Promise

Culdee Creek Christmas
All Good Gifts
The Christkindl's Gift

Guardians of Gadiel Series
Giver of Roses

These Highland Hills Series
Child of the Mist

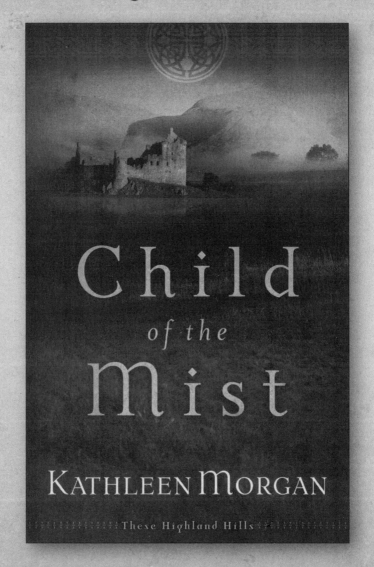